Reproductive Medicine

Editor

VLADIMIR JEKL

VETERINARY CLINICS OF NORTH AMERICA: EXOTIC ANIMAL PRACTICE

www.vetexotic.theclinics.com

Consulting Editor
JÖRG MAYER

May 2017 • Volume 20 • Number 2

ELSEVIER

1600 John F. Kennedy Boulevard • Suite 1800 • Philadelphia, Pennsylvania, 19103-2899
http://www.vetexotic.theclinics.com

VETERINARY CLINICS OF NORTH AMERICA: EXOTIC ANIMAL PRACTICE Volume 20, Number 2
May 2017 ISSN 1094-9194, ISBN-13: 978-0-323-52866-5

Editor: Katie Pfaff
Developmental Editor: Meredith Madeira

Veterinary Clinics of North America: Exotic Animal Practice (ISSN 1094-9194) is published in January, May, and September by Elsevier, Inc., 360 Park Avenue South, New York, NY 10010-1710. Subscription prices are $265.00 per year for US individuals, $460.00 per year for US institutions, $100.00 per year for US students and residents, $311.00 per year for Canadian individuals, $554.00 per year for Canadian institutions, $347.00 per year for international individuals, $554.00 per year for international institutions and $165.00 per year for Canadian and foreign students/residents. To receive student/resident rate, orders must be accompanied by name of affiliated institution, date of term, and the *signature* of program/residency coordinator on institution letterhead. Orders will be billed at individual rate until proof of status is received. Foreign air speed delivery is included in all *Clinics* subscription prices. All prices are subject to change without notice. **POSTMASTER:** Send address changes to *Veterinary Clinics of North America: Exotic Animal Practice*, Elsevier Health Sciences Division, Subscription Customer Service, 3251 Riverport Lane, Maryland Heights, MO 63043. **Customer Service: Telephone: 1-800-654-2452** (U.S. and Canada); **1-314-447-8871** (outside U.S. and Canada). **Fax: 1-314-447-8029. E-mail: journalscustomerservice-usa@elsevier.com (for print support); journalsonlinesupport-usa@elsevier.com (for online support).**

Reprints. For copies of 100 or more of articles in this publication, please contact the Commercial Reprints Department, Elsevier Inc., 360 Park Avenue South, New York, New York 10010-1710. Tel.: 212-633-3874; Fax: 212-633-3820; E-mail: reprints@elsevier.com.

Veterinary Clinics of North America: Exotic Animal Practice is covered in *MEDLINE/PubMed (Index Medicus).*

Contributors

CONSULTING EDITOR

JÖRG MAYER, Dr med vet, MSc
Diplomate American Board of Veterinary Practitioners (Exotic Companion Mammals); Diplomate European College of Zoological Medicine (Small Mammals); Diplomate American College of Zoological Medicine; Associate Professor of Zoological Medicine, Department of Small Animal Medicine and Surgery, College of Veterinary Medicine, University of Georgia, Athens, Georgia

EDITOR

VLADIMIR JEKL, DVM, PhD
Diplomate, European College of Zoological Medicine (Small Mammal Medicine and Surgery); Associate Professor, Avian and Exotic Animal Clinic, Faculty of Veterinary Medicine, University of Veterinary and Pharmaceutical Sciences Brno, Brno, Czech Republic

AUTHORS

TOM A. BAILEY, BVSc, MRCVS, CertZooMed, MSc, PhD
RCVS Specialist in Zoo and Wildlife Medicine; Diplomate, European College of Zoological Medicine; Origin Vets, Goetre Farm, Nr Narberth, Pembrokeshire, United Kingdom

HANA BANDOUCHOVA, MVDr, PhD
Diplomate, European College of Zoological Medicine (Wildlife Population Health); Department of Ecology and Diseases of Game, Fish and Bees, University of Veterinary and Pharmaceutical Sciences Brno, Brno, Czech Republic

DANIEL CALVO CARRASCO, LV CertAVP(ZooMed), MRCVS
Great Western Exotics, Vets-Now Referrals, Swindon, United Kingdom

EVA CERMAKOVA, DVM
Avian and Exotic Animal Clinic, Faculty of Veterinary Medicine, University of Veterinary and Pharmaceutical Sciences Brno, Brno, Czech Republic

NORIN CHAI, DVM, MSc, PhD
Diplomate, European College of Zoological Medicine (Zoo Health Management); Ménagerie du Jardin des Plantes, Muséum national d'Histoire naturelle, Paris, France

NICOLA DI GIROLAMO, DMV, MSc(EBHC), PhD
Diplomate, European College of Zoological Medicine(Herpetology); Clinica per Animali Esotici, Centro Veterinario Specialistico, Rome, Italy

MICHAELA GUMPENBERGER, Dr med vet
Assistant Professor, Clinical Unit of Diagnostic Imaging, Department for Companion Animals and Horses, University of Veterinary Medicine (Vetmeduni Vienna), Vienna, Austria

FRANCES MARGARET HARCOURT-BROWN, BVSc, FRCVS
Crab Lane Vets, North Yorkshire, United Kingdom

KAREL HAUPTMAN, DVM, PhD
Avian and Exotic Animal Clinic, Faculty of Veterinary Medicine, University of Veterinary and Pharmaceutical Sciences Brno, Brno, Czech Republic

GIANNI INSACCO, MNatSc
Scientific Curator, Museo Civico di Storia Naturale, Comiso (Ragusa), Sicily, Italy

VLADIMIR JEKL, DVM, PhD
Diplomate, European College of Zoological Medicine (Small Mammal Medicine and Surgery); Associate Professor, Avian and Exotic Animal Clinic, Faculty of Veterinary Medicine, University of Veterinary and Pharmaceutical Sciences Brno, Brno, Czech Republic

CATHY A. JOHNSON-DELANEY, DVM
Board of Directors, Washington Ferret Rescue & Shelter, Kirkland, Washington

KRISTA A. KELLER, DVM
Diplomate, American College of Zoological Medicine; Vida Veterinary Care, Denver, Colorado

ZDENEK KNOTEK, DVM, PhD
University Professor; Diplomate, European College of Zoological Medicine (Herpetology); European Recognized Veterinary Specialist in Zoological Medicine (Herpetology), Avian and Exotic Animal Clinic, Faculty of Veterinary Medicine, University of Veterinary and Pharmaceutical Sciences Brno, Brno, Czech Republic

LEONIE KONDERT, Dr med vet
Department of Small Animal Medicine and Surgery, College of Veterinary Medicine, University of Georgia, Athens, Georgia

VERONIKA KOVACOVA, MSc
Department of Ecology and Diseases of Game, Fish and Bees, University of Veterinary and Pharmaceutical Sciences Brno, Brno, Czech Republic

ANGELA M. LENNOX, DVM
Diplomate, American Board of Veterinary Practitioners-Avian, Exotic Companion Mammal; Diplomate, European College of Zoological Medicine-Small Mammals; Avian and Exotic Animal Clinic of Indianapolis, Indianapolis, Indiana

MICHAEL LIERZ, DZooMed
Diplomate, European College of Zoological Medicine (Wildlife Population Health); Diplomate, European College of Poultry Veterinary Science; Clinic for Birds, Reptiles, Amphibians and Fish, Justus-Liebig-University Giessen, Giessen, Germany

PETR LINHART, MSc
Department of Ecology and Diseases of Game, Fish and Bees, University of Veterinary and Pharmaceutical Sciences Brno, Brno, Czech Republic

JAUME MARTORELL, DVM, PhD
Diplomate, European College of Zoological Medicine (Small Mammal); Professor, Departament de Medicina I Cirurgia Animals, Facultat de Veterinaria, Universitat Autònoma de Barcelona, Bellaterra, Spain

JÖRG MAYER, Dr med vet, MSc
Diplomate American Board of Veterinary Practitioners (Exotic Companion Mammals); Diplomate European College of Zoological Medicine (Small Mammals); Diplomate American College of Zoological Medicine; Associate Professor of Zoological Medicine, Department of Small Animal Medicine and Surgery, College of Veterinary Medicine, University of Georgia, Athens, Georgia

MARK A. MITCHELL, DVM, MS, PhD
Diplomate, European College of Zoological Medicine (Herpetology); Department of Veterinary Clinical Sciences, Louisiana State University, School of Veterinary Medicine, Baton Rouge, Louisiana

MANUEL MORICI, DVM, PhD
Department of Veterinary Science, Polo Didattico Annunziata, Veterinary Teaching Hospital, University of Messina, Sicily, Messina, Italy

MATTEO OLIVERI, DVM
Avian and Exotic Animal Clinic, Faculty of Veterinary Medicine, University of Veterinary and Pharmaceutical Sciences Brno, Brno, Czech Republic

SEAN M. PERRY, DVM
Department of Veterinary Clinical Sciences, Louisiana State University, School of Veterinary Medicine, Baton Rouge, Louisiana

VLADIMIR PIACEK, MVDr
Department of Ecology and Diseases of Game, Fish and Bees, University of Veterinary and Pharmaceutical Sciences Brno, Brno, Czech Republic

JIRI PIKULA, MVDr, PhD
Diplomate, European College of Zoological Medicine (Wildlife Population Health); Professor, Department of Ecology and Diseases of Game, Fish and Bees, University of Veterinary and Pharmaceutical Sciences Brno, Brno, Czech Republic

MIKEL SABATER GONZÁLEZ, LV CertZooMed
Diplomate, European College of Zoological Medicine (Avian); Avian, Reptile and Exotic Pet Hospital, University of Sydney, Brownlow Hill, New South Wales, Australia

MARIO SANTORO, DVM, PhD
Diplomate, European College of Zoological Medicine (Wildlife Population Health); Istituto Zooprofilattico Sperimentale del Mezzogiorno, Portici (Naples), Italy

ALYSSA M. SCAGNELLI, DVM
Zoological Medicine Intern, Veterinary Clinical Sciences, School of Veterinary Medicine, Louisiana State University, Baton Rouge, Louisiana

PAOLO SELLERI, DMV, PhD
Diplomate, European College of Zoological Medicine (Herpetology & Small Mammals); Clinica per Animali Esotici, Centro Veterinario Specialistico, Rome, Italy

FILIPPO SPADOLA, DVM, PhD
Associate Professor, Department of Veterinary Science, Polo Didattico Annunziata, Veterinary Teaching Hospital, University of Messina, Sicily, Messina, Italy

THOMAS N. TULLY Jr, DVM, MS
Diplomate, American Board of Veterinary Practitioners (Avian); Diplomate, European
College of Zoological Medicine; Professor of Zoological Medicine, Veterinary Clinical
Sciences, School of Veterinary Medicine, Louisiana State University, Baton Rouge,
Louisiana

JAN ZUKAL, PhD
Associate Professor, Institute of Vertebrate Biology, Academy of Sciences of the Czech
Republic, Brno, Czech Republic

Contents

Reproduction of amphibians includes ovulation, spermiation, fertilization, oviposition, larval stage and development, and metamorphosis. A problem at any stage could lead to reproductive failure. To stimulate reproduction, environmental conditions must be arranged to simulate changes in natural habits. Reproductive life history is well documented in amphibians; a thorough knowledge of this subject will aid the practitioner in diagnosis and treatment. Technologies for artificial reproduction are developing rapidly, and some protocols may be transferable to privately kept or endangered species. Reproductive tract disorders are rarely described; no bacterial or viral diseases are known that specifically target the amphibian reproductive system.

Diagnostic imaging of the reproductive tract in reptiles is used for gender determination, evaluation of breeding status, detection of pathologic changes, and supervising treatment. Whole-body radiographs provide an overview and support detection of mineralized egg shells. Sonography is used to evaluate follicles, nonmineralized eggs, and the salpinx in all reptiles. Computed tomography is able to overcome imaging limitations in chelonian species. This article provides detailed information about the performance of different imaging techniques. Multiple images demonstrate the physiologic appearance of the male and female reproductive tract in various reptile species and pathologic changes. Advantages and disadvantages of radiography, sonography, and computed tomography are described.

Sea turtles' reproductive disorders are underdiagnosed, but potentially, there are several diseases that may affect gonads, genitalia, and annexes. Viruses, bacteria, and parasites may cause countless disorders, but more frequently the cause is traumatic or linked to human activities. Furthermore, veterinary management of the nest is of paramount importance as well as the care of newborns (also in captivity). This article gives an overview on the methods used to manage nests and reproductive activities of these endangered chelonians species.

Chelonian reproductive medicine is an extremely important facet to ensuring captive populations for the pet trade and conservation efforts around the globe. This article covers basic chelonian reproductive anatomy and physiology, natural history, behavior, and sexing chelonians, in addition to discussing reproductive disorders that are commonly seen by veterinarians. Reproductive disorders covered include infertility, dystocia, follicular stasis, egg yolk coelomitis, phallus prolapse, and reproductive neoplasia. It is hoped that this information will allow clinicians to recognize, understand, and successfully treat reproductive disorders in chelonians, thus providing the best available care for our chelonian patients.

 Video content accompanies this article at http://www.vetexotic. theclinics.com.

Reproduction of snakes is one of the challenging aspects of herpetology medicine. Due to the complexity of reproduction, several disorders may present before, during, or after this process. This article describes the physical examination, and radiographic, ultrasonographic, and endoscopic findings associated with reproductive disorders in snakes. Surgical techniques used to resolve reproductive disorders in snakes are described. Finally, common reproductive disorders in snakes are individually discussed.

Common reproductive problems in captive male lizards are hemipenile plugs in hemipenial sac, unilateral prolapse of hemipenis, or bilateral prolapse of hemipene. Although the orchiectomy is performed as a treatment for testicular disease, the effectiveness in reducing aggressive behavior is unclear. Female captive lizards suffer from cloacal prolapse, preovulatory follicular stasis, or dystocia. The veterinarian must differentiate between the disorders because the treatment differs. Mating, physical, or visual contact with the male stimulates ovulation and prevents preovulatory follicular stasis. Surgical intervention is usually required for dystocia. This article discusses selected procedures and use of ultrasonography and diagnostic endoscopy.

Reptile perinatology refers to the time period surrounding hatching for oviparous species, and immediately after birth for viviparous species. Veterinarians working in myriad conservation and breeding programs require knowledge in this area. This article reviews anatomy and physiology of the amniotic egg, the basics of artificial incubation, when manual pipping is indicated, and basic medicine of the reptile hatchling or neonate.

Video content accompanies this article at http://www.vetexotic.
theclinics.com.

Captive breeding has contributed to successful restoration of many species of birds of prey. Avicultural techniques pioneered by raptor breeders
include double clutching, direct fostering, cross-fostering, hatch and
switch, hacking, imprinting male and female falcons for semen collection,
and artificial insemination techniques. However, reproductive failure occurs related to management problems, including hygiene measures,
food quality issues, breeding flock structure, or individual health issues
of breeding birds. These may result in non–egg laying females, low-
quality eggs, or infertile eggs caused by male infertility. Veterinary care
of breeding collections is extremely important. This article provides an
overview of veterinary involvement in raptor breeding projects.

Disease affecting the reproductive tract of the companion parrot is often
impacted by physiologic and environmental stimuli. In conjunction with
appropriate medical management, some birds diagnosed with reproductive disorders may be successfully treated. Once the bird is diagnosed
with a disease condition affecting the reproductive tract, therapeutic measures are focused on stabilizing and supporting the patient, and surgical
intervention is required only in the most severe cases. Hormonal therapy
with synthetic, long-acting GnRH agonists should be considered for
chronic reproductive disease conditions in which decreasing ovarian activity can help alleviate certain disease processes.

Backyard poultry and other commonly kept fowl species are often kept for
their ability to lay eggs. Reproductive disease is common in fowl species.
Despite being classified as food-producing species, they can be considered valuable pets, and the demand for adequate veterinary care is
constantly increasing. The clinician should be familiar with the different abnormalities and the potential treatment options. Fowl species have been
traditionally an anatomic, physiologic, and experimental model for avian
medicine; however, information about treatment options is often limited
and extrapolated from other species.

Marsupial reproduction differs significantly in anatomy and physiology
from that of placental mammals. The gastrointestinal and urogenital tracts
empty into a cloaca. Reproductive parameters include gestation and
pouch time, as the fetus develops outside of the uterus. Captive marsupials discussed include sugar gliders), short-tailed opossums, Virginia

opossums, and Tammar and Bennett's wallabies. Common disease conditions include joey eviction, pouch infections, mastitis, metritis, prostatitis, penile necrosis, and neoplasia. Common surgeries include penile amputation, castration, and ovario-vaginal-hysterectomy or ovario-hysterectomy. Therapeutics used for these conditions are presented.

Disorders of the reproductive tract are common in rabbits. Conditions are different in rabbits that are farmed for their meat or fur and those that are kept as pets. Farmed rabbits suffer from infections and diseases associated with pregnancy. Congenital abnormalities are more likely to be recognized and treated in pet rabbits. Pet rabbits suffer from age-related changes to their genital tract (hyperplasia, neoplasia, or hernias). Neutering is an important part of prevention and treatment of reproductive disorders. Knowledge of normal male and female reproductive anatomy is essential to prevent complications. These are described and illustrated.

Reproduction diseases are common presentations in small rodents. Some can be presented to the clinician as an emergency where a fast and effective treatment is required. This article presents an overview of reproductive disorders in these species. Diseases affecting the ovary, uterus, testicles, and mammary gland are developed in rats, mice, hamsters, and gerbils: inflammatory, infectious, and neoplasia. Clinical signs, diagnosis, and treatment information are included. Some specific indications about the surgical reproduction procedures are described. Literature regarding reproductive disorders exists for squirrels and prairie dogs. Brief information about the normal anatomy of the reproductive system is given.

Guinea pigs, chinchillas, and degus are hystricomorph rodents originating from South America. They are commonly presented as exotic pets in veterinary practice. Reviewing the anatomy and physiology of their reproductive tract helps to offer better client education about preventive medicine and helps to act faster in emergency situations. Choosing the right anesthetic protocol helps to prevent complications. This article should aid as a guideline on the most common reproductive problems of these 3 species and help in making decisions regarding the best treatment options.

In the United States, desexing is performed routinely in ferrets at the age of 6 weeks, therefore reproductive tract diseases are not so common. However, in Europe most ferrets are desexed when they are several months old, or they are kept as intact animals. For this reason, diseases of the reproductive organs and a prolonged estrus are far more frequent in Europe than in the United States. This article summarizes and reviews the anatomy, reproductive physiology, management of reproduction (including surgical and hormonal contraception) and reproductive tract diseases in male and female ferrets.

Jiri Pikula, Hana Bandouchova, Veronika Kovacova, Petr Linhart, Vladimir Piacek, and Jan Zukal

Long-term conservation and educational activities of numerous nongovernmental organizations have greatly increased public awareness about bats and their lifestyle. As a result, there is growing public concern about threats to bat populations. Many species of bats declined over recent decades and there is great demand for medical services to help injured or diseased bats. Veterinary clinicians dealing with such cases have to consider many issues, including ethical issues associated with the delayed fertilization reproduction strategy of temperate insectivorous bats. An outline of veterinary and physiologic requirements for treatment of and keeping vespertilionid bats in captivity is highlighted.

VETERINARY CLINICS OF NORTH AMERICA: EXOTIC ANIMAL PRACTICE

THE CLINICS ARE NOW AVAILABLE ONLINE!
Access your subscription at:
www.theclinics.com

Preface

Reproductive Medicine in Exotic Animal Species

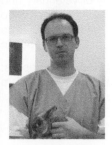

Vladimir Jekl, DVM, PhD
Editor

It is indeed an honor and a pleasure to introduce the new issue of *Veterinary Clinics of North America: Exotic Animal Practice*. This issue focuses not only on the reproductive disorders of commonly kept exotic companion animals but also on the reproductive management of endangered species, as captive breeding has contributed to the successful restoration of many exotic animals.

Within the past few years, quality research has delved into the anatomic and physiologic soundness of procedures, response to therapy, and development of the associate diseases. Of particular relevance is the assessment of short- and long-term responses to certain drugs and reproductive techniques (eg, long-acting synthetic gonadotropins as contraceptive drugs).

This issue intended to review the most current and up-to-date knowledge about reproductive tract anatomy, physiology, diagnostics, reproductive tract diseases, and management of reproduction of selected groups of exotic companion and wild animals (eg, amphibians, reptiles, birds of prey, and bats).

I sincerely thank the authors, who are specialists with considerable routine experience with the animal species they write about, for sharing their knowledge and valuable time. I hope the amount and depth of information supplemented with high-quality images will be of interest and value to practitioners, researchers, veterinary students, and zoologic conservation. All information is given in an easy-to-read style and can be readily applicable in the clinical and zoologic practice. I would also like to

Vet Clin Exot Anim 20 (2017) xiii–xiv
http://dx.doi.org/10.1016/j.cvex.2016.11.017
1094-9194/17/© 2016 Published by Elsevier Inc.

vetexotic.theclinics.com

thank Meredith Madeira, Developmental Editor, for her assistance during preparation of this issue.

Vladimir Jekl, DVM, PhD
Avian and Exotic Animal Clinic
Faculty of Veterinary Medicine
University of Veterinary and
Pharmaceutical Sciences Brno
Palackeho tr. 1946/1, 61242 Brno
Czech Republic

E-mail addresses:
jeklv@vfu.cz; VladimirJekl@gmail.com

Reproductive Medicine in Amphibians

Norin Chai, DVM, MSc, PhD, DECZM (Zoo Health Management)

KEYWORDS

- Amphibians • Reproduction • Anatomy • Artificial reproduction • In vitro fertilization
- Reproductive surgery • Reproductive disorder

KEY POINTS

- In general, to stimulate reproduction, environmental conditions have to be arranged to simulate changes in natural habits.
- Reproductive life history is well documented in amphibians; a thorough knowledge of this subject will aid the practitioner in diagnosis and treatment.
- Reproductive disorders are rarely described in amphibians.
- Some protocols of artificial reproduction were developed with research models and may be transferable to privately kept or endangered species.

INTRODUCTION

Amphibians are globally distributed except in the polar regions of Antarctica. They display a diversity of life history and reproductive strategies to suit almost all habitats, from rainforests to deserts. New species continue to be discovered. There are 3 orders of amphibians: Anura, Caudata, and Gymnophiona. The AmphibiaWeb database currently contains 7546 amphibian species.[1] Each year more veterinarians are seeing amphibian patients, and the knowledge of how to manage these animals is increasing at a rapid pace. If reproductive disorders are rarely described in private practice or zoo collections, it may be a future common topic in research facilities or some breeding program for conservation initiatives to fight against declining populations.

Reproduction of amphibians includes ovulation, spermiation, fertilization, oviposition, larval stage and development, and metamorphosis. Thus, a problem at any stage could lead to reproductive failure. To stimulate reproduction, environmental conditions have to be arranged to simulate changes in natural habits: raining, cooling, heating, varying photoperiod, varying amount of food, and so forth. Optimal reproduction in captivity of one species is linked to the extensive knowledge of its natural biology (examples in **Table 1**).

The author has nothing to disclose.
Ménagerie du Jardin des Plantes, Muséum national d'Histoire naturelle, 57 Rue Cuvier, Paris 75005, France
E-mail address: norin.chai@mnhn.fr

Table 1
Reproductive life history of selected species of amphibians

Family	Sexing	Life History, Habitat	Reproduction Biology
Fire-bellied toad (*Bombina bombina*, Bombinatoridae)	Male has resonators, a slightly larger head, and, during the breeding season, black nuptial pads on the 1st and 2nd fingers and on the inner surface of his forearm	Eurasia. Temperature usually at 18–20°C. Activity in the daytime, but the maximum calling by males occurs at dusk Tadpoles consume mainly algae and higher plants; lower animals frequently are eaten. Adults consume mainly various insects	Breeding season: May to the end of summer. Male vocalizes floating on the water surface (also able to call from under the water). Amplexus is pelvic
Toads (*Bufo* sp, Bufonidae)	Male differs from female in having nuptial pads on 1st finger (during the breeding season on 1st, 2nd, and/or 3rd fingers), smaller body size and in some body proportions	Eurasia. Active mainly in twilight. Adults are voracious and eat wood lice, slugs, beetles, caterpillars, flies, earthworms, and even small mice. They need spacious terrarium (100 L for a pair of *B bufo*), deep litter of leaf and important hygrometry maintained by vaporization. Temperature never above 23°C	Breeding season: March to June (usually late April to May). No vocalization. A few males often clasp one female, and in many instances several males try to clasp the same female. Amplexus is pectoral
Dendrobates (*Dendrobates* spp, *Phyllobates* spp, Dendrobatidae)	Difficult; sometimes variation in colors	Central and South America. Need a terrarium from at least 60 cm × 40 cm × 40 cm for 4 animals maximum with high temperature (26–28°C) and hygrometry (near 100%). Diet with small arthropods: drosophilas, micro-crickets, plant louses, ants, termites, very small insects	Diurnal, they lay eggs on land. Males are highly territorial (vocalization, wrestling competitions) and display cephalic amplexus (grasping the female around the head during mating, unique among anurans). Example in *Dendobates tinctorius*: Mating behavior starts with the male calling. The male then leads the female to his chosen spot, where a clutch of 2–6 eggs are laid. The eggs hatch within 14–18 d, and the tadpoles are carried to water pools within a plant leaf by both the female and the male

(*continued on next page*)

Table 1 (continued)			
Family	Sexing	Life History, Habitat	Reproduction Biology
Bullfrogs (*Rana catesbeiana*, Ranidae) "True frogs"	Males are smaller with yellow throats and tympani larger than their eyes. The tympani in females are about the same size as the eyes	Largest ranges of any North American amphibian. They are aquatic and terrestrial. They need aqua terrarium with emerged area. Bull frog can live in large temperature range, but is better grown between 20–25°C.	Breeding takes place in spring and early summer and is earliest in southern latitudes. Male will aggressively defend oviposition sites. Females select a mate by entering his territory. Older females sometimes vocalize within male choruses, which may elicit higher levels of male-male competition. Eggs are laid in thin sheets on the water surface. Bullfrogs are extremely prolific, producing up to 20,000 eggs/clutch
Tiger Salamander (*Ambystoma tigrinum*, Ambystomatidae)	Difficult; males typically have significantly longer and taller tails, but females are longer	Most widespread salamander species in North America. The environment must be terrestrial subtropical forester. The breeding is easy, between 15 and 25°C.	Typically spring breeders with migrations to breeding sites occurring at night during rainy weather. Breeding is aquatic. Males compete for access to females, who then choose. Upon spermataphore deposition by the male, a female quickly decides whether to induct. Tiger salamanders show a wide range of clutch sizes, from an average of 421 ova to 7631 eggs

NORMAL ANATOMY, SEXING

Sexual dimorphism is present in almost all species from all orders of amphibians except the caecilians (**Fig. 1**). In the "true" salamanders and newts (Urodela: Salamandridae), sexual dimorphism is common. In most cases, the dimorphisms are discrete and have been demonstrated qualitatively, such as the presence of male secondary sexual characteristics or differences in head size or tail length. For instance, the male great crested newt (*Triturus cristatus*) has a swollen and dark cloaca, and during the breeding season, it has a deeply notched middorsal crest, which extends from the level of eyes to the base of tail. The female lacks these characters, and its cloaca is flattened with a tail presenting a longitudinal reddish or orange band from below (**Fig. 2**). The most common method used to sex anurans is to identify differences between sexes in nuptial pads, tympanum size and color, throat and body color, and

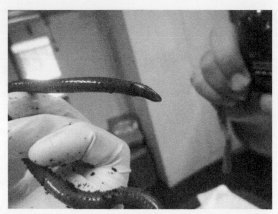

Fig. 1. In caecilians, there is no sexual dimorphism. The specimen here is a *Geotrypetes seraphini*. (*Courtesy of* Norin Chai, DVM, MSc, PhD, DECZM (ZHM), Paris, France.)

vocalization. The thumbs present hypertrophies in males (nuptial pads) to help the male to hold the female during mating (amplexus; **Fig. 3**A, B). Nuptial pads tend to be more prominent in aquatic spawning compared with terrestrial spawning amphibians. In some species, nuptial pads are absent, like in midwife toads (*Alytes* sp) or apparently in Dendrobatidae species. The tympanic membrane is larger in the males of some frogs, and it is used it to amplify vocalizations.[2] In males of some species, the vocal sac may clearly be seen (**Fig. 3**C, D). Throats of male frogs are generally darker and more colored than those of the females. The throats of females are often pale or white, but not in all species (**Fig. 3**E–G). Some species have dramatic color and pattern differences between males and females. For instance, the common toad (*Bufo bufo*) tends to be sexually dimorphic with the females being browner and the males being grayer. In the Chiriqui harlequin frog (*Atelopus chiriquiensis*), sexual dimorphism is clearly obvious with the female larger than the male with highly variable colors (uniformly yellow, lime green in males and orange or orange-red striped in females). In female marsupial frogs, a "pouch" may be seen, a sac underlying the dorsal integument (**Fig. 4**). This pouch is absent in the male and juvenile female. In general, only males

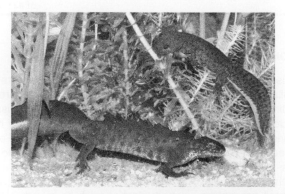

Fig. 2. Sexual dimorphism in the great crested newt (*T cristatus*). During the breeding season, the male has a deeply notched middorsal crest that extends from the level of eyes to the base of tail. (*Courtesy of* Françoise Serre-Colet, France; with permission.)

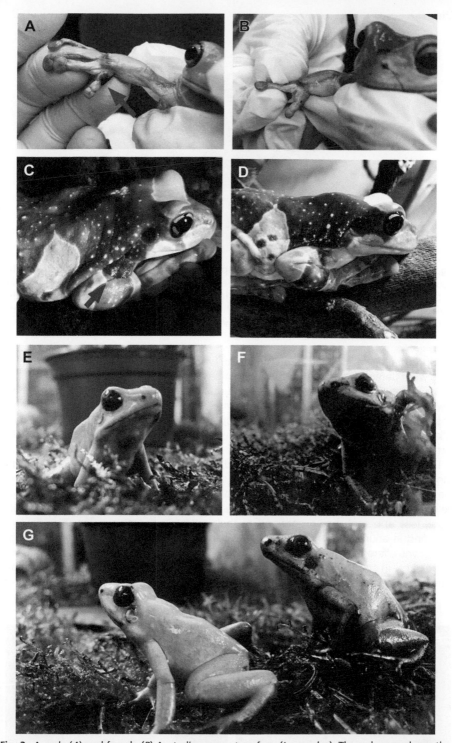

Fig. 3. A male (*A*) and female (*B*) Australian green tree frog (*L caerulea*). The red arrow shows the nuptial pads (often melanic) of the male. A male (*C*) and female (*D*) Amazon milk frog (*Trachycephalus resinifictrix*). The red arrow shows the vocal sac of the male. A female (*E*) and a male (*F*) golden poison frog (*Phyllobates terribilis*). (*G*) Throats of male frogs are generally darker and more colored than those of the females. The throats of females are often pale or white (this is not in all species and even in not all populations). (*Courtesy of* Norin Chai, DVM, MSc, PhD, DECZM (ZHM), Paris, France.)

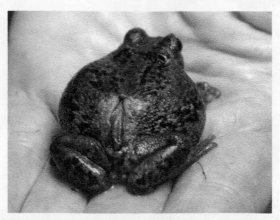

Fig. 4. Maternal pouch of an Andean marsupial tree frog (*Gastrotheca riobambae*). The pouch is a sac underlying the dorsal integument, but is essentially independent of it except at the aperture. It is absent in the male and juvenile female. After the eggs leave the female's cloaca, the male places them inside the pouch, where the embryos develop until the tadpole stage. (*Courtesy of* Norin Chai, DVM, MSc, PhD, DECZM (ZHM), Paris, France.)

produce mating calls. However, in Australian green tree frogs (*Litoria caerulea*), mating calls were detected by the author in both male and female. The range of reproductive characteristics in salamanders includes nuptial pads, which can form on the digits, lower forearm, and mouth. The crests of many newts prominently reflect permanent or seasonal changes in the intensity and display of coloration.[3] It is difficult to sex caecilians by external morphology or color; however, a sign of breeding in this taxa is the formation of cloacal glands on the males.[4]

The testis is an elongated organ located posteriorly in the pleuroperitoneal cavity lying ventral and connected to the kidney by the mesorchium. In adult caecilians, the paired testes are elongated and lobulated. In salamanders, additional lobes may be added with each breeding season. The small, ovoid testes of the male frogs are much less apparent, being confined to their relatively dorsal position (**Fig. 5**). One may find in anurans pigmented testes. Sperm reach nephric collecting tubules by way of vas efferentes, which lead into the Wolfian duct. The Wolfian duct empty sperm into cloaca. In caudata like the common mudpuppy (*Necturus maculosus*), the narrow anterior part of the kidney is genital in function, while the wider posterior portion is

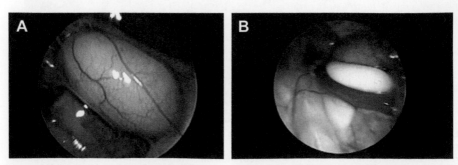

Fig. 5. (*A*) Testis of an American bullfrog (*L catesbeiana*). (*B*) Testis of giant monkey frog (*P bicolor*). (*Courtesy of* Norin Chai, DVM, MSc, PhD, DECZM (ZHM), Paris, France.)

urinary.[5] The nephric collecting duct carries sperm from the testis as well as urine from the urinary portion of the kidney. Sperm reach the duct by way of ductules efferentes, which lead into the genital portion of the kidney and thence to the Wolfian duct.[6] In male caudata, a vestigial oviduct can be seen as a dark threadlike structure along the lateral edge of the nephric duct. It has no connection with the latter and continues anteriorly on its own.

In male salamander, the margins of the cloaca bear numerous cloacal papillae, which engorge during the breeding season and consist of numerous tiny tubules and are involved in clumping sperm to form spermatophores. The spermatophore is a gelatinous structure that encapsulates the sperm to protect it from the environment before it is taken up by the female's cloaca. In caecilians, an intromittent organ, the phallodeum, is present, which allows for internal fertilization.[6] Internal fertilization has evolved independently several times in frogs. In *Ascaphus*, the "tailed frogs" from western North America, the cloaca of the male has been modified to form a copulatory organ that is inserted into the cloaca of the female for mating. These frogs are the only species with internal fertilization that have true inguinal amplexus.

In females, the elongated ovary, supported by the mesovarium (**Fig. 6A**), may be quite large. The presence of numerous eggs within follicles gives the ovary a lobulated or granular appearance (**Fig. 6B**), in contrast to the more regular surface of the testes. The follicles and eggs vary in size depending on their stage of maturity, being quite large in some specimens and smaller in others. The nephric duct in the female carries only urine from the kidney. The oviduct is the long, prominent, and convoluted tube lying between the ovary and kidney and extending nearly the length of the peritoneal cavity. At its anterior end is the open, funnel-shaped ostium, into which the eggs pass after they have been released into the coelom by the ovary.[5,6] Cloacal glands and papillae are absent in the female salamanders.

In both sexes, each gonad is associated with a conspicuous fat body, which is subdivided into numerous digitiform lobes that are often pressed up against the sides of the pleuroperitoneal cavity. Stored nutrients in the fat bodies are primarily used to nourish the developing gametes. The size of the fat bodies thus varies greatly with the stage of reproductive cycle.[5]

Bidder's organ is an ovarylike structure, which develops from the anterior part of the gonadal ridge in anuran amphibians belonging to the Bufonidae family. Because of similarity with the undeveloped ovary, Bidder's organ was, in early literature, described inaccurately, as a structure present only in males. In fact, Bidder's organs are present in males and females of most bufonid species. They usually disappear in females during the lifetime. Because Bidder's organ contains female germ cells (oocytes), the bufonid males are de facto hermaphrodites. Bidder's organs grow and resume oogenesis after the removal of testes and grow when the testosterone level is low, which occurs depending on the species during a reproductive or nonreproductive season.[7]

If sexual dimorphisms are not obvious, sexing may also be achieved by ultrasound or endoscopy (**Fig. 6C–F**).[8]

REPRODUCTIVE LIFE HISTORY

Amphibians are unique among vertebrates in the variety of ways in which they reproduce. There have been many attempts to classify amphibian reproductive modes. Only for Anurans, 29 reproductive modes had been listed.[4] This classification was based on features such as site of egg deposition (in water, on land, or retained in the oviducts), type of eggs (small aquatic eggs, large terrestrial eggs, foam nests, and so forth), and mode of development (feeding or nonfeeding aquatic larvae, nonaquatic

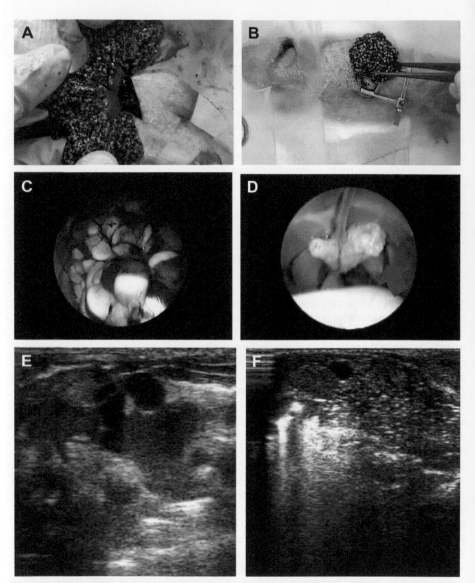

Fig. 6. (*A*) The mesovarium supports the ovary, here in an African clawed frog (*X laevis*). (*B*) Ovary of an axolotl (*A mexicanum*). Amphibian coelioscopy in (*C*) an African clawed frog of giant and (*D*) in immature great crested newt (*T cristatus*) where one can note the immature ovaries that are dorsally located (*red arrow*). Sexing 2 cururu toads (*Bufo paracnemis*) by ultrasound: male (*E*) and female (*F*). In the female, the irregularly shaped ovaries are generally conspicuous, "speckled" structures containing developing follicles that are usually visible. (*Courtesy of* Norin Chai, DVM, MSc, PhD, DECZM (ZHM), Paris, France.)

larvae, or direct development of eggs into small froglets). This list has been updated, bringing the total to 39.[9] All of the modes of egg deposition and development found in urodeles have been described in anurans.[10] The reproductive mechanisms of amphibians are as varied as their phylogeny, microhabitats, and life histories. Extensive reviews on amphibian reproduction can be found in excellent reviews.[4,10]

Typically, anurans are oviparous; salamanders and newts are ovoviviparous, and caecilians are viviparous, although there are some exceptions to these categorizations, especially in anurans. Most caecilians and salamanders spawn annually, although some spawn biannually or intermittently. For instance, in the Japanese clawed salamander (*Onychodactylus japonicus*), 2 spawning periods at a single breeding site: in May-July and October-December, have been described. Temperate and some mountain anurans tend to spawn annually. For instance, the common frog (*Rana temporaria*) will spawn generally in April. Tropical anurans in wet habitats spawn multiple clutches throughout the year, like the dwarf tree frog (*Hyla nana*) or the Uruguay harlequin frog (*Lysapsus limellus*). Anurans from arid areas often aestivate and spawn immediately after flooding rains, which may not occur for years. Clutch size also varies widely among species. Some amphibians like the dyeing poison frog (*Dendrobates tinctorius*) or the yellow-headed poison frog (*Dendrobates leucomelas*) may have as low as 2 eggs per clutch (sometimes until 6–10), whereas some anurans such as the bullfrog (*Rana catesbeiana*) spawn many thousands. All caecilians and most salamanders use internal fertilization. Except in the genus *Ascaphus*, fertilization is external in anurans. Eggs are usually laid in water or moist locations (**Fig. 7**). Anurans generally have an aquatic tadpole or larval stage and undergo metamorphosis to produce the radically different adult form. However, some members of the Pipidae produce eggs that develop directly into juvenile frogs. Some species of Nectophrynoides (*Bufonidae*) are viviparous. In *Gastrotheca* sp (Hylidae), the juvenile frogs develop directly in pouches in the female's skin. In *Rhinoderma darwini* (Rhinodermatidae), the tadpoles complete their development in the vocal sacs of the male and in female stomachs in *Rheobatrachus silus*.[11] The author refers interested readers to a review of current amphibian biology and conservation, which includes reproduction protocols for a range of species.[1,4,10]

REPRODUCTIVE PHYSIOLOGY

The age of sexual maturity in amphibians is generally lower in males than in females. Males of some species regularly mature in less than 4 months, whereas females often first spawn in their second year.[4,12] In most amphibians, egg numbers increase with female weight. Like in other vertebrates, external environmental cues are responsible for the production of primary hormones in the hypothalamus, pituitary gland, and gonads. The hormonal systems in anurans, urodeles, and caecilians are similar, and hormonal pathways can be found elsewhere.[11]

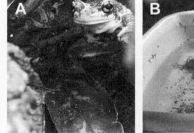
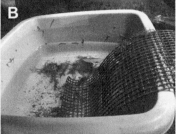
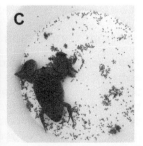

Fig. 7. Eggs are usually laid in water or moist locations. (*A*) Egg laying on a leaf of an Amazon milk frog. (*B*) A pool/water nest before the cleaning (water must be changed every day). (*C*) African clawed frog lays eggs easily in water. (*Courtesy of* Norin Chai, DVM, MSc, PhD, DECZM (ZHM), Paris, France.)

REPRODUCTION IN CAPTIVITY

Any breeding program requires adequate environmental conditioning of both females and males. Even the use of hormonal induction may be ineffective if amphibians are not in good condition. Variables include temperature, nutrition, and light. Water qualities including temperature, depth, and dispersion often induce the final stages of reproduction.[4] In some species, including Xenopus laevis and Pipa parva, vocalizations are paramount in inducing ovulation, and such calls can induce ovulation and even oviposition.[13] A seasonal cycling of temperature and humidity is essential for the maturation of follicles in some species. This cycling of temperature can include hibernation, aestivation, and slow and rapid temperature changes. For captive breeding, it is necessary to program the cycle to the same magnitude and duration as that in the wild.[14] Temperature may also affect both ovarian maturation and the maturation of testes. Red-backed salamanders (Plethodon cinereus) require low temperatures to induce spermiation.[4] In contrast, the testes of the marbled newt (Triturus marmoratus marmoratus) or the northern leopard frog (Rana sylvatica) do not mature at low temperatures.[4] The ingestion of large amounts of feed can accelerate the maturation of the ovaries of some amphibians, clearly seen in the toad, B bufo.[14] Females in particular should receive a continuous surplus of food for the last 6 to 8 weeks before reproduction. However, consumption of a diet in excess of an animal's energy needs can cause obesity and related disease (eg, corneal lipidosis, fatty liver). As the photoperiod affects the reproductive cycles of some caudates and anurans, it is advisable to follow the natural day/light cycle when providing light for captive species, particularly with species from high latitudes. However, for most species, the photoperiod requirements are not known.[15] The cycling of reproduction follows rainfall in some species, and aestivation protocols can be a useful tool to bring some amphibians into breeding condition. Species that respond to rainfall as a cue to induce calling in males and spawning in females can be amenable to the use of simulated rain events for promoting reproduction.[11] For instance, the breeding migration of the Mexican spadefoot (Spea multiplicata) is triggered when monsoon rainfall fills temporary pools, usually in July. The rain tank should have a design and a program to produce intermittent simulated heavy rainfall. The simulated rain should cycle with dry periods with a suggested duration of 30 to 60 minutes 2 or 3 times a day. For small arboreal species from tropical forests, a cycling from a dry environment to a wet and humid environment may induce spawning like with Leptodactylus macrosternum. Small sheltered pools, raising water levels, or the provision of large plastic leaves provides specialized spawning sites.[11] Consequently, because of the number of affecting factors and the complexity of their interaction, the success of either natural entrainment or the artificial induction of ovulation can be unpredictable.

ARTIFICIAL FERTILIZATION

Technologies for the reproduction of amphibians in captivity are developing rapidly, and particular techniques for sperm cryopreservation and for the induction of ovulation are undergoing improvement. The literature reflects the development of reliable techniques for the cryopreservation of sperm and for the short-term storage of oocytes for a range of amphibians in research and conservation.[16] A review has summarized valuable technological achievements in amphibian artificial fertilization that need to be considered when developing artificial fertilization techniques for species conservation.[17] A recent article describes a reliable protocol for gamete collection from live axolotl and in vitro fertilization for urodele amphibians that may be transferable to endangered urodeles.[18]

In the author's institution, they use in vitro fertilization in *X laevis*, especially for research purposes. The method is standardized. Here are the basic steps. The research facility uses 12:12-hours light:dark cycles, an ambient temperature of 18°C to 19°C, dechlorinated and filtered water, and a commercial diet (TetraRubin granules). Males are not necessarily injected with human chorionic gonadotropin (hCG); if so (when they are to full sexual maturity), 300 units of hCG are used. Male frogs are sacrificed with a 40-minute bath of tricaine methanesulfonate (1 g/L; MS-222) followed by decapitation. Their testes are removed and placed in Petri dishes with cold 1× Marc's modified Ringers (MMR: 0.1 M NaCl, 2.0 M KCl, 1 mM $MgSO_4$, 2 mM $CaCl_2$, 5 mM HEPES [pH 7.8], 0.1 mM EDTA) at 4°C. Testis can be kept for up to 2 weeks in the refrigerator. Ovulation is induced by injection of hCG. Females are injected (generally in the evening) with 500 to 1000 units of hCG (depending on the size) into the dorsal lymph sac (**Fig. 8**A) and placed in a large tank containing good-quality water at a depth of approximately 15 cm. Egg laying starts quickly in the middle of the night. After 12 hours, eggs are collected manually by gentle lateral and vertical pressure on the caudal part of the female (**Fig. 8**B) (the idea is to mimic the actions of the male frog) and put in Petri dishes with 1× MMR at room temperature. Then, using a 1000-μL tip, eggs are moved into a single layer. Meanwhile, the testis is cut off and chopped (**Fig. 8**C, D) and put in 0.4× MMR at room temperature. Then, with a sterile forceps, the author teases a piece of testis apart and rubs the tissue over the waiting eggs (**Fig. 8**E). After contact with sperm, the eggs are flooded with 0.1× MMR (**Fig. 8**F). Shortly after fertilization, a transient contraction of the highly pigmented animal cap occurs, and a region of denser pigmentation on the ventral side of the embryo becomes discernible. It is the cortical cytoplasmique rotation, meaning that fertilization was successful (**Fig. 8**G, H). The embryos are removed to a small beaker, and dechlorinated water with 2% cysteine is used to dejelly the embryos. The dejellied embryos are then washed with 0.1× MMR and placed in a Petri dish with 0.1× MMR and 1% agarose in water at the bottom. Petri dishes are incubated at 16°C until ready to use for research or at 23°C for production of tadpoles. This description gives the practitioner the basis of in vitro fertilization. The technique can be a very good start for further studies aiming to improve the yield of reproduction and to introduce the IVF technique in assisted breeding programs adapted to endangered amphibian populations.

INFECTIOUS AND PARASITIC DISEASES

Bacterial organisms may be the primary cause of disease, or they may be secondary invaders, taking advantage of a breach in the amphibian's integument or compromise of its immune system, common consequences of other problems such as traumatic injury in unsanitary captive situations. Most of bacterial environmental agents become pathogens in stressed animals. Most pathogenic bacteria are gram-negative organisms, yet gram-positive bacteria may also produce significant disease. Despite the high incidence of septicemias, involvement of the gonads in cases of bacterial septicemia is relatively rare. No bacterial infections are known that specifically target the amphibian reproductive system. Infection of the pouch of female *Gastrotheca* sp is more a dermatologic issue than a reproductive disorder (**Fig. 9**A). In the author's experience, the only bacterial disease that involves the reproductive system as sole macroscopic lesion is systemic mycobacterial infections. Mycobacteriosis is predominately a chronic granulomatous infection. Although insidious chronicity with no clinical signs is the rule, peracute and acute cases may occur, reflecting the heterogeneous biological behavior of the various mycobacterial species as well as the heterogeneity of host responses. An increasingly diverse array of *Mycobacterium* spp has been isolated from

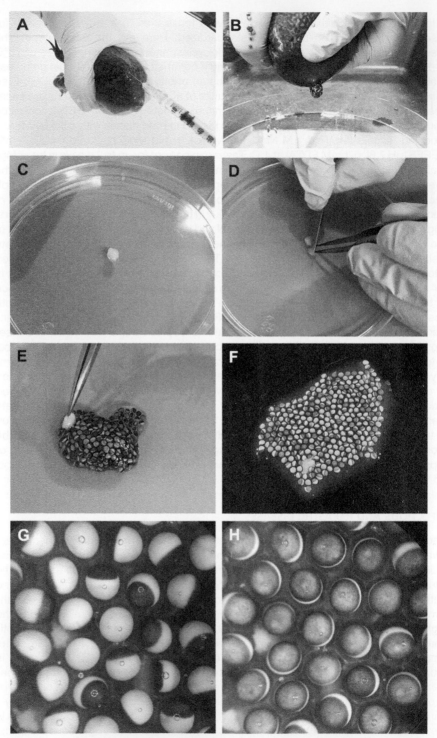

Fig. 8. In vitro fertilization in African clawed frog. (*A*) Females are injected (generally in the evening) with 500 to 1000 units of hCG (depending on the size) into the dorsal lymph sac.

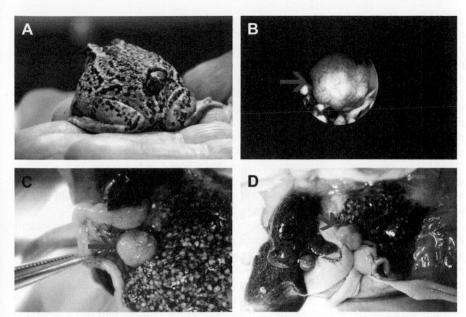

Fig. 9. (A) Abscess of the maternal pouch of an Andean marsupial tree frog. (B) Ovarian abscess in a western clawed frog (X tropicalis) caused by M szulgaï observed by endoscopy (red arrow). (C, D) Two cases of M szulgaï infection in the western clawed frog, where the only lesion was a granuloma in the ovary (red arrow). (Courtesy of Norin Chai, DVM, MSc, PhD, DECZM (ZHM), Paris, France.)

frogs in recent years, supplanting the paradigm of Mycobacterium marinum, Mycobacterium fortuitum, and Mycobacterium xenopi as the only causing agents adequately described. Several mycobacteria species have been isolated (eg, Mycobacterium abscessus, Mycobacterium chelonae, M fortuitum, M marinum, Mycobacterium gordonae, Mycobacterium ranae, Mycobacterium thamnospheos, Mycobacterium avium, M xenopi, Mycobacterium szulgaï). In the last 10 years, a Mycobacterium spp closely related to Mycobacterium ulcerans and M marinum, has been isolated from Xenopus tropicalis: Mycobacterium liflandii, characterized by the presence of insertion sequences IS2404 and IS2606, as well as by the production of the toxin, mycolactone. The author has diagnosed and managed multiple outbreaks of mycobacterial infections in laboratory-reared X laevis and X tropicalis. In 2 cases of M szulgaï infection, the only lesion seen was a granuloma in the ovary (Fig. 9B–D). A review on Mycobacteriosis in amphibians can be found elsewhere.[19]

The most significant and well-studied anurans viruses are Ranaviruses (Iridoviridae). A review on ranaviruses has been published recently.[20] In amphibians, outbreaks of ranaviral disease are most often observed in larvae and recently metamorphosed

---

(B) Eggs are collected manually by gentle lateral and vertical pressure on the caudal part of the female. (C, D) The testis is cut off and chopped. (E) With a sterile forceps, a piece of testis is rubbed over the waiting egg (it is important to touch every egg with the testis). (F) After contact with sperm, the eggs are flooded with MMR. (G, H) Shortly after fertilization, a transient contraction of the highly pigmented animal cap occurs, and a region of denser pigmentation on the ventral side of the embryo becomes discernible. It is the cortical cytoplasmique rotation, meaning that fertilization was successful. (Courtesy of Norin Chai, DVM, MSc, PhD, DECZM (ZHM), Paris, France.)

animals (outbreaks that include adult animals are recognized as well).[21] It has been demonstrated that ranavirus-associated mortality of larvae or metamorphs was sufficient to cause population declines in highly susceptible species. Mortality events often present as sudden and massive deaths across multiple species.[22] Deaths may continue for weeks, with later deaths due to individuals succumbing to secondary bacterial or fungal infections. The appearance of disease in individual animals reflects the systemic distribution of the virus and associated host response. Internally, hemorrhage and necrosis are common findings, especially in the spleen, pronephros and mesonephros (kidney), and liver. Even if necrosis may present in several organs, the reproductive system is rarely involved. To the author's knowledge, only one study clearly describes a lesion in gonads with ranaviral disease. In this outbreak associated with mass mortality in wild amphibians in France, moderate to severe lesions were noted in the skin, kidney, lung, intestinal tract, spleen, and liver, and mild lesions were noted in the testes and, in one animal, in skeletal muscle.[23]

Fungi and fungallike organisms represent relatively common pathogens, particularly in aquatic environments. In many instances, these agents are ubiquitous in nature and affect stressed, injured, or immunocompromised amphibians. Saprolegniasis is a disease of aquatic amphibians, mostly urodeles and premetamorphic anurans. *Saprolegnia ferax* infects egg masses and has been linked with amphibian decline along the Pacific coast of the United States. *Saprolegnia* is typically an opportunistic invader of traumatized or devitalized tissue. It may ascend the oviduct causing infection.[15] Death of embryos within egg masses is a result of fungal invasion through the eggshell and possibly impaired oxygen exchange through the mycelial mat covering the mass.[24] Microsporidians that parasitize amphibian hosts have a tropism for muscle, connective tissues of various organs, or oocytes. Vertical transmission of the microsporidian, *Microsporidium schuetzi*, from ovary to eggs in the northern leopard frog (*R pipiens*) has been described.[25]

The ciliate *Tetrahymena*, although a frequent gastrointestinal commensal in many amphibians, has contributed to mortality among salamanders, including eggs and embryos.[26] Myxozoan parasites are relatively common parasites; however, morbidity and mortality are uncommon in amphibians. The genus *Myxobolus* has been identified as a gonadotropic myxozoa in anurans with varying degrees of testicular damage.[27,28]

Interestingly, several studies explore the relationship between infection and amphibian reproductive investment. In the face of infection, illness, or immune challenge, animals can increase their reproductive investment (measured through efforts in mating, parental care, and gametogenesis), which is one outcome of terminal investment. Indeed, increased resistance is not the only mechanism by which a species can respond to infection, and a shift in life history, such as reproductive fitness, can also explain population persistence in the face of large disease-induced mortality. Three studies have explored reproductive fitness in animals with *Batrachochytrium dendrobatidis* infection. Infected *R* (*Lithobates*) *pipiens* males had larger testicular size with more mature sperm, which suggests that exposed animals invest in more spermatogenesis.[29] Infected wild *Litoria rheocola* in good body condition were more likely to be found calling than uninfected males.[30] In *Pseudophryne corroboree* and *Litoria verreauxii alpina*, gametogenesis, both oogenesis and spermatogenesis, increased when animals were experimentally infected with *B dendrobatidis*.[31]

NEOPLASIA

Testicular and ovarian neoplasms have been described in research and captive amphibians, and reports of spontaneous neoplasia in wild amphibians are rare. Research has shown that at least some anuran species possess inherent anticancer secretory products and cytoprotective devices and are relatively resistant to some mammalian carcinogens. The remarkable regenerative capacity of urodeles is hypothesized to reduce tumor susceptibility.[32] To date, neoplasia has not been reported in caecilians. In males, reports of neoplasia are limited to Sertoli cell tumors in both anurans and urodeles. These tumors are considered an incidental finding at necropsy. They have been described in *Ambystoma mexicanum*, a Hellbender (*Cryptobranchus alleganiensis*), and in an *R pipiens–R palustris* hybrid.[33,34]

In females, ovarian tumors are identified as epithelial neoplasia or carcinomas. Use of nonspecific classification schemes makes it difficult to draw firm conclusions regarding specific tissue of origin, biologic behavior, and similarities with primary ovarian tumors in other species. One cystadenocarcinoma was reported in an *R pipiens*. Dysgerminomas are not documented in amphibians.[33]

In the author's experience, it is not that uncommon to find neoplasia in amphibians. The physiopathology is unclear, but the author has seen general symptoms like lethargy or acute death with gonadal neoplasia in *X laevis*. In the case of cachexia in a *Phyllomedusa bicolor* seen by the author, the only lesion found was an ovarian tumor (**Fig. 10**). The author considers gonadal neoplasia whenever an amphibian presents with abdominal distension.

The most reliable way to diagnose gonadal neoplasms is via a laparoscopic endoscopy. Noninvasive diagnostic techniques including radiography, ultrasonography, and computed tomography (CT) may also be used. Once the diagnosis of a gonadal tumor is made, the best treatment is surgical removal of the mass. All tumors seen by the author have not metastasized.

DYSTOCIA

Egg retention, or dystocia, normally occurs when captive gravid females are exposed to a lack of appropriate environmental parameters or physiologic/natural stimuli for release. All types of stress before or during oviposition may lead to a failure to lay eggs. One of the problems facing the clinician is when to make the definitive diagnosis of dystocia. In many cases, it is a subjective decision, as it is in other egg-laying animals. Medical treatment would include correcting any environmental problems. As seen previously, natural history of amphibian reproduction is well documented. A thorough knowledge of this subject will aid the amphibian practitioner in diagnosis and treatment. The clinician might use several protocols of hormonal manipulation for

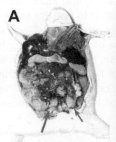
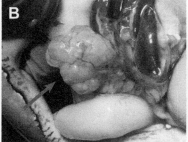
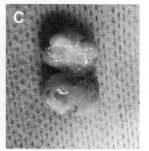

Fig. 10. Neoplastic diseases (*A*) in African clawed frog. (*B*) Ovarian neoplasia in a giant monkey frog (*arrow*). (*C*) The ovary of the frog cut out. (*Courtesy of* Norin Chai, DVM, MSc, PhD, DECZM (ZHM), Paris, France.)

artificial reproduction to stimulate ovulation. Whitaker[15] gives a detailed table of hormonal manipulation of selected amphibian species. The author injected 500 to 1000 units of hCG (depending on the size) into the dorsal lymph sac to induce ovulation in *X laevis*. This injection should be used only if the ova are mature or hypermature. Digital palpation and noninvasive diagnostic techniques including radiography, ultrasonography, and CT may be used to characterize the ovaries and search for any condition that may cause blockage of the oviduct or cloaca. These causes may also include neoplastic, congenital, or infectious condition.[15]

ASCITES AND REPRODUCTIVE ISSUE

Some dendrobatid and hylid frogs will accumulate large amounts of fluid in the coelomic and subcutaneous tissues. As the fluid builds up, egg production declines. Removing the fluid via aspiration is the first step of diagnostic and palliative treatment. Ascites in amphibians is common and may be caused by lymph heart failure, cardiac failure, renal, gastrointestinal, or hepatic disease, neoplasia, microbial infection, parasitism, toxicosis, and/or improper environmental conditions. It may also occur due to anorexia, metabolic bone disease, or retained ova.[35] In those conditions, the fluid should be typically transudate in nature. The cause of ascites related to reproduction is generally unknown.[15] The stressors of folliculogenesis and the reproductive cycle in general may contribute to the increased prevalence of hydrocoelom and/or lymphedema in females from dendrobatid species. Aspiration may be associated with soaking the animal 20 to 30 minutes in a concentrate of "amphibian Ringers": 6.6 g NaCl, 0.15 g $CaCl_2$, 0.15 g KCl, and 0.2 g $NaHCO_3$ per 900 mL of fresh dechlorinated water, instead of 1 L. If amphibian Ringer is not available, then a solution composed of 3 parts lactated Ringer solution to 1 part 5% glucose may be used. The author has managed several cases with regular fine-needle aspiration of the coelom and hypertonic solution bath. Diuretics such as furosemide (1–2 mg/kg intramuscularly every 24 hours) may be used with random success to remove fluids from affected amphibians. The specific treatment plan for each case should be based on the primary cause (if known) for the edema.

CLOACAL PROLAPSE

Prolapse of the cloaca, rectum, colon, stomach, bladder, or oviduct is common in amphibians. A prolapse is often secondary to gastrointestinal nematodes or obstruction, but can also occur as the result of enteritis, peritonitis, retained ova, recent egg laying, or neoplasia. The first important step is to determine the origin/identity of prolapsed tissue. Most cases of cloacal prolapse are not complicated and can be treated by gentle tissue reduction and its replacement after thorough cleaning and lubrication. The underlying cause of the prolapse must be identified and treated to prevent recurrence. Stay sutures placed across the vent may help to prevent recurrence. Cloacal prolapse may involve the reproductive system (**Fig. 11**). Prolapse of the ovary through the genital pore may be concurrent with dystocia. In such a case, the necrotic tissue should be removed surgically, and the eggs should be carefully moved from the coelomic cavity of the amphibian. If gentle manual pressure along the sides of the amphibian does not dislodge the eggs, then a celiotomy may be required to remove the ovaries. Treatment by cloacopexy has been described.[36]

HYPOVITAMINOSIS A

Hypovitaminosis A refers to the condition of squamous metaplasia of mucus-secreting epithelia with concomitant low levels of retinol (vitamin A) in the liver. In captive

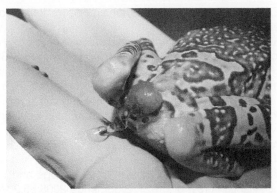

Fig. 11. Cloacal prolapse in Amazon milk frog that involves reproductive system. Eggs may be observed. (*Courtesy of* Norin Chai, DVM, MSc, PhD, DECZM (ZHM), Paris, France.)

amphibians, hypovitaminosis A is increasingly recognized as a significant disease. Secondary reproductive disease may be observed, such as low reproductive success with low fertilization rates, low numbers of eggs produced, early deaths of larvae, and failure of larvae to complete metamorphosis.[37] In amphibians, hypovitaminosis A specifically causes lingual squamous metaplasia, or short-tongue syndrome. Other disorders include squamous metaplasia of the conjunctiva and bladder mucosa, renal insufficiency, hydrocoelom, and chronic immune suppression with outbreaks of infectious disease.[38,39]

REPRODUCTIVE SURGERY

A review on amphibian surgery, reproductive surgery included, has been published recently.[36] Ovariectomy is a common method used in various frog species for obtaining oocytes for embryologic studies. In the male, unilateral orchiectomy may be a good option for artificial insemination without sacrifice of the animal. Endoscopic orchiectomy in a bullfrog (*Lithobates catesbeianus*), as an example of minimal invasive surgery, has been also described.[36]

ACKNOWLEDGMENTS

The author especially thanks Lindsey Marshall, PhD student of the Muséum National d'Histoire Naturelle for her help in writing the artificial fertilization article; and our colleague, Françoise Serre-Colet, for **Fig. 2**. A profound thanks is extended for their great work to all the keepers of the Reptiles and Amphibians Department of the Menagerie du Jardin des Plantes, France.

REFERENCES

1. AmphibiaWeb: Information on amphibian biology and conservation. Berkeley (CA). Available at: http://amphibiaweb.org. Accessed July 29, 2016.

2. Purgue AP. Tympanic sound radiation in the bullfrog Rana catesbeiana. J Comp Physiol A 1997;181:438–45.

3. Dan C. Reproduction twice a year of the crested newt in captivity. In: Townson S, editor. Breeding reptiles and amphibians. London: British Herpetological Society; 1983. p. 209–11.

4. Duellman WE, Trueb L. Biology of amphibians. London: Johns Hopkins University Press Ltd; 1986. p. 13–197.
5. De Iuliis G, Pulerà D. The dissection of vertebrates. A laboratory manual. 1st edition. Burlington (MA): Academic Press, Elsevier; 2007. p. 113–30.
6. Wright KM. Anatomy for the clinician. In: Wright KM, Whitaker BR, editors. Amphibian medicine and captive husbandry. Malabar (FL): Krieger; 2001. p. 15–30.
7. Piprek RP, Kloc M, Kubiak JZ. Bidder's organ–structure, development and function. Int J Dev Biol 2014;58:819–27.
8. Chai N. Anurans. In: Miller E, Fowler ME, editors. Fowler's zoo and wild animal medicine, vol. 8. St Louis (MO): Elsevier Saunders; 2014. p. 1–13.
9. Haddad CFB, Prado CPA. Reproductive modes in frogs and their unexpected diversity in the Atlantic Forest of Brazil. BioScience 2005;55:207–17.
10. Wells KD. The ecology and behavior of amphibians. Chicago: The University of Chicago Press; 2007. p. 451–515.
11. Browne RK, Zippelv K. Reproduction and larval rearing of amphibians. ILAR J 2007;48(3):214–34.
12. Horton P. Precocious reproduction in the Australian frog Limnodynastes tasmaniensis. Herpetologica 1982;38:486–9.
13. Rabb GB. Evolutionary aspects of the reproductive behavior of frogs. In: Vial JL, editor. Evolutionary biology of the anurans: contemporary research on major problems. Columbia (MO): University of Missouri Press; 1973. p. 213–27.
14. Jørgensen CB. Factors controlling the ovarian cycle in a temperate zone anuran, the toad Bufo bufo: food uptake, nutritional state, and gonadotrophin. J Exp Zool 1982;224:437–43.
15. Whitaker BR. Reproduction. In: Wright KM, Whitaker BR, editors. Amphibian medicine and captive husbandry. Malabar (FL): Krieger; 2001. p. 285–307.
16. Sargent MG, Mohun TJ. Cryopreservation of sperm of Xenopus laevis and Xenopus tropicalis. Genesis 2005;41:41–6.
17. Kouba AJ, Vance CK, Willis EL. Artificial fertilization for amphibian conservation: current knowledge and future considerations. Theriogenology 2009;71:214–27.
18. Mansour N, Lahnsteiner F, Patzner RA. Collection of gametes from live axolotl, Ambystoma mexicanum, and standardization of in vitro fertilization. Theriogenology 2011;75:354–61.
19. Chai N. Mycobacteriosis in amphibians. In: Fowler M, Miller R, editors. Zoo and wild animal medicine. 8th edition. St Louis (MO): WB Saunders; 2011. p. 224–30.
20. Miller DL, Pessier AP, Hick P, et al. Comparative pathology of ranaviruses and diagnostic techniques. In: Gray MJ, Gregory Chinchar V, editors. Ranaviruses. Lethal pathogens of ectothermic vertebrates. New York: Springer International Publishing AG; 2015. p. 171–208.
21. Cheng K, Jones MEB, Jancovich JK, et al. Isolation of a Bohle-like iridovirus from boreal toads housed within a cosmopolitan aquarium collection. Dis Aquat Organ 2014;111(2):139–52.
22. Wheelwright NT, Gray MJ, Hill RD, et al. Sudden mass die-off of a large population of wood frog (Lithobates sylvaticus) tadpoles in Maine, USA, likely due to ranavirus. Herpetol Rev 2014;45:240–2.
23. Miaud C, Pozet F, Curt Grand Gaudin N, et al. Ranavirus causes mass die-offs of alpine amphibians in the southwestern alps, France. J Wildl Dis 2016;52(2): 242–52.
24. Paré JA. Fungal diseases of amphibians: an overview. Vet Clin North Am Exot Anim Pract 2003;6:315–26.

25. Schuetz AW, Selman K, Samson D. Alterations in growth, function and composition of Rana pipiens oocytes and follicles associated with microsporidian parasites. J Exp Zool 1978;204:81–94.
26. Pessier AP. An overview of amphibian skin disease. Semin Avian Exot Pet Med 2002;11:162–74.
27. Browne RK, Scheltinga DM, Pomering M, et al. Testicular myxosporidiasis in anurans, with a description of Myxobolus fallax n. sp. Syst Parasitol 2002;52: 97–110.
28. Eiras JC. An overview on the myxosporean parasites in amphibians and reptiles. Acta Parasitol 2005;50:267–75.
29. Chatfield MW, Brannelly LA, Robak MJ, et al. Fitness consequences of infection by Batrachochytrium dendrobatidis in northern leopard frogs (Lithobates pipiens). Ecohealth 2013;10(1):90–8.
30. Roznik EA, Sapsford SJ, Pike DA, et al. Condition-dependent reproductive effort in frogs infected by a widespread pathogen. Proc Biol Sci 2015;282:1810.
31. Brannelly LA, Webb R, Skerratt LF, et al. Amphibians with infectious disease increase their reproductive effort: evidence for the terminal investment hypothesis. Open Biol 2016;6(6):150251.
32. Prehn RT. Regeneration versus neoplastic growth. Carcinogenesis 1997;18(8): 1439–44.
33. Green DE, Harshbarger JC. Spontaneous neoplasia in amphibia. In: Wright KM, Whitaker BR, editors. Amphibian medicine and captive husbandry. Malabar (FL): Kreiger; 2001. p. 335–400.
34. Humphrey RR. Tumors of the testis in the Mexican axolotl (Ambystoma, or Siredon, mexicanum). In: Mizell M, editor. Biology of amphibian tumors. New York: Springer-Verlag; 1969. p. 220–8.
35. Hadfield CA, Whitaker BR. Amphibian emergency medicine and care. Semin Avian Exot Pet Med 2005;14(2):79–89.
36. Chai N. Surgery in Amphibians. Vet Clin North Am Exot Anim Pract 2016;19(1): 77–95.
37. Yun LS, Elinson RP. Abnormalities of forelimb and pronephros in a direct developing frog suggest a retinoic acid deficiency. Appl Herpetol 2008;5:33–46.
38. Li H, Vaughan MJ, Browne RK. A complex enrichment diet improves growth and health in the endangered Wyoming toad (Bufo baxteri). Zoo Biol 2009;28: 197–213.
39. Rodríguez CE, Pessier AP. Pathologic changes associated with suspected hypovitaminosis A in amphibians under managed care. Zoo Biol 2014;33(6):508–15.

Diagnostic Imaging of Reproductive Tract Disorders in Reptiles

Michaela Gumpenberger, Dr med vet

KEYWORDS

- Reproductive tract • Radiography • Ultrasonography • Computed tomography
- Chelonian • Snake • Lizard • Reptile

KEY POINTS

- Radiographs serve as a cheap and widely available imaging tool for getting an overview of the general condition in reptiles. Mineralized egg shells are differentiated in most species.
- Sonography allows the evaluation of the whole reproductive tract in lizards and snakes; however, the examination of chelonians is limited by the shell.
- Computed tomography is the perfect imaging tool for the visualization of all organ systems in chelonians.
- Diagnosis of dystocia should always be supported by diagnostic imaging, especially in chelonians where the shell hampers proper palpation.

Diagnostic imaging of the reptilian reproductive tract may be helpful for determining gender (particularly in monomorphic species),[1] for evaluating the breeding status,[2] for finding pathologic conditions, and for supervising treatment.[3] This article demonstrates the most commonly used imaging techniques, including their advantages and disadvantages (**Table 1**). Physiologic appearance and pathologic findings of male and female reproductive tract are described and illustrated.

INTRODUCTION TO DIFFERENT DIAGNOSTIC IMAGING METHODS IN REPTILE MEDICINE
Radiography

Radiography is the most popular imaging method in reptiles because of its worldwide availability, ease of use, and predictable costs. Usually-whole body radiographs are performed. For chelonians, small and large lizards, and snakes dorsoventral and laterolateral views normally provide sufficient information for the reproductive tract. In chelonian species craniocaudal views may be used in addition, but are usually of

Disclosure Statement: The author has nothing to disclose.
Clinical Unit of Diagnostic Imaging, Department for Companion Animals and Horses, University of Veterinary Medicine (Vetmeduni Vienna), Veterinärplatz 1, Vienna 1210, Austria
E-mail address: Michaela.Gumpenberger@vetmeduni.ac.at

Vet Clin Exot Anim 20 (2017) 327–343
http://dx.doi.org/10.1016/j.cvex.2016.11.003
1094-9194/17/© 2016 Elsevier Inc. All rights reserved.

Table 1
Comparison of the value of radiography, sonography, and plain computed tomography in differentiating various reproductive conditions

	Chelonians, Turtles			Lizards, Iguanas, Chameleons			Snakes		
	RX	US	CT	RX	US	CT	RX	US	CT
Ovary	0	+	++	0	+/++	+/++	0	+	+
Follicles, eggs with noncalcified shells	0/+	++/+++	+++	++	+++	+++	+/++	+++	+++
Eggs, poorly calcified shells	++	+++	+++	++	+++	+++	++	+++	+++
Eggs, well-mineralized shells	+++	+	+++	+++	++	+++	+++	+++	+++
Salpinx	0	+/++	+++	0	+	+	0	0/++	n.i.
Testes	0	++	+/++	0	+/++	+/++	0	+	n.i.

Abbreviations: 0, no value/organ not visible; +/++/+++, little/moderate/high value; CT, computed tomography; n.i., no information available; RX, radiography; US, ultrasound.

main interest for diagnosing respiratory tract disorders. Lateral views in turtles should be performed in horizontal view to minimize organ displacement and to ensure symmetric views. The animal is placed on a wooden block or a paper box for proper positioning (**Fig. 1**A). Small lizards should be done in a similar way, but rather be confined in a radiolucent box (**Fig. 1**B). Manual restraint in tiny species might hurt the patient and result in compromised images because of superimposition. Chameleons may be offered a kind of (preferably radiolucent) perch (**Fig. 1**C, D). For larger lizards and snakes either horizontal or vertical beam imaging is applied. Usually large lizards are restrained and positioned in a similar way to dogs or cats.[4]

One disadvantage of radiology is artifacts caused by superimposition. This can at least to some extent be overcome by always performing two radiographs in perpendicular directions. Restricting oneself to only one view results in considerable loss of information (discussed later).

Another disadvantage in reptile radiography is the lack of coelomic fat between the organs. Therefore differentiation of ovaries, follicles, or testes is difficult or even completely impossible, especially in chelonians. Mineralized egg shells are usually defined when proper imaging techniques are used. Superimposition of the shell hampers the visualization of eggs with poorly mineralized shells, especially in underexposed images. The easily applicable digital radiography might tempt to an excessive use of milliampere and/or kilovolt to overcome this problem, which is certainly unacceptable for reasons of radiation protection.

Sonography

Sonography may be used more often in diagnosing reproductive disorders than radiography, particularly in snakes and lizards (eg, iguanas).[5] The main advantage of sonography is the possibility to evaluate the inner architecture of soft tissues. Sonography is therefore a perfect supplement to radiography.[3] Although radiographs serve the purpose of being documents that are evaluated anytime, sonographic diagnoses are made during the examination of patients. Even if videos are taken it is difficult to form a trustworthy second opinion about somebody else's images. Thorough training and detailed knowledge of different species and their sometimes unique anatomy are therefore prerequisites for performing sonography.

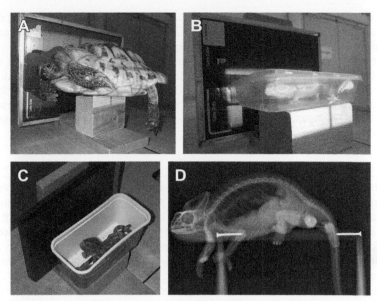

Fig. 1. (*A*) Positioning of a Hermann's tortoise (*Testudo hermanni*) in sternal recumbency on a wooden block for a lateral radiograph in horizontal beam. Note that there is less super-imposition if the animal's legs are protruded from the shell. The beam is centered between the costal and marginal shields. (*B*) The same device is used when performing a lateral radio-graph in horizontal beam in a Leopard gecko (*Eublepharis macularius*). The animal is placed in a radiolucent plastic box to prevent escape. There may be some superimpositioning of the animal's legs on the radiograph. Nevertheless, usually a good overview is obtained sufficient enough to diagnose mineral imbalances and presence of eggs. (*C*) Chameleons prefer a kind of perch (in this case a branch) within the positioning device. In this case numerous eggs could be visualized on the radiograph. (*D*) Lateral radiograph of a chameleon that was offered a wooden perch that was screwed together. Radiolucent or at least metal-free posi-tioning devices should always be preferred to avoid artifacts. (*Courtesy of* Michaela Gum-penberger, Dr med vet, Austria.)

Transducers should always feel comfortable for the examiner. In general, microcon-vex transducers with a high frequency (7.5–12 MHz) and superior spatial resolution are the best choice for smaller turtles up to 5 kg body weight, whereas larger species may require convex or linear transducers (3.5–5 MHz). The frequency depends on actual patient size and the organ of main interest. Sonography in turtles is usually performed through the natural shell openings (mediastinale, axillary, and inguinal window) but can sometimes be performed through the shell, when the plastron lacks proper mineral-ization. Most aquatic species have large inguinal windows (also known as prefemoral fossa) so that the genital tract is more easily accessible.

Lizards and snakes are usually scanned with high-frequency linear transducers (the author still prefers a microconvex transducer). Images do not need to be "pretty," but should rather be diagnostic. Hence there is hardly a restriction in transducer choice. Sometimes the use of several transducers in one animal is legitimate to achieve desired results.

It is crucial to aim for good transducer-skin contact in all sonographic examinations, which is achieved by the use of sonographic gel. Dysecdysis may compromise sono-graphic imaging as soon as gas is entrapped between transducer and skin. This is partially overcome by soaking the patient in warm water. However, performing sonography during soaking often results in undesirable movements and splashing as soon as the animal starts to struggle and is therefore considered less advisable.

A simple stand-off pad, made from a gel-filled finger of an examination glove, can be helpful for sonography performed via the prefemoral window in turtles (**Fig. 2**A). In tiny patients the stand-off pad is also useful for obtaining proper imaging of superficial organs whenever an adequate high-frequency transducer is not available. In general, all patients are restrained only as much as necessary and in the most comfortable way possible (**Fig. 2**B, C).

Computed Tomography

Computed tomography (CT) is a radiographic, cross-sectional imaging method that overcomes superimposition artifacts of plain radiographs. Reading CT images is comparatively easier to learn than reading MR images , because the different tissue densities resemble those of radiographs. Some advantages are the opportunity to do multiplanar and three-dimensional reconstructions, volumetry, densitometry, or virtual endoscopy. CT examinations are admittedly more expensive than radiography or sonography and require special equipment and premises. That is why CT is still not available for all veterinarians. Nevertheless, if available and used in complement to radiography and sonography valuable information is gained that leads to a better understanding of all imaging techniques.

Usually chelonian species need no anesthesia. Lizards and snakes are restrained in cardboard boxes and plastic rolls. For rapid multislice CT machines, sedation is increasingly dispensable. In general there is no need for intravenous contrast media application for further evaluation of the reproductive tract. If needed a dosage of 600 mg iodine/kg body weight should be administered intravenously.[6]

MRI

In general all soft tissues can be evaluated perfectly with MRI. Because of their different signal even their quality is evaluated further. T2-weighted images highlight fluid and are therefore often addressed as "pathology scans," whereas T1-weighted images offer further details on anatomy in which fluid appears hypointense and fat hyperintense. Variations of these sequences help to differentiate between liquor, hemorrhage, and plain cysts. Solid bone and air appear in all sequences dark without a signal. Because MRI examinations are easily depreciated by movement artifacts, sedation is usually necessary.

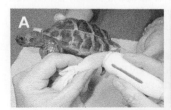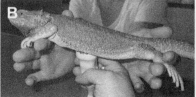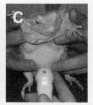

Fig. 2. Sonographic examination of a (A) Hermann's tortoise (*Testudo hermanni*) and (B, C) two Bearded dragons (*Pogona vitticeps*). The examiner tries to place the patient in a most convenient and physiologic position. (A) A simple stand-off pad, made from a gel-filled finger of a glove, is used to achieve optimal skin contact within the prefemoral window. (*Courtesy of* Michaela Gumpenberger, Dr med vet, Austria.)

Although the author has access to MRI, all diagnoses are perceived to be gained much faster with CT for the reproductive tract in reptiles (sometimes complemented with sonography). Because MRI examinations are more time consuming, require sedation, and are much more expensive, the author's clinic prefers other imaging methods for diagnosing reproductive tract disorders.

APPEARANCE OF REPRODUCTIVE ORGANS IN DIAGNOSTIC IMAGING IN REPTILES
Testes

Radiographically testes may only be properly differentiated when surrounded by gas or huge amounts of fat. Therefore the best chance of visualization is in chameleons, whereas testes in turtles, snakes, and most lizards remain invisible, although they may become large during breeding season.

The ovoid testes appear mildly to moderately hypoechoic in comparison with the kidneys in sonography, which certainly depends on the species and the equipment. They are homogeneous and finely granulated (**Fig. 3**). The right one may be positioned a little bit cranial to the left one.

The testes are differentiated as homogeneous organs cranioventral to the kidneys in chelonians in CT, if the organs are not too much compressed because of the legs being retracted into the shell or other organ enlargement (eg, huge urinary bladder). They are clearly visible after intravenous contrast media application. In snakes and lizards differentiation is more difficult.

Pathologic changes of testes are rare and most likely caused by neoplastic disease. Heterogenity of the parenchyma and asymmetric or unilateral enlargement may be found in sonography, CT, and MRI.[3] Severely enlarged testes may cause distortion of the otherwise horizontal borderline between coelomic organs and the lung in turtles on lateral radiographs or they may even compromise the liver.[7]

Penis and Hemipenes

Hemipenes in some lizard species (eg, some varanids) are known to have mineralized foci (hemibacula) that are visualized radiographically and are therefore apt for sexing. Otherwise the penis is hardly an object for diagnostic imaging.

Ovary, Follicles, Eggs

The ovary and low numbers of (small) follicles cannot be differentiated in any reptile radiographically. When large numbers of follicles are present, the contour between the soft tissues of the abdominal organs and the lung seems to be elevated to caudal on lateral radiographs (horizontal beam) in chelonians (**Fig. 4**). In lizards and snakes

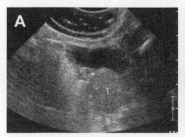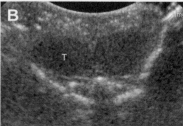

Fig. 3. Sonography of testes (T) of a (*A*) Hermann's tortoise (*Testudo hermanni*, sagittal view) and a (*B*) Bearded dragon (*Pogona vitticeps*, transverse view, comparing left and right organ). The spherical to oval testicles have a homogenous parenchyma. (*Courtesy of* Michaela Gumpenberger, Dr med vet, Austria.)

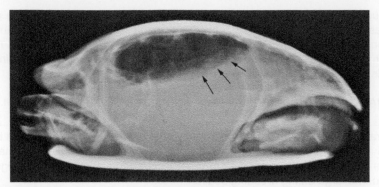

Fig. 4. Lateral radiograph of an adult female Red Eared Slider turtle (*Trachemys scripta elegans*). The lung fields are narrowed. The borderline between the lung and the other coelomic organs has risen to caudally (*arrows*). A vast number of follicles was identified sonographically as cause. (*Courtesy of* Michaela Gumpenberger, Dr med vet, Austria.)

follicles and eggs may be differentiated as roundish or oval soft tissue opacity objects, often accumulating in a grapelike manner in lizards.[8,9] Mineralized shells should appear of similar shape, size, and density in one clutch, although number, size, shape, and shell density are species-dependent (**Fig. 5**). For example, Box turtles produce exceptionally large eggs. Tortoises have radiographically denser shells than most aquatic species. However, the shell of the two large eggs (in comparison with body size) is hardly visible in leopard geckos (**Fig. 6**). A clear visibility of the shell indicates dystocia in these geckos.[4]

The visibility of poorly mineralized egg shells in chelonians significantly depends on proper image settings. If the shell is not penetrated on dorsoventral views, the thin shells cannot be differentiated (see **Fig. 5A**). Differentiation of follicles or thin-shelled eggs on radiographs of lizards and snakes is easier due to lack of a bony shell.

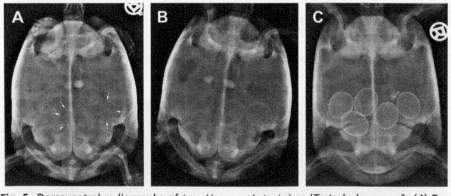

Fig. 5. Dorsoventral radiographs of two Hermann's tortoises (*Testudo hermanni*). (*A*) Two thin-shelled eggs that are barely visible (*arrows*). (*B*) On a follow-up examination 5 days later those eggs are not fully but better mineralized. The shell is mildly demineralized. (*C*) Shell and skeleton are perfectly mineralized in another individual. Five fully mineralized eggs of similar shape and size are visible. Radiographically the clutch appears normal (and was delivered on the next day). (*Courtesy of* Michaela Gumpenberger, Dr med vet, Austria.)

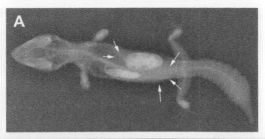

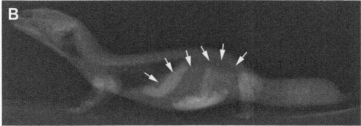

Fig. 6. Dorsoventral (*A*) and lateral (*B*) radiograph of a Leopard gecko (*Eublepharis macularius*) showing relatively poor mineralization of the skeleton. Nevertheless, two thin shells are visible (*arrows*), partially superimposed by ingesta and some radiopaque material of unknown origin (there was no history of contrast media application). This female showed difficulties in delivering the eggs, which might be caused by mineral imbalances. (*Courtesy of* Michaela Gumpenberger, Dr med vet, Austria.)

The appearance of follicles and eggs in CT is in general similar to that of radiographs, because both use x-rays for imaging (**Figs. 7** and **8**). Since CT offers a much larger gray scale and is not limited by superimposition, each follicle and egg is detected and clearly evaluated.[6]

Sonographically normal, nonovulated follicles appear spherical, homogeneous, and hyperechoic in chelonians, but anechoic to hypoechoic in all other reptiles (**Fig. 9**). The larger they become the more artifacts may arise in chelonians (see **Fig. 9**B). Distal shadowing hinders further examination of other follicles, especially in case of small prefemoral windows. Proper counting is then impossible. Follicle size can be an indicator for ovulation (eg, in Mediterranean chelonians, follicles larger

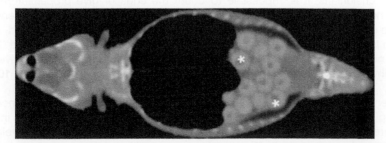

Fig. 7. Coronal CT in soft tissue window of a Bearded dragon (*Pogona vitticeps*) at the level of the ovaries. Unremarkable, hyperdense follicles (*asterisks*) with a less dense center are visible. The animal suffered from obstipation, which was not related to the follicles. (*Courtesy of* Michaela Gumpenberger, Dr med vet, Austria.)

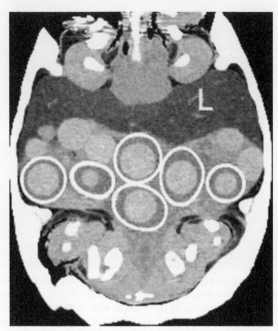

Fig. 8. Coronal CT in soft tissue window of a Hermann's tortoise (*Testudo hermanni*). Several normal-shaped eggs of unremarkable density and structure are present. The liver (L) is mildly enlarged (not clearly seen at this level) and shows decreased density (lipidosis). (*Courtesy of* Michaela Gumpenberger, Dr med vet, Austria.)

than 2.2–2.4 cm are prone to ovulation).[10] Premordial follicles may undergo atresia. Then they become heterogenous with hypoechoic to anechoic zones.[10] As soon as follicles are ovulated they are hyperechoic and tend to elongate, especially in lizards and snakes.[8] A small peripheral anechoic rim is built, representing the albumen (see **Fig. 9**E). A poorly mineralized shell appears as curvilinear echoic thin line. The better mineralized the shell the more hyperechoic it becomes (see **Fig. 14**A). Well-mineralized shells even cause distal shadowing, depending on species and grade of mineralization. Then the albumen and yolk can no longer be differentiated and the eggs superimpose each other in sonography. Therefore using sonography, especially in chelonians, it is impossible to count the eggs or give proper information about their position. Visibility of follicles or eggs in chelonians not only depends on the size of the inguinal acoustic window, but also on bowel loop contents and, especially in larger individuals, on the cooperation of the patient. Radiography and CT are less or not at all hampered by the previously mentioned circumstances. However, sonography can easily detect cardiac action in fetus in viviparous snakes (**Fig. 10**) and lizards.

Depending on the species and developmental status horizontal and concentric layering of various intensities is observed in follicles and eggs in reptiles in MRI. The preovulatory follicles of lizards appear hyperintense in T2-weighted sequences. In case of eggs, the albumen appears hyperintense, the yolk hypointense, and the calcified shell very hypointense in T2-weighted sequences, whereas in T1-weighted images the yolk appears of similar intensity as muscle.[3,11]

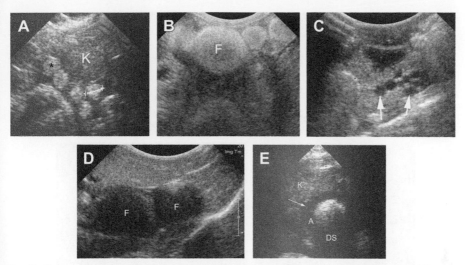

Fig. 9. Comparison of sonographic appearance of normal follicles in chelonians and lizards, demonstrating the difference in echogenicity. Chelonians show exceptional hyperechoic follicles right from the beginning. (*A*) Small primordial, hyperechoic follicles (one marked with *measurement tags*, one with an *asterisk*) representing previtellogenesis at the ovary of a Hermann's tortoise (*Testudo hermanni*), projecting in front of the homogeneous kidney (K). (*B*) Large mature, hyperechoic follicle (F) with typical distal shadowing in a Red Eared Slider turtle (*Trachemys scripta elegans*) close to ovulation. (*C*) Small hypoechoic follicles (*arrows*) on the ovary of a Bearded dragon (*Pogona vitticeps*). (*D*) Preovulatory hypoechoic follicles (F) in a Frill Necked lizard (*Chlamydosaurus kingii*). (*E*) Postovulatory hyperechoic follicle or yolk in a Hermann's tortoise (*T hermanni*), projecting in front of the homogeneous kidney (K). The yolk is causing typical distal shadowing (DS). The albumen (A) is represented by a hypoechoic rim. There is even a thin line (*arrow*) around the albumen visible, indicating the arising mineralized shell. In the far field a second egg is seen. (*Courtesy of* Michaela Gumpenberger, Dr med vet, Austria.)

Salpinx

The salpinx cannot be visualized radiographically, but it is clearly seen as a narrow folded, tubular, hyperechoic or hyperdense structure in the caudal part of the shell in turtles in sonography and CT, respectively (**Fig. 11**). In lizards and snakes it is hardly visible when nonaffected and not filled with fluid.

Pathologic Imaging Findings in the Female Reproductive Tract

Dystocia (postovulatory egg stasis)

Common imaging findings in dystocia include absolutely enlarged eggs (**Figs. 12** and **13**), broken shells, rarely malpositioned eggs (into the urinary bladder; **Figs. 14** and **15**[6]), and follicular stasis (**Fig. 16**). Thickened shells or layered contents with a gas pocket on top (**Fig. 17**) are an indicator for a chronic and long-standing process, whereas a broken shell does not necessarily indicate dystocia (**Fig. 18**).[6]

The diagnosis of dystocia also depends on the clinical signs (**Fig. 19**).[12] A broken egg may be delivered without further pathologic events. Nevertheless, a follow-up radiograph helps to ensure that no shell fragments have remained in the salpinx. In the author's opinion, a correct and sufficient diagnosis of a clutch or suspected dystocia in turtles and tortoises is only possible with a combined clinical and radiographic examination.[12] Sometimes additional imaging techniques help to further

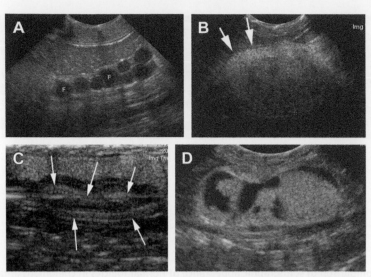

Fig. 10. Sonographic images of various breeding status in snakes. (*A*) Small hypoechoic follicles (F) are present on the normal ovary in a Tiger python (*Python molurus*). (*B*) Normal egg with a barely distinguishable shell (*arrows*) and hyperechoic contents of a Tiger python (*P molurus*). Measuring points indicate the size (4.7 × 3 cm). (*C*) A hockey-stick linear transducer was used for this examination. The vertebrae and spine (*arrows*), surrounded by soft tissues, of a fetus in a Garter snake (*Thamnophis sirtalis*) are visible. In live view the heartbeat proved this animal to be alive. (*D*) In the dead fetus inside a Dumeril boa (*Acrantophis dumerili*) there is no need to find a heartbeat because of the obviously degenerated status. (*Courtesy of* Michaela Gumpenberger, Dr med vet, Austria.)

evaluate any suspicious or uncertain diagnoses. In viviparous species the heartbeat of the fetus in sonography helps to distinguish between vivid and dead individuals and can therefore support further treatment (see **Fig. 10**C, D). Radiography is also valuable in detecting secondary causes for dystocia, such as an old pelvic or shell fracture, obstipation, or urinary calculi.

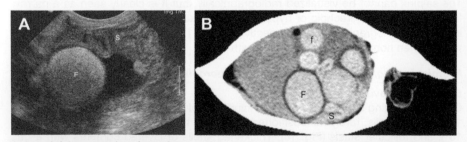

Fig. 11. (*A*) Sonography of a Red Eared Slider turtle (*Trachemys scripta elegans*). The hyperechoic follicle (F) measures more than 2.4 cm in diameter and may ovulate soon. Distal shadowing is present, which is typical for large follicles in chelonians. Right next to the follicle some part of the unremarkable urinary bladder is visible. In the near field the hyperechoic, tubular, serpentine salpinx (S) is seen. (*B*) Right lateral sagittal CT in soft tissue window of a Hermann's tortoise (*Testudo hermanni*), the head is to the left. Small hyperdense follicles (f) and large ones with a hypodense peripheral rim (F) are present. The salpinx is a hyperdense tubular structure folded between them (S). (*Courtesy of* Michaela Gumpenberger, Dr med vet, Austria.)

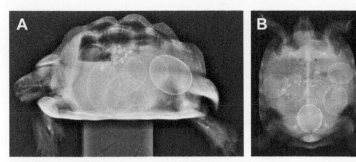

Fig. 12. Lateral (*A*) and dorsoventral (*B*) radiograph of a Hermann's tortoise (*Testudo hermanni*). One egg has already entered the pelvis but could not pass the shell opening. This is only seen on the lateral radiograph. Another indication for dystocia is the different density of the shells; the egg that got stuck in the cloaca has a much denser shell than the other eggs. (*Courtesy of* Michaela Gumpenberger, Dr med vet, Austria.)

Follicular stasis (preovulatory follicular stasis)

Follicular stasis is a common diagnosis that may occur more often in lizards than in turtles and snakes. Atrophic follicles appear heterogeneous with hypoechoic to anechoic zones sonographically. In lizards and snakes they tend to show an onion shell–like appearance of moderate to increased echogenity more often. Several follow-up sonographic examinations may help to reassess the condition (**Fig. 20**). Additionally, clear horizontal leveling of the contents of the follicle or egg is seen in CT, typically as soon as degeneration starts.

Preovulatory follicles are said to appear more uniform, round, and anechoic to hypoechoic in lizards and snakes. They tend to become more heterogenous and rough, and

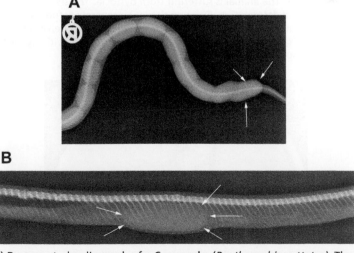

Fig. 13. (*A*) Dorsoventral radiograph of a Corn snake (*Pantherophis guttatus*). The egg positioned at the cloaca (*arrows*) seems a little bit larger than the others. Moreover, a swelling was found at the cloaca during physical examination, most likely responsible for the dystocia. (*B*) Lateral radiograph of a Mandarin Rat snake (*Euprepiophis mandarinus*) that was pregnant with a single egg (*arrows*) and showed symptoms of dystocia. (*Courtesy of* the Section of Reptiles and Birds, Vetmeduni Vienna, Austria.)

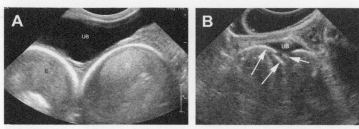

Fig. 14. Sonography of a Red Eared Slider turtle (*Trachemys scripta elegans*) (*A*) and a Hermann's tortoise (*Testudo hermanni*) (*B*). Two eggs (E) of the Red Eared Slider turtle are clearly positioned outside of the urinary bladder (UB). Even a thin bladder wall is visible. In (*B*) shell fragments (*arrows*) are present within the urinary bladder. This egg-displacement was caused by improper manual therapy resulting in shell fracture and in additional pneumoperitoneum and peritonitis, which was fatal for the patient. Compare with **Fig. 15**A, B. Note that in a poorly mineralized shell the yolk (hyperechoic) and albumen (hypoechoic) are seen (*A*). The shell is represented by a thin hyperechoic curvilinear reflex (*A*). As soon as the shell is fully mineralized only the surface of the shell is visualized (*B*). (*Courtesy of* Michaela Gumpenberger, Dr med vet, Austria.)

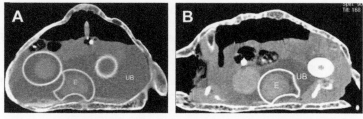

Fig. 15. Transverse (*A*) and sagittal (*B*) CT of a Hermann's tortoise (*Testudo hermanni*), modified soft tissue window. The animal is suffering from dystocia. The shell and skeleton show poor mineralization and deformation. One egg shell (E) is severely deformed and positioned within the urinary bladder (UB). Another shell is obstructing the pelvis and has a mildly thickened shell and a gas cap (not visible in these levels). Compare with **Fig. 14**A, B. (*Courtesy of* Michaela Gumpenberger, Dr med vet, Austria.)

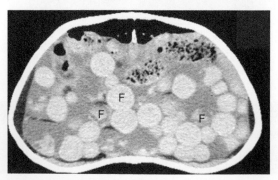

Fig. 16. Transverse CT (soft tissue window) in the middle of the coelomic cavity of a 60-year-old Spur-thighed tortoise (*Testudo graeca*). Multiple follicles (F) of various sizes and densities cause severe lung compression. Some show horizontal layering with a hypodense dorsal cap. The connective tissue in between the follicles is hypodense with irregular hyperdense areas, indicating coelomitis. Surgery proved severe follicular stasis with peritonitis and multiple adhesions. (*Courtesy of* Michaela Gumpenberger, Dr med vet, Austria.)

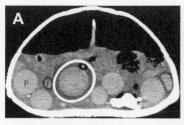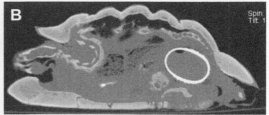

Fig. 17. (*A*) Transverse CT image (soft tissue window) of a Hermann's tortoise (*Testudo hermanni*). A normally calcified shell with an unremarkable yolk is seen. A tiny dorsal gas cap suggests dystocia (*asterisk*). Adjacent to the egg some follicles (F) are visible. One small follicle (f) shows a hypodense peripheral rim indicating atrophy. (*B*) Sagittal CT image (bony window) of another Hermann's tortoise. A thickened egg-shell (being denser than the skeleton) with a rough spiculated surface is positioned within the pelvis. The egg is wider than the maximal diameter of the shell opening near the cloaca. Chronic dystocia is not only indicated because of the egg-shell formation but also by the loss of proper egg contents, a gas cap within the egg-shell, and multiple gas pockets around the egg-shell. Surgery proved severe inflammation and adhesion of the egg-shell to the oviduct (compare **Fig. 22**). Note the thickened heterogenous shell and the pyramid-shaped neural bony plates indicating long-standing mineral imbalances and improper feeding and keeping. (*Courtesy of* Michaela Gumpenberger, Dr med vet, Austria.)

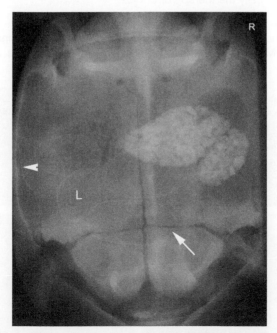

Fig. 18. Dorsoventral radiograph of a Spur-thighed tortoise (*Testudo graeca*). During a routine check several malshaped eggs were found: one was lemon-shaped (L), one showed some impressions (*arrowhead*), and another one was missing one pole (*arrow*). Nevertheless the animal produced this clutch without further help 2 weeks later. Some shells were broken when the clutch was delivered. Therefore a follow-up radiograph was taken, but no shell fragments could be found. (*Courtesy of* Michaela Gumpenberger, Dr med vet, Austria.)

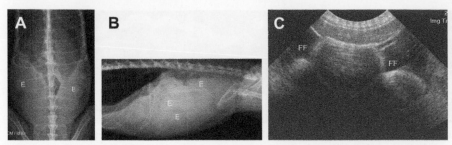

Fig. 19. Dorsoventral (*A*) and lateral (*B*) radiograph of a Green iguana (*Iguana iguana*) Multiple soft tissue–dense oval structures (E) indicate pregnancy. Poor serosal detail would be normal under these circumstances. Sonographic examination (*C*) of the same animal shows normal, thin-shelled eggs, causing some distal shadowing surrounded by free fluid (FF). Ascites in combination with typical clinical symptoms led to the diagnosis of dystocia. (*Courtesy of* Michaela Gumpenberger, Dr med vet, Austria.)

several layers may appear, depending on the duration of the disorder. Retained follicles often become friable and can rupture, leading to egg yolk coelomitis.[13] Free fluid is therefore an indicator for aggravation of the process (**Fig. 21**). In the post-ovulatory stage the ova should appear more elliptical and of increased echogenicity.[3,9,14] According to the author's experience, these two conditions may sometimes be difficult to differentiate. Actually, no matter if there is a preovulatory or postovulatory follicular stasis, surgery is usually the therapy of choice.

Salpingitis

In rare circumstances one may be able to identify a fluid-filled salpinx in sonography (**Fig. 22**) or CT (or MRI if used) that is most likely caused by salpingitis. An inflammation

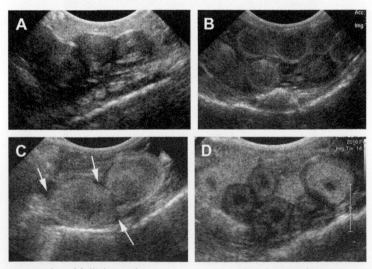

Fig. 20. Sonography of follicles and eggs in various Bearded dragons (*Pogona vitticeps*). (*A*) Normal, hypoechoic, mildly layered, seemingly ovulated follicles. (*B–D*) Cases suffering from follicular stasis that were proved surgically. Mild peritoneal effusion is present (*arrows in C*). (*D*) Different densities and sizes of layered follicles. (*Courtesy of* Michaela Gumpenberger, Dr med vet, Austria.)

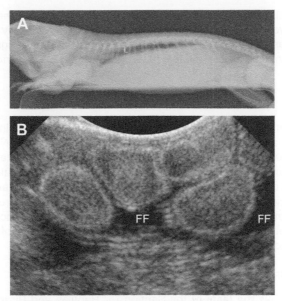

Fig. 21. Lateral radiograph (*A*) and sonography (*B*) of a Bearded dragon (*Pogona vitticeps*). Ascites may be better seen on horizontal lateral radiographs than on dorsoventral views. Note the small and compressed lung fields (L). The abdominal organs appear as a broadened homogeneous soft tissue density. Sonographically the easily detectable fluid (FF) surrounds the layered, hyperechoic ova, which appear mildly oval and deformed. Although the shape and inner architecture of the ova already indicate follicular stasis, the ascites (especially when containing hyperechoic particles) is indicative for an inflammatory process most of the time. In addition, the appearance of the follicles has hardly changed in several follow-up examinations whereas ascites has progressed. (*Courtesy of* Michaela Gumpenberger, Dr med vet, Austria.)

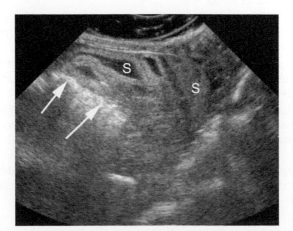

Fig. 22. Sonographic image of the same animal shown in **Fig. 17**B. The right salpinx (S) is fluid filled, indicating salpingitis. It is differentiated from the bowel loops because of position and different wall-layering. A hyperechoic egg shell with multiple spicules (*arrows*) is seen in the far field. (*Courtesy of* Michaela Gumpenberger, Dr med vet, Austria.)

or firm manual palpation (especially in snakes) may cause rupture of the oviduct, which can lead to egg yolk coelomitis.[13] In sonography free fluid additionally to degenerated follicles and eggs is seen. In CT the contours of follicles and eggs may become blurred. The connective tissue appears heterogenous and often of increased density (see **Fig. 16**).

SUMMARY

CT provides the most thorough information of the reproductive tract in chelonian species. The salpinx and all reproductive products can clearly be seen. Nevertheless, radiographs are much easier and cheaper to obtain and therefore remain the preferred first choice imaging technique for a first overview. In lizards and snakes sonography seems to be the most appropriate imaging technique. Being quick and noninvasive, it enables satisfying diagnoses and can be applied anywhere, whereas radiography and CT are restricted to dedicated locations. Still, more experience is needed to correctly interpret sonographic images with the additional difficulty of getting second opinions on found diagnoses.

ACKNOWLEDGMENT

The author thanks the team of the Section for Reptiles and Birds of the Clinical Department for Small Animals and the team of the Department for Pathology and Forensic Medicine of the University of Veterinary Medicine in Vienna (Vetmeduni Vienna), Austria for their great cooperation and support.

REFERENCES

1. Morris PJ, Alberts AC. Determination of sex in white-throated monitors (*Varanus albigularis*), Gila monsters (*Heloderma suspectum*), and Beaded lizards (*H. horridum*) using two-dimensional ultrasound imaging. J Zoo Wildl Med 1996;27(3):371–9.
2. Kuchling G. Ultrasound scanning as an effective tool in the conservation of chelonians. IZY 2015;49:22–30.
3. Pees M, Kiefer I, Ludewig E. Reptiles. In: Krautwald-Junghanns M-E, Pees M, Reese S, et al, editors. Diagnostic imaging of exotic pets: birds, small mammals, reptiles. Hannover (Germany): Schlütersche; 2010. p. 309–439.
4. Gumpenberger M, Schumacher J, Souza M. Reptilien. In: Hecht S, editor. Röntgendiagnostik in der kleintierpraxis. 2nd edition. Stuttgart (Germany): Schattauer; 2012. p. 439–63.
5. Lance VA, Rostal DC, Elsey RM, et al. Ultrasonography of reproductive structures and hormonal correlates of follicular development in female American alligators, *Alligator mississippiensis*, in southwest Louisiana. Gen Comp Endocrinol 2009; 162:251–6.
6. Gumpenberger M. Chelonians. In: Schwarz T, Saunders J, editors. Veterinary computed tomography. 1st edition. Chicheter (United Kingdom): Wiley-Blackwell; 2011. p. 533–44.
7. Pees M, Ludewig E, Plenz B, et al. Imaging diagnosis: seminoma causing liver compression in a Spur-thighed tortoise (*Testudo graeca*). Vet Radiol Ultrasound 2014;56(2):E21–4.
8. Spörle H, Kramer M, Göbel TH, et al. Sonographische graviditäts- und ovarialdiagnostik bei schlangen. Prakt Tierarzt 1991;4:286–90.

9. Love NE, Douglass JP, Lewbart G, et al. Radiographic and ultrasonographic evaluation of egg retention and peritonitis in two Green iguanas (*Iguana iguana*). Vet Radiol Ultrasound 1996;37(1):68–74.
10. Gumpenberger M, Hittmair K. Möglichkeiten der bildgebenden diagnostik beim urogenitaltrakt von schildkröten. Verh. Ber. Erkrg. Zootiere 1997;1997(38):77–85.
11. Kummrow MS, Smith DA, Crawshaw G, et al. Characterization of fecal hormone patterns associated with the reproductive cycle in female veiled chameleons (*Chamaeleo calyptratus*). Gen Comp Endocrinol 2010;168:340–8.
12. Gumpenberger M, Filip T. Bildgebende diagnostik verschiedener formen von legenot bei schildkröten und deren therapie: fallbeispiele. Wien Tierarztl Monatsschr 2001;88:70–9.
13. Rivera S. Health assessment of the reptilian reproductive tract. J Exot Pet Med 2008;17(4):259–66.
14. Hochleithner C, Holland M. Ultrasonography. In: Divers M, editor. Current therapy in reptile medicine & surgery. 1st edition. St Louis (MO): Elsevier Saunders; 2014. p. 107–27.

Reproductive Disorders and Perinatology of Sea Turtles

Filippo Spadola, DVM, PhD[a], Manuel Morici, DVM, PhD[a],*,
Mario Santoro, DVM, PhD, Dipl ECZM (Wildlife Population Health)[b],
Matteo Oliveri, DVM[c], Gianni Insacco, MNatSc[d]

KEYWORDS

- Sea turtles • Nest • Reproduction • Hatchling • Newborns

KEY POINTS

- Veterinary management is of paramount importance in the conservation of sea turtle species.
- Several disorders by virus, bacteria, parasites, or traumatic causes can affect the reproductive tract of sea turtles. The most common are the infections by herpesvirus and the cloacal prolapse.
- Useful diagnostic techniques are ultrasound, computed tomography, and cloacoscopy.
- Veterinary nest management and pediatrics of sea turtles includes several methodologies, such as nest translocation or captive hatchlings.

INTRODUCTION

Sea turtles are taxonomically part of the superfamily Chelonioidea and divided in 2 families (Dermochelyidae and Cheloniidae) and 7 species. The first family has just one species, the leatherback sea turtle (*Dermochelys coriacea*). The Cheloniidae family comprises the following species: the loggerhead sea turtle (*Caretta caretta*), the Kemp's ridley sea turtle (*Lepidochelys kempii*), the olive ridley sea turtle (*Lepidochelys olivacea*), the green sea turtle (*Chelonia mydas*), the hawksbill sea turtle (*Eretmochelys imbricata*), and the flatback sea turtle (*Natator depressus*). Cheloniidae species are

Disclosure Statement: The authors have nothing to disclose.
[a] Department of Veterinary Science, Polo Didattico Annunziata, Veterinary Teaching Hospital, University of Messina, Sicily, Messina 98168, Italy; [b] Istituto Zooprofilattico Sperimentale del Mezzogiorno, Portici (Naples) 80055, Italy; [c] Faculty of Veterinary Medicine, Avian and Exotic Animal Clinic, University of Veterinary and Pharmaceutical Sciences Brno, 1-3 Palackeho Street, Brno 612 42, Czech Republic; [d] Museo Civico di Storia Naturale, Via degli Studi 9, Comiso (Ragusa), Sicily 97013, Italy
* Corresponding author.
E-mail address: mmorici@unime.it

Vet Clin Exot Anim 20 (2017) 345–370
http://dx.doi.org/10.1016/j.cvex.2016.11.002
1094-9194/17/© 2016 Elsevier Inc. All rights reserved.

hard-shelled turtles with paddlelike limbs and a depressed body but streamlined. The shell is covered with horny scutes, and the limbs and head are partially covered with rather thin scales.

Species recognition is of paramount importance for a sea turtle veterinarian practitioner. Apart from the unique morphology of *D coriacea*, Cheloniidae species possess distinguishable anatomic features. An elliptical carapace covered by imbricate scutes and a hawklike beak tomium is typical of the hawksbill sea turtle, whereas a nearly oval carapace with no imbricate scutes, blunt head, and the preorbital distance visibly smaller than the orbital length are typical morphologic features of the green sea turtle. The flatback sea turtle has a round and flattened carapace, with an upward-folded edge. In the loggerhead sea turtle, the carapace is cardiform; its length is always greater than the width because of the presence of one more lateral scutes (5 lateral scutes). Five lateral scutes are also reported in *Lepidochelys* spp; these species have a round carapace with length similar to the width, and they possess a unique cutting tomium provided with an internal alveolar rim. Obviously the body color is greyolive or olive-yellowish. Because of the worldwide distribution and the authors' experiences, the loggerhead sea turtle is used as a model for the present article.

The species of this family have a pantropical distribution, with periodic or occasional migrations into temperate waters for feeding. In detail, apart from loggerhead and green sea turtles having a worldwide distribution, Kemp's ridley sea turtle is present just in the Gulf of Mexico, with some aberration findings,[1] whereas the olive ridley sea turtle occurs in all tropical waters[2] but never in the Mediterranean Sea. Flatback sea turtles can be found just along the coastal waters of Northern Australia and Papua New Guinea.[3]

The leatherback sea turtle is one of the largest living reptiles, with spindle-shaped huge bodies and leathery, unscaled carapaces. Furthermore, *D coriacea* has unique anatomic and physiologic features, such as the presence of vascularized growth, epiphyseal cartilages and a kind of endothermy similar to that of marine mammals.[4] Thanks to this exclusive feature, adult leatherbacks are more adapted to colder water than other sea turtles; as a result of this, the leatherback is the most widely distributed of all sea turtles, covering most all the salt-water surfaces.[5]

Sea turtle species have different diets: the loggerhead, Kemp's ridley, olive ridley, hawksbill, flatback, and leatherback sea turtles are omnivorous; but some species may specialize on certain prey, depending on the living area (for example, the hawksbill sea turtle is highly specialized on sponge eating). Green sea turtles are exclusively herbivorous during the adult ages, with omnivorous stages during the juvenile phases.[6] The leatherback turtles feed almost exclusively on jellyfish.

LIFE BIOLOGY

Because the loggerhead is the most widely distributed sea turtle, detailed data found in the literature regard mainly this species. It is used here as a model for the life biology. However, the life biology of the others species are similar without excessive differences. Loggerhead sea turtles, during their life, may inhabit several different ecosystem based on life phases: the terrestrial zone, the coastal waters, and the oceanic area. The terrestrial phase is typical of the nesting female turtles and of the hatchlings. After the hatch, newborn loggerheads start a swim frenzy for several days. In this phase the posthatchlings, carried by the currents, reach the oceanic area where they spend several years in seaweed (*Sargassum* spp) zones.[7] When they reach the 40 cm of curved carapace length (CCL; length of the turtles carapace measured from the notch at the anterior of the carapace to the tip of the last posterior marginal scute), they move in the coastal waters where they complete the maturation to the adult and reproductive age.[8] The adult loggerhead may migrate for thousands of kilometers and feed on diving in shallow waters, whereas juvenile and posthatchlings do not perform long diving phases and spend most of their time on superficial water.[9]

REPRODUCTIVE BIOLOGY AND MORPHOLOGY
Ontogeny of Reproductive Tract and Temperature Sex Determination

The gonads and genitalia of sea turtles develop from the gonadal ridge. The gonadal ridge derives from epithelial, mesothelial, and mesenchymal cells located between the mesonephric tubules and the dorsal mesentery.[10] During days 16 to 18 of incubation, the primordial germ cells accumulate at the base of the gonadal ridges to start the development of gonads.[11] The structure of the embryonic gonads is similar in both sexes, and the sexual differentiation occurs during embryonic stages 24 to 29.[12] In female sea turtles, the ovary results from the synchronized multiplication of the cortical cells (cortex) and from the regressive modification of the medullar cells. The oviduct, on the other hand, develops from the mullerian ducts (paramesonephric ducts), which are paired ducts that run down the lateral side of the urogenital ridge and terminate at the sinus tubercle in the primitive urogenital sinus. In male sea turtles, the testis results from the simultaneous regression of the cortex and from the differentiation of the seminiferous tubules in the medulla. At the same time, the vas deferens is derived from the wolffian duct. Mullerian (paramesonephric) ducts are present and developed in both sexes. They are functional in female sea turtles (oviducts) and vestigial in male sea turtles. In inspected male loggerhead turtles (through necropsy or coelioscopy), the mullerian ducts may be visibly linked to the testis; but they end within the caudal mesentery and are not directly connected to the cloaca.[13]

As in the other chelonian species, loggerhead turtles show temperature sex determination. In this species, the sex of the embryo is determined during a specific thermosensitive period of incubation.[14,15] The temperature during the incubation period (IP) is the most important factor in the gonadal differentiation of sea turtles.[16] As a general rule, incubation greater than 30°C results in female hatchlings, whereas eggs incubated at less than 28°C will result in male hatchlings.[17] Incubation temperature between 28°C and 30°C will result in a mixed clutch whereby both sexes are expressed. Recent research suggests that a high mortality rate occurs when the temperature of the nest reaches 32°C.[18]

Secondary Sexual Characteristics and Sex Identification

Sexual dimorphism is usually apparent in adult sea turtles. Male sea turtles present a longer tail with a more distal cloacal opening compared with female sea turtles (**Fig. 1**). Moreover, male sea turtles have large curved claws in the front limbs (flippers) and show a shorter plastron and a wider head.[19] As in other chelonians species, the sexual determination through secondary sexual characteristics is not possible in juvenile individuals. Accurate sex identification may be accomplished through necropsy, ultrasonography (in some cases), endoscopy,[20,21] or testosterone/estrogen assay from biological fluids or eggshell.[22–24]

Male Morphology and Reproductive Cycle

The male reproductive system is composed of the testicles, the vasa deferens, the urogenital papillae, and the phallus (**Fig. 2**). The testicles are located dorsally in the coelom, caudally to the lungs, and ventrally to the kidney. They are attached on the peritoneal wall, and they show an elongated appearance (**Fig. 3**). The epididymis is

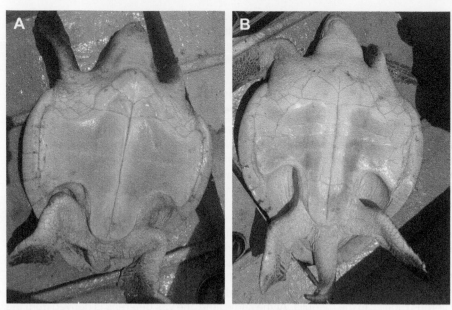

Fig. 1. Olive ridley sea turtle (*L olivacea*). Sexual dimorphism is evident in adult individuals. Female sea turtles show a short tail (*A*). Male sea turtles present a longer tail with a more distal cloacal opening compared with female sea turtles (*B*).

distinctly visible in adult male sea turtles; it is connected to the testis and transports the sperm to the vas deferens. The vas deferens finally ends in the urogenital papilla.

The urogenital papillae are located in the urodeum; they show a cauliflower shape and are directly involved in the copula. During mating, the sperm leaks from the papilla on the sulcus spermaticus and is directed by the phallus into the female cloaca. The phallus is composed of the 2 corpora cavernosa, the corpora fibrosa, and the glans. The corpora cavernosa begin from the urogenital papillae and continue on the floor of the proctodeum. During the erection, they become engorged

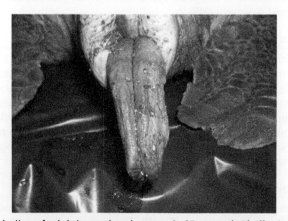

Fig. 2. Exposed phallus of adult loggerhead sea turtle (*C caretta*). Phallus is composed of the 2 *corpora cavernosa*, the *corpora fibrosa*, and the glans. During the erection, the *sulcus spermaticus* is formed in the dorsal part of the phallus.

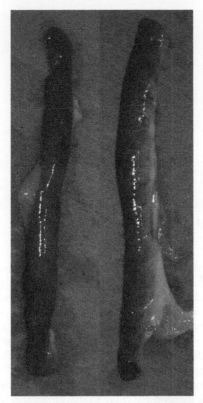

Fig. 3. Testicles of an adult loggerhead sea turtle (*C caretta*). Testicles present an elongated appearance.

with blood proceeding from the iliac veins. With the organ erect, the sulcus spermaticus is formed in the dorsal part of the phallus. The chelonian phallus also contains the corpora fibrosa; these bow the penis ventrally and then anteriorly during the full erection.[25]

Spermatogenesis lasts approximately 9 months in loggerhead sea turtles.[26] In adult male sea turtles, only a short quiescent period (2–3 months) exists between the peak of the spermiogenesis (during the courtship) and the beginning of the next spermatogenic cycle.[27] Male sea turtles are promiscuous seasonal breeders. They exhibit migratory behavior and show strong fidelity to both courtship areas and foraging sites.[28] Courtship seems to occur during a short period before the nesting season. Male-to-male aggressiveness has been recorded during the courtship period.[29,30] After the courtship period and once the mating occurred, male sea turtles return to their foraging areas. Female sea turtles will then proceed to the nesting sites. The cessation of male courtship is characterized by a significant decrease in body condition score, lower plasma triglyceride level (from a normal average of 2.41 mg/dL to an average of 0.77 mg/dL), and increased plasma proteins (from a normal average of 3.38 mg/dL to an average of 4.90 mg/dL).[27]

Female Morphology and Reproductive Cycle

The female reproductive tract is composed of the ovaries, the oviducts, the suspensory ligaments (or mesovarium), the genital papillae, and the clitoris (**Figs. 4** and **5**).

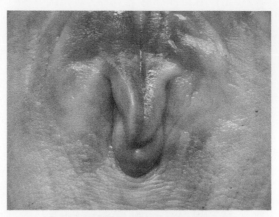

Fig. 4. Clitoris of a nesting green sea turtle (*C mydas*).

The clitoris is a vestigial organ, anatomically similar to the phallus but obviously smaller in size. Genital papillae are located in the urodeum (grossly in the same position as in the male), and they lead to the 2 oviducts. In the adult female loggerhead, oviducts are extremely long and convoluted (**Figs. 6** and **7**). They can reach the length of 4 to 6 m. They run ventrally to the kidneys and are suspended into the coelomic cavity through the mesosalpinx. Specialized sperm storage areas were not identified in sea turtles; evidence of the capability of female sea turtles to store sperm was, however, confirmed by Chaves and colleagues[31] in the *L olivacea*; however, evidence regarding how long female sea turtles may store sperm is still missing. The ovaries are located caudally to the lungs and inside the coelom. They are bonded to the peritoneum and suspended through the *mesovarium*. Another fibrotic structure connects the ovaries with the oviducts; this is the *mesotubarium*. Ovulated follicles enter the oviduct through the *ostium*. There is no direct connection between the ovary and the oviduct (**Fig. 8**A). In juvenile female sea turtles, the follicles are not easily visualized; the ovaries, however, show a rough surface that helps in distinguishing the immature ovaries from the testicles (**Fig. 8**B). In adult female sea turtles, yellow vascularized vitellogenic follicles may be present in the ovaries. Once

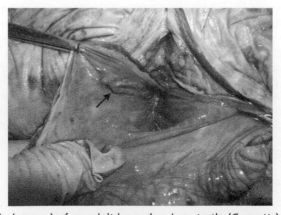

Fig. 5. Clitoris (*black arrow*) of an adult loggerhead sea turtle (*C caretta*).

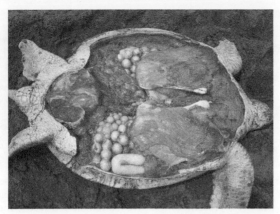

Fig. 6. A nesting green sea turtle (*C mydas*) killed by jaguar (*Panthera onca*) attack while he was coming ashore to nest in the Tortuguero National Park, Caribbean coast of Costa Rica.

ovulated, the formed eggs are stored into the oviduct until the deposition (see **Figs. 6** and **7**). Thus, shelled eggs may be present in the oviduct of adult female sea turtles approaching the coast.[32] As for other reptiles, vitellogenin is involved in the vitellogenesis and in the development of the follicles. Ovarian changes have been abundantly described in *C mydas*. In this species, the ovarian cycle is linked to the climatic conditions at the foraging area and the abundance of food availability.[33,34] According to Jessop and colleagues,[27] sea turtles may decide whether to start the reproductive activity (folliculogenesis and ovulation or spermatogenesis) or not according to the availability of food resources and the temperature. If the requirements in terms of energy intake are not fulfilled in a certain year, the reproduction activity can be procrastinated to the next year. However, other investigators suggest that the climate conditions are not directly correlated with the reproduction of most carnivores/omnivores sea turtles.[32,33] In *Lepidochelys* spp, an increase in follicle size occurs between the 8 and 10 months before the breeding season.[27,35] Sea turtles, as many other reptiles, have induced ovulation. Thus, once the follicles reached the proper size for ovulation, they remain quiescent until the mating. Female sea turtles show polyandrous behavior.[36]

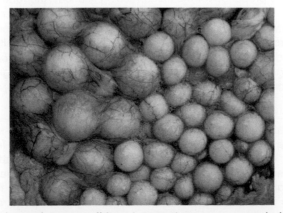

Fig. 7. Eggs, follicles, and *corpora albicans* in a nesting green sea turtle (*C mydas*).

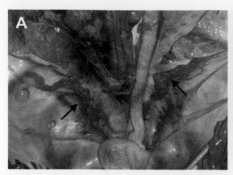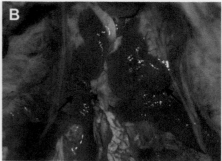

Fig. 8. Appearance of ovaries and *mesovarium* of 2 juvenile loggerhead sea turtles (*C caretta*). Ovaries (*black arrows*) are dorsally located in the pelvic region (*A*). No connection between ovaries and oviduct is present. In the juvenile female sea turtle, the follicles are still not easily visualized; the ovaries, however, show a rough surface that helps in distinguishing the immature ovaries from the testicles (*B*).

Nesting

Nesting occurs on average 34.7 days after mating in captive *C mydas*.[37] Gravid female sea turtles may show anorexia, and after the nesting they show a decrease in body weight of an average of 0.9 kg.[38] Polyphagia has been recorded after nesting[27] and is likely meant to provide female sea turtles with the sufficient energy for the next breeding season. A proper energetic balance will result in an improved reproductive success. The nesting success (NS), which can be described as the percentage of nesting attempts that results in successful delivery of the eggs, is in fact one of the most important expressions of reproductive success in female sea turtles. The NS may differ among species and populations and is often lower than 100%.[30,39] Once female sea turtles reach the proper nesting site (on a beach), they start digging with the hind flippers. The nest is ultimately covered with sand (the moister and last moved) and then compacted (**Fig. 9**).[40]

Sea turtles of *Lepidochelys* spp may show a spectacular synchronism in nesting. Female sea turtles of this species may emerge to nest in an event known as the arribada (**Fig. 10**). The arribada occurs during the night or the early morning, when hundreds of female *Lepidochelys* reach the beaches of Central America to nest simultaneously. The event lasts for several days and may occur again after 1 month.[30] After nesting season, female sea turtles return to their foraging areas. There they will accumulate energy preparing for the next breeding season. After one migration (from the foraging area to the nesting area and back), female sea turtles may remain in a quiescent period whereby no reproductive activity is noticed. Once female sea turtles are ready again to reproduce, they will return to the same nesting site showing high fidelity. Published data suggest that 98% of Australian female *C caretta* return to the same nesting site.[32] According to Miller and colleagues,[41] migratory cycles in *C caretta* occur on average every 3 years (ranging from 1 to 9 years).

Mating

Courtship and mating occur in the water (**Fig. 11**). The male sea turtle starts to swim in circles around the female sea turtle. The courtship includes biting the female sea turtle around the neck area and on the shoulders (**Fig. 12**) and several attempts to stud. Once the male sea turtle is in the correct position (on the female carapace and fixed with the forelimbs), he will slide the long tail beneath the female plastron (see **Fig. 11**). As the cloacae are in line, the erected phallus penetrates the female sea turtle and the mating occurs.[41]

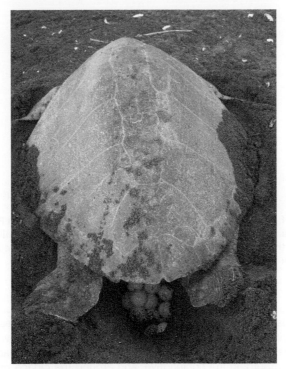

Fig. 9. An adult *L olivacea* during egg laying. Once the female sea turtle reaches the proper nesting site, she starts digging with the hind flippers; the nest is finally covered with sand and then compacted.

REPRODUCTIVE DISORDERS

Reports of illnesses specifically related to the reproductive tract of sea turtles are scarce in the literature. However, bacterial, viral, mycotic, parasitic, mechanical, and traumatic diseases localized or related to the genital tract may potentially affect sea turtles.

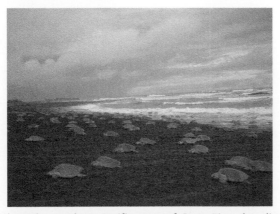

Fig. 10. In Ostional on the northern Pacific coast of Costa Rica, the olive ridley sea turtle shows a characteristic synchronous massive nesting aggregation, termed *arribada*, which occurs approximately once a month throughout the year.

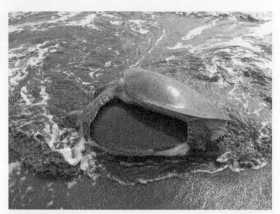

Fig. 11. Mating of green sea turtles (*C mydas*) at the Tortuguero National Park (Costa Rica). Once the male sea turtle is in the correct position, he will slide the long tail beneath the female plastron. As the cloacae are in line, the erected phallus penetrates the female sea turtle and the mating occurs.

Viral Diseases

Fibropapillomatosis is probably the most common viral disease in sea turtles. Particularly in the Caribbean Sea populations, this pathogen shows a very high prevalence.[42] It is characterized by the formation of tumor masses (papilloma) on the skin, around the mouth, in the conjunctiva, and around the cloaca of sea turtles. All the species are sensitive to the infection.[43] Fibropapillomatosis spreads through horizontal transmission and is caused by the Chelonid fibropapilloma–associated herpesvirus (C-FPTHV).[44] However, the simple presence of the pathogen in the environment seems to be insufficient for the disease to spread. A multifactorial cause was suggested for the fibropapillomatosis; predisposing factors may include parasites (marine leeches [*Ozobranchus* spp]), bacteria, pollution, biotoxins (lyngbyatoxin produced by cyanobacterium *Moorea producens*, formerly *Lyngbya majuscule*; okadaic acid from a

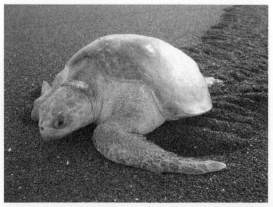

Fig. 12. An adult female olive ridley sea turtle (*L olivacea*) during the arribada in Ostional. The courtship includes biting the female sea turtle around the neck and on the shoulders, as it is possible to see in this adult female sea turtle.

dinoflagellate), adverse environmental conditions (eg, microalgae proliferation), and immunosuppression.[45–49]

The C-FPTHV causes the proliferation of the papillary cells, dermal fibroblasts and epidermal keratinocytes.[50] According to Campbell[51] the masses may involve also the internal organs including the reproductive tract (*proctodeum,* and *urodeum*). The involvement of other areas of the reproductive tract (oviduct and ovaries) is likely, but actual reports are lacking.

Stacy and others[52] have described the loggerhead genital and respiratory herpesvirus. This pathogen causes lesions in the trachea and around the cloaca. Ulcers on the phallus and clitoris of necropsied specimens are reported as well. Most of the described lesions were found on necropsy in juvenile subjects, but the presence in adult reproductive specimens is likely. Horizontal transmission through contact (mating) and marine leeches (mechanical vectors) has been proposed.

Bacterial and Fungal Diseases

Several bacterial and fungal diseases have been diagnosed in sea turtles but never specifically in the reproductive tract.

Parasites

Chelonacarus elongatus is a parasite mite that lives in the cloacal wall of sea turtles, often producing a stressful cloacitis.[53] Cardiovascular flukes belonging to the family Spirorchiidae represent a major threat for sea turtle health, considered among the most important parasitic cause of its stranding and mortality worldwide. Adult flukes live in the cardiovascular system of their host and produce vast numbers of eggs, which penetrate the gut wall and move into the intestinal lumen and are eliminated into the external environment with the host's feces. However, many eggs become lodged in body organs and tissues, including oviducts, leading to a severe granulomatous response.[54]

Others

Columbus crabs (*Planes minutus*) are often found living on sea turtles,[55] especially on loggerheads (**Fig. 13**). It is now thought to fill a cleaning role but in the past was thought to feed on feces, living near cloaca, also causing cloacitis and distress.

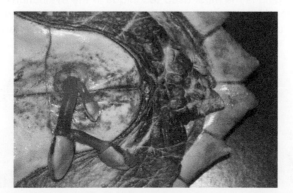

Fig. 13. Pericloacal region of a subadult female loggerhead sea turtle (*C caretta*). A Columbus crab (*Planes minutus*) is present on the left of the tail. This crab is often found living in sea turtles. Living near cloaca can also cause cloacitis and distress. In this turtle, an infestation of barnacles (*Lepas spp*) was also found.

Urolithiasis is thought to cause cloacal damage.[56] Dystocia is probably underdiagnosed in sea turtles. Nutter and colleagues[57] described an oviduct prolapse, evolved in necrotic oophoritis with retained eggs in a loggerhead sea turtle. The animal was treated surgically (mono lateral ovario-salpingectomy), and the recovery was uneventful. The reproductive function was not compromised, and the female sea turtle was able to lay eggs during the following season.

Frutchey and colleagues[58] reported 2 distinct cases of oviduct detachment. The disconnected tissue was found in both cases on the nest in conjunction with several nonvital eggs.

Otherwise, prolapse of the cloaca (or penis \ clitoris, **Fig. 14**) may be common. During the authors' veterinary practice (F.S, G.I.), all cloacal prolapses were related to gastrointestinal impaction or ingested fish lines. A penile prolapse was diagnosed in an adult male loggerhead (**Fig. 15**). The prolapse was secondary to gastrointestinal impaction due to the ingestion of a plastic bag. Once the primary issue was resolved, the prolapse spontaneously reduced. Most of the prolapses involving the lower genital tract (cloaca, caudal oviduct, and genitalia) are in fact related to the ingestion of plastic bags and fishing lines.[50] Thus, accidental foreign-bodies ingestion shall always be considered when dealing with prolapses in sea turtles.

Two cases of *pseudohermaphroditism* in *C caretta* have been diagnosed.[59] These loggerheads have been found with precocious masculine external sex features, not confirmed by hormonal assay and coelioscopy. Further, heavy metal toxicosis can also lead to gonadal diseases, with possible embryo development abnormalities.[50]

DIAGNOSTIC TECHNIQUE

Physical examination of sea turtles did not differ from other aquatic chelonian species. Specific attention should be paid on turtles' ability to swim, in order to guarantee a further releasing. Even the excessive presence of cutaneous symbionts can alter the ability of turtles to move, both in the water and during the nesting phases. For the duration of every diagnostic technique, of paramount importance is to cover the eyes with a wet towel in order to avoid excessive excretion of mucus from the salt gland.

Diagnostic imaging is the most used technique in the evaluation of the sea turtle reproductive tract. Most sea turtles are collaborative animals; a gentle contention helps during the diagnostic technique. However, care must be taken when working

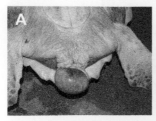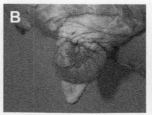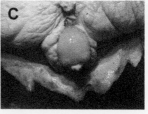

Fig. 14. Prolapse of the cloaca in 3 subadult loggerhead sea turtles. At the authors' veterinary practice (F.S., G.I.), all cloacal prolapses were related to gastrointestinal impaction or ingested fish lines. Once the primary issue was resolved, the prolapse spontaneously reduced.

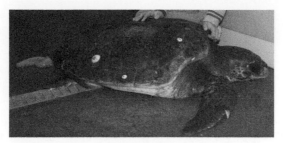

Fig. 15. Penile prolapse in a mature male loggerhead sea turtle (*C caretta*).

close to the head because bites can be decidedly dangerous for the operator. In extremely strong and active turtles, sedation is mandatory to perform radiographic or ultrasonographic examinations. Ultrasonography through the prefemoral area **(Fig. 16)** is the best option for wide visualization of the genital tract.[60–62] In female sea turtles, the early and late preovulatory stage and the postovulatory stage are noticeable by means of ultrasound exploration of the ovaries.[60] During the early nesting season (preovulatory), ovaries are filled with vitellogenic follicles (large and hyperechoic). Otherwise, when ovulation (and nesting) occurs, the ovaries are generally quiescent, with no preovulatory follicles. A few hyperechoic atresic follicles may be visible in the quiescent ovaries.[63] Radiographs and computed tomography may also be useful to diagnose neoplasia, egg development, and pregnancy **(Fig. 17)**.

A more invasive technique for the visualization of the reproductive tract is coelioscopy. Approach is preferably performed from the prefemoral fossa, which is larger in sea turtles compared with the common captive species (*Testudo* spp and *Trachemys* spp). The endoscope is inserted into the coelom for a broad visualization of the internal organs. Coelioscopy is a relatively safe procedure; it requires, however, a strong knowledge of the anatomy of sea turtles and the proper skill. This technique entails the incision and the inflation of the coelom with air. Thus, the animal shall be anesthetized and ventilated during the procedure; the whole recovery must be

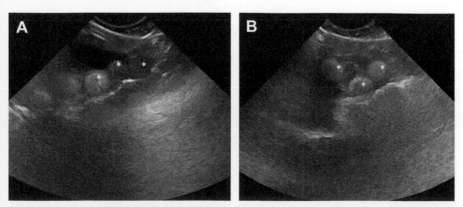

Fig. 16. Ultrasonography through the prefemoral area in 2 subadult female loggerhead sea turtles (*C caretta*). In these animals, ovaries were occupied by a few vitellogenic follicles (hyperechoic, *white asterisks*).

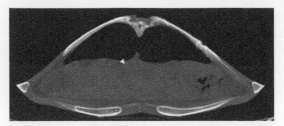

Fig. 17. Computed tomography of stranded subadult female loggerhead sea turtle (*C caretta*). In this image it is possible to see a few follicles (*white arrowhead*).

carefully monitored.[64] Being wild animals, sea turtles are easily stressed by invasive techniques.[65,66] Thus, it is important to reduce contact with humans as much as possible.

Cloacoscopy, as for other chelonians, may be used for minor procedures, such as the removal of foreign bodies[67] or the study of cloaca and annexed reproductive organs.[68] Cloacoscopy allows for the exploration of the phallus \ clitoris (**Fig. 18**), the urethral orifice, the urogenital sinus, and the distal colon. The urethral orifice may be overcome, allowing the direct visualization of the urinary bladder. In juvenile turtles, it is possible to visualize the coelomic organs through the diaphanous wall of the urinary bladder.[69] The authors (F.S., M.M.) generally use a 10-mm diameter laparoscope with 0° optics.

Captive Breeding

Historically, 3 facilities in 3 countries attempted the captive breeding of sea turtles: Grand Cayman Island, Reunion Island, and Australia. Nowadays only the Grand Cayman Island facility (GCIf) persists. All of the aforementioned were breeding *C mydas*, and GCIf has been the only one capable to produce a second generation of turtles. Recently, in the GCIf a first generation of the endangered *L kempii* has been obtained, proving that the sustainable captive breeding for commercial purpose is a noticeable (and essential) tool in the conservation of endangered reptile species.

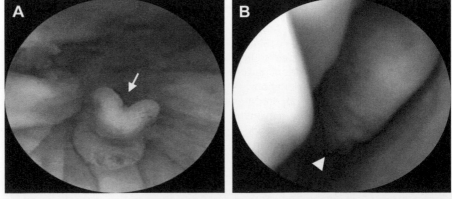

Fig. 18. Cloacoscopy of male and female adult loggerhead sea turtles (*C caretta*). Clitoris (*A, white arrow*) and phallus (*B, white arrowhead*) are visible.

VETERINARY NEST MANAGEMENT AND PEDIATRICS

If, for adults, the anthropogenic threats have a significant effect, for newborns, such phenomena have to be considered even more impactful, such as the following:

- Collisions with boats
- Oil poisoning
- Impact with fishing tool nets
- Ingestion of foreign bodies (abandoned waste, such as plastic fragments and other floating objects, and so forth)
- Devastation of marine habitats and environmental integrity of the nesting beaches (eg, passage of mechanical machines for beaches cleaning)[70]
- Human presence (For example, presence during the night on nesting beaches disturbs and reduces nesting attempts and artificial light sources interfere with orientation of newborns at hatching time.)[71]

Nesting Area Monitoring, Nest Management, and Husbandry

The deposition area must be regularly monitored by direct supervision or by video surveillance systems. In any case, maintaining a low sound level is mandatory.[71] Until the end of the deposition, operators must keep at least 4 m from the turtle, staying at the rear of the turtle. A small number (maximum of 4) of operators can stay during the nesting phase.[72]

Translocation of nests menaced by flooding must occur within 2 hours of laying[73] and only in cases of extreme risk within 12 hours.[74] Alternatively, in order to not cause high mortality induced by egg movement, translocation can be performed belatedly (after 25 days have passed).[75] Nest translocation can be necessary when laying is in exceptionally visited and inhabited beaches.

During nest translocation, it is important that this takes place when the temperature of the nest is the same as the external temperature. The choice of the new area to recompose the nest is crucial; the same grain size of the sand must be maintained.

For egg removal from the nest firstly is indispensable to measure the depth of the first and the last layer of eggs; consequently, the eggs can be collected and ordered by layers, marked at the upper pole, and keeping them in an upright position. The eggs then have to be placed in a casing with a few centimeters of the original nest sand. Subsequently, the new nest can be dug, and the eggs relocated with the same scheme as the original nest, maintaining the same depth, layers, and egg disposition.

Concerning the closure of the nest chamber, the sand of the original nest should be used, also to cover areas adjacent to the new nest.[76] Assessment of the internal temperature of the nest is an important parameter in order to establish the goodness of the place of deposition and translocation.[77]

Nests must be protected from predators with fences (**Fig. 19**). In case of the nest of loggerheads, the authors used a cylindrical-shaped sturdy metal net, with 2 × 2-cm mesh, inserted in the sand with a depth of 10 cm and equipped with a removable cover. Obviously, the choice depends on the site of deposition and on the type of predators present in the environment. Such protection in any case requires continuous monitoring. For nests that were not subjected to continuous surveillance, fencing must allow the exit of newborns (a horizontal net must be commensurate with the size of newborns). For collecting biometric data of newborns, these are held into a plastic box with 5 cm of moistened sand, protected from sunlight, and released in close

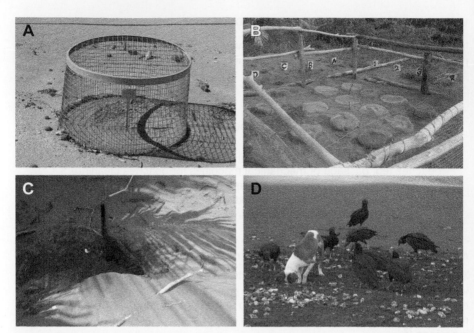

Fig. 19. Sea turtles' nest protection is of paramount importance against possible predators. A metal-net basket protection was placed on a nest of *C caretta* in San Lorenzo beach, Siracusa, Sicily Island (*A*). Leatherback sea turtle hatchery on the Caribbean coast of the Costa Rica (*B*). Depredation by white-nosed coati (*Nasua narica*) on a green turtle (*C mydas*) nest in the Caribbean coast of Costa Rica (*C*). Depredation by a dog and black vultures (*Coragyps atratus*) on nests of olive ridley sea turtle (*L olivacea*) in Ostional (Costa Rica) (*D*).

proximity to the nest immediately after the collection of relevant data. If the beach is exposed to anthropic threats, it will be necessary to ensure that newborns reach the sea even by direct action. Inspection of the nest can be made after at least 3 nights since the last hatching. The discovery of unhatched eggs, but with the presence of embryo on candling, requires the repositioning of the same into the same original position. Nests must be recomposed, as explained earlier, while awaiting the further hatchings.

Incubation of Egg and Captive Hatching

When necessary, captive incubation of egg can be accomplished. Several investigators have described incubation methods for sea turtle eggs.[78,79] A plastic container may be used; in the investigators' experiences, at the start of incubation, 65 +10 mL of water was added to moisten the foam sponge base. In the abovementioned technique, the eggs were surrounded by wet vermiculite. The authors' experience with captive incubation regards the hatching of loggerhead eggs (**Fig. 20**). The mother laid 79 eggs in a popular seaside, and removing the eggs was considered necessary. Eggs were collected and marked and placed in a professional reptile incubator. The temperature was set at 31°C, with humidity ranging from 80% to 90%. Instead that vermiculites the eggs were incubated, surrounded by the nest sand. After 55 days, 8 broken eggs have been removed (false eggs, without embryo). Because of

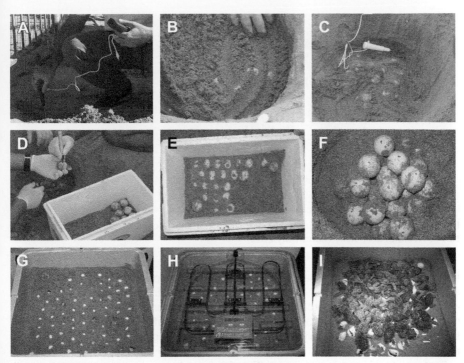

Fig. 20. During nest translocation, or eggs transport in captive incubator, several phases must be performed. In this case a flooded-risk nest of *C caretta* was found in a beach of Marina di Ragusa, Sicily Island. First translocation phases regard checking the external nest temperature (*A*); the following eggs may be exposed (*B*). Internal nest temperature must be recorded (*C*). Further, the egg's pole must to be marked in order to no change the position. The tank for the transport must to be filled with nest sand (*E*). Following the new area location, the eggs must be replaced in the same order of the collection (*F*). In captive hatching, the authors suggest the use of nest sand (*G*) instead of moist vermiculite. The incubator was set up at 31°C with 80% to 90% humidity (*H*). Seventy of 71 eggs hatched (*I*). Captive hatching has been performed at the Regional Rescue Center of Wildlife in Comiso, Ragusa, Sicily Island.

the high percentage of hatching (70 of 71), the use of the sand instead of vermiculites can be suggested.

Nest and Embryo Health

The most important threat for the nests is related to the alteration of chemical-physical and geo-morphologic beach characteristics. The imbalance between erosion and accumulation can change the slope of the beaches and the sand size with consequences for both deposition and embryonic development.[71] Embryos are also vulnerable to changes in temperature, salinity, moisture, and ventilation of nest substrate; such conditions can also affect the growth of the clutch.[80] The optimal temperature (OT) of the nesting beaches typically ranges from 24°C to 33°C; therefore, eggs incubated at lower or higher temperatures (especially in the period close to hatching and for prolonged periods) will hardly hatch.[41] The IP varies depending on the temperature. Normal development of the offspring is described at an OT of 25°C for 13 weeks.[41,77,81] A change of 1° in OT increases or decreases the IP of about 5 days.[82] Newborns usually rise to the surface from 2 to 15 days after hatching (**Fig. 21**); the compactness of

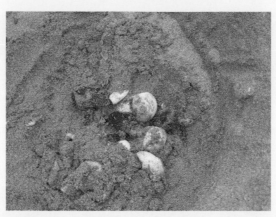

Fig. 21. Submerging from the nest of several posthatchling loggerhead sea turtles (*C caretta*) in Avola beach, Sicily Island (July 2010).

the sand, depth, and especially all the difference in temperatures between nest and external surface may influence the success of the exit from the nest[41]; in fact, it is recorded that a small percentage of newborns are unable to emerge from the nest.[41] Sizes of newborns vary according to species, but regularly the weight is half the egg weight (eg, averagely a loggerhead egg is 32.7 g, whereeas the newborn is averagely 20 g).[83]

Bacteria, fungi, and insect larvae (**Fig. 22**) have been shown in association with reduced hatchling success.[84–88] The bacterial cloacal flora of nesting sea turtles that are apparently healthy is composed of a very wide microbe spectrum, including several potential pathogens; however, the finding of potential pathogenic bacteria is not synonymous with illness and/or hatchling mortality[85–87] and should be evaluated relative to the environmental biotic and abiotic factors of the nesting beach. Deprivation of oxygen and exposure to higher temperatures resulting from microbial decomposition in the nest have been suggested as the main causes of reduced hatchling success.[89] For instance, high levels of bacterial species inside the eggs of *C caretta* have been correlated with lower hatchling success,[88] whereas egg mortality has been found to increase with the presence of fungi.[90,91] Contrariwise, *Pseudomonas aeruginosa*, *Bacillus* spp, *Aspergillus* spp, *Penicillium* spp, and *Cladosporium* spp do not cause embryo death but may invade eggs opportunistically after they have already lost their protective antimicrobial mechanisms.[92–94] Pathogenicity, however, may vary by strain or beach location. Microorganisms may contaminate eggs during (cloacal fluids) and after disposition (meiofauna, protozoans, zooplankton, crabs, humans, and other predatory animals).[93] In some cases genetic deformities could be found (**Fig. 23**).

Newborn Management

If eggs were incubated in captivity, newborns must be released into nature no later than 2 to 4 days after hatching (**Fig. 24**). General clinical examination must be performed gently. In exceptional cases, for debilitated or too-small hatchlings, it can be necessary to hospitalize them in temperature-controlled salt-water aquariums to an optimum temperature around 26°C, with UVA/UVB light control (8–10 hours of light in the authors' facilities [F.S., G.I.]). During hospitalization, hematologic and chemistry analyses may be performed. The authors note that the hatchlings of loggerhead sea

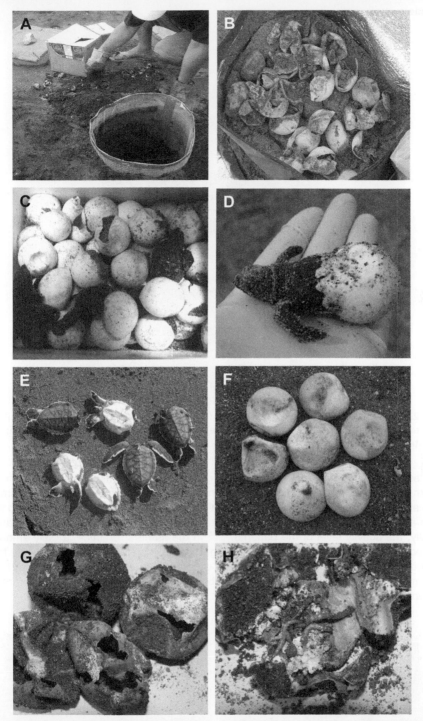

Fig. 22. Several cases of unsuccessful hatching. A researcher is evaluating hatching success in olive ridley nests in Ostional (A). Sometimes the nest can be found flooded, with death of all embryos and newborns (Sicily Island, Italy, B–D). Depredation by black vultures (C atratus) on newborns of green sea turtles in Tortuguero National Park (Costa Rica) (E). Unviable eggs of olive ridley sea turtles (L olivacea) (F). Depredation by insect larvae on olive ridley sea turtle (L olivacea) eggs in Ostional, Costa Rica (G, H).

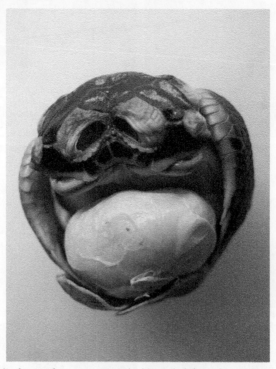

Fig. 23. A dicephalic fetus of green sea turtle (*C mydas*) found in Tortuguero National Park (Costa Rica). Developmental anomalies may be related to genetic, mutagenic, and environmental causes, such as inappropriate incubation temperature.

turtles hospitalized in the aquarium have a great fondness for fish eggs, and they can be maintained on this diet for the first few months of life and then weaned with small fish and shrimp (**Fig. 25**). Feeding of hospitalized newborns must vary according to the size and weight of the animal, the caloric and nutritional values of used food, and, finally, the activity level of the patients.[65,66] In the authors' practice, a daily amount of food equal to 5% to 10% of body weight is administered in posthatchlings. The diet of sea turtles in the authors' practice is constituted of marine animals (eg, fish, shrimps, jellyfish, and so forth) in eating patients, whereas in rehab patients, common veterinary carnivore care is used.

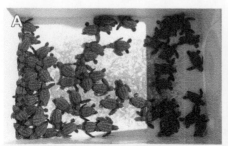
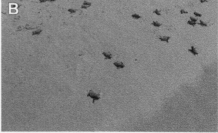

Fig. 24. Captive hatching of loggerhead sea turtles (*C caretta*). Twelve hours after the hatching in captivity, the newborns were released in an isolated beach in Sicily Island.

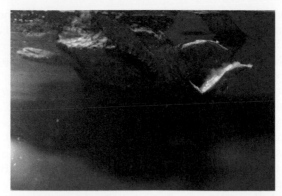

Fig. 25. Captive-bred juvenile loggerhead sea turtle (*C caretta*) at Regional Rescue Center of Wildlife in Comiso, Ragusa, Sicily Island. In this case, it was necessary to hospitalize the newborn for some weeks in a salt-water tank with controlled temperature (22°C–24°C). Hospitalization was necessary because, on physical examinations after hatching, the newborn showed weakness, poor skeletal development, and reluctance to move. After some months of critical care feeding, the juvenile loggerhead started to eat fishes and shrimps and it was further releases.

REFERENCES

1. Insacco G, Spadola F. First record of Kemp's ridley sea turtle, *Lepidochelys kempii* (Garman, 1880) (Cheloniidae), from the Italian waters (Mediterranean Sea). Acta Herpetol 2010;5(1):113–7.
2. Pritchard PC. Evolution, phylogeny, and current status. In: Lutz PL, Musick JA, editors. The biology of sea turtles. Boca Raton (FL): CRC Press Inc; 1996. p. 1–29.
3. Limpus CJ, Parmenter CJ, Baker V, et al. The flatback turtle, *Chelonia depressa*, in Queensland: post-nesting migration and feeling ground distribution. Wildl Res 1983;10(3):557–61.
4. Davenport J, Holland DL, East J. Thermal and biochemical characteristics of the lipids of the leatherback turtle *Dermochelys coriacea*: evidence of endothermy. J Mar Biol Assoc UK 1990;70(1):33–41.
5. Marquez R. Sea turtles of the world. FAO Fish Synopsis 1990;125(11):53–8.
6. Arthur K, Boyle M, Limpus C. Ontogenetic changes in diet and habitat use in green sea turtle (*Chelonia mydas*) life history. Mar Ecol Prog Ser 2008;362: 303–11.
7. Musick JA, Limpus C. Habitat utilization and migration in juvenile sea turtles. In: Lutz PL, Musick JA, editors. The biology of sea turtles. Boca Raton (FL): CRC Press Inc; 1996. p. 140–2.
8. Dodd CK. Synopsis of the biological data on the loggerhead sea turtle *Caretta caretta* (Linneaus 1758). U.S. Fish Wildl Serv Biol Rep 1988;88(14):35–82.
9. Plotkin PT, Wicksten MK, Amos AF. Feeding ecology of the loggerhead sea turtle *Caretta caretta* in the Northwestern Gulf of Mexico. Mar Biol 1993;115(1):1–5.
10. Miller JD, Limpus C. Ontogeny of marine turtle gonads. In: Lutz PL, Musick JA, Wyneken J, editors. Biology of sea turtle, vol. II. Boca Raton (FL): CRC Press Inc; 2002. p. 199–224.
11. Fujimoto T, Ukeshima A, Miyayama Y, et al. Observations of primordial germ cells in the turtle embryo (*Caretta caretta*): light and electron microscopic studies. Dev Growth Differ 1979;21:3–10.

12. Merchant-Larios H, Villalpando I, Centeno B. Gonadal morphogenesis under controlled temperature in the sea turtle *Lepidochelys olivacea*. Herpetol Monogr 1989;3:128–57.

13. Limpus CJ, Miller JD, Reed P. Intersexuality in a loggerhead sea turtle, *Caretta caretta*. Herpetol Rev 1982;13:32–3.

14. Miller JD. Embryology of marine turtles. In: Gans C, Billet F, Madderson PFA, editors. Biology of the reptilia, vol. 14. New York: John Wiley & Sons; 1985. p. 270–328.

15. Yntema CL, Mrosovsky N. Sexual differentiation in hatching loggerheads (*Caretta caretta*) incubated at different controlled temperatures. Herpetologica 1980;36:33–6.

16. Ackerman RA. The nest environment and the embryonic development of sea turtles. In: Lutz PL, Musick JA, editors. The biology of sea turtles. Boca Raton (FL): CRC Press Inc; 1996. p. 83–106.

17. Georges A, Limpus CJ, Stoutjesijk R. Hatchling sex in the marine turtle *Caretta caretta* is determined by proportion of development at a temperature, not daily duration of exposure. J Exp Zool 1994;270:432–44.

18. Sim EL, Booth DT, Limpus CJ. Incubation temperature, morphology and performance in loggerhead (*Caretta caretta*) turtle hatchlings from Mon Repos, Queensland, Australia. Biol Open 2015;4(6):685–92.

19. Pritchard PC, Mortimer JA. Taxonomy, external morphology, and species identification. In: Eckert KL, Bjorndal KA, Abreu-Grobois FA, et al, editors. Research and management techniques for the conservation of sea turtles. Washington, DC: IUCN/SSC Marine Turtle Specialist Group; 1999. p. 21–38. Publication No 4.

20. Hernandez-Divers SJ, Stahl SJ, Farrell R. An endoscopic method for identifying sex of hatchling Chinese box turtles and comparison of general versus local anesthesia for coelioscopy. J Am Vet Med Assoc 2009;234(6):800–4.

21. Martínez-Silvestre A, Bargalló F, Grífols J. Gender identification by cloacoscopy and cystoscopy in juvenile chelonians. Vet Clin North Am Exot Anim Pract 2015;3:527–39.

22. Owens DW, Hendrickson JR, Lance V, et al. A technique for determining sex of immature *Chelonia mydas* using radioimmunoassay. Herpetologica 1978;34: 270–3.

23. Wellins DJ. Use of an H-Y antigen assay for sex determination in sea turtles. Copeia 1987;1:46–52.

24. Wibbels T, Owens DW, Limpus CJ. Sexing juvenile sea turtles: is there an accurate and practical method? Chelonian Conserv Biol 2000;3:756.

25. Innis CJ, Boyer TH. Chelonian reproductive disorders. Vet Clin North Am Exot Anim Pract 2002;5(3):555–78.

26. Wibbels T, Owens DW, Limpus CJ, et al. Seasonal changes in serum gonadal steroids associated with migration, mating, and nesting in the loggerhead sea turtle (*Caretta caretta*). Gen Comp Endocrinol 1990;79:154.

27. Jessop TS, Hamman M, Limpus C. Body condition and physiological changes in male green turtles during breeding. Mar Ecol Prog Ser 2004;276(1):281–8.

28. Jessop TS, FitzSimmons NN, Limpus CJ, et al. Interactions between behavior and plasma steroids within the scramble mating system of the promiscuous green turtle, *Chelonia mydas*. Horm Behav 1999;36(2):86–97.

29. Owens DW, Morris YA. The comparative endocrinology of sea turtles. Copeia 1985;3:723–35.

30. Miller JD. Reproduction in sea turtles. In: Lutz PL, Musick JA, editors. The biology of sea turtles. Boca Raton (FL): CRC Press Inc; 1996. p. 51.

31. Chaves A, Arana M, du Toit L. Primary evidence of sperm storage in the ovaries of the olive ridley marine turtle (*Lepidochelys olivacea*). In: proceedings 18th international sea turtle symposium. Sinaloa (Mexico), March 3-7, 1998. p. 123.
32. Limpus CJ, Limpus DJ. The biology of the loggerhead turtle, Caretta caretta, in the southwest Pacific Ocean foraging areas. In: Bolten A, Witherington B, editors. Loggerhead sea turtles. Washington, DC: Smithsonian Institution Press; 2002. p. 93–113.
33. Limpus CJ, Nicholls N. The southern oscillation regulates the annual numbers of green turtles (*Chelonia mydas*) breeding around northern Australia. Aust Wild Res 1988;15(2):157–61.
34. Chaloupka M. Historical trends, seasonality and spatial synchrony in green sea turtle egg production. Biol Conserv 2001;101(3):263–79.
35. Rostal DC, Grumble J, Byles R, et al. Nesting physiology of Kemp's ridley sea turtles, *Lepidochelys kempii*, at Rancho Nuevo, Tamaulipas, Mexico, with observations on population estimates. Chelonian Conserv Biol 1997;2(4):538–47.
36. FitzSimmons NN. Male marine turtles: gene flow, philopatry and mating systems of the green turtle *Chelonia mydas*. Brisbane (Queensland): The University of Queensland; 1997. p. 241.
37. Wood JR, Wood FE. Captive reproduction of Kemp's ridley *Lepidochelys Kempi*. Herpetol J 1988;1:247–9.
38. Limpus CJ, Carter D, Hamann M. The green turtle, *Chelonia mydas*, in Queensland: the Bramble Cay rookery in the 1979–1980 breeding season. Chelonian Conserv Biol 2001;4(1):34–46.
39. Godley BJ, Broderick AC, Hays GC. Nesting of green turtles (*Chelonia mydas*) at ascension Island. South Atlantic Biol Conserv 2001;97:151.
40. Hailman JP, Elowson AM. Ethogram of the nesting female loggerhead (*Caretta caretta*). Herpetologica 1992;48:1–30.
41. Miller JD, Limpus C, Godfrey M. Nest site selection, oviposition, eggs, development, hatching, and emergence of loggerhead turtles. In: Bolten AB, Witherington BE, editors. Biology of loggerhead turtles. Washington, DC: Smithsonian Books; 2003. p. 125–43.
42. Alfaro-Núñez A, Bertelsen M, Bojesen AM, et al. Global distribution of Chelonid fibropapilloma-associated herpesvirus among clinically healthy sea turtles. BMC Evol Biol 2014;14:206.
43. Huerta P, Pineda H, Aguirre A, et al. First confirmed case of fibropapilloma in a leatherback turtle (*Dermochelys coriacea*). In: Mosier A, Foley A, Brost B, editors. Proceedings of the 20th Annual Symposium on Sea Turtle Biology and Conservation. National Oceanic and Atmospheric Administration technical memorandum NMFS-SEFSC-477. Washington, DC: U.S. Department of Commerce; 2002. p. 193.
44. Jacobson ER. Viruses and viral diseases of reptiles. In: Infectious diseases and pathology of reptiles. Boca Raton (FL): CRC Press; 2007. p. 395–460.
45. Arthur K, Limpus C, Balazs GH, et al. The exposure of green turtles (*Chelonia mydas*) to tumour promoting compounds produced by the cyanobacterium *Lyngbya majuscula* and their potential role in the aetiology of fibropapillomatosis. Harmful Algae 2008;7(1):114–25.
46. Herbst LH, Klein PA. Green turtle fibropapillomatosis: challenges to assessing the role of environmental cofactors. Environ Health Perspect 1995;103(4):27–30.
47. Aguirre AA, Lutz PL. Marine turtles as sentinels of ecosystem health: is fibropapillomatosis an indicator? Ecohealth 2004;1:275–83. http://dx.doi.org/10.1007/s10393-004-0097-3.

48. Greenblatt RJ, Work TM, Balazs GH, et al. The Ozobranchus leech is a candidate mechanical vector for the fibropapilloma-associated turtle herpesvirus found latently infecting skin tumors on Hawaiian green turtles (Chelonia mydas). Virology 2004;321(1):101–10.

49. Van Houtan KS, Hargrove SK, Balazs GH. Land use, macroalgae and a tumour-forming disease in marine turtles. PLoS One 2010;5(9):e12900.

50. Russo G, Di Bella C, Loria GR, et al. Notes on the influence of human activities on sea chelonians in Sicilian waters. J Mt Ecol 2014;7:37–41.

51. Campbell TW. Sea turtle rehabilitation. In: Mader DR, editor. Reptile medicine and surgery. Philadelphia: W. B. Saunders; 1996. p. 427–36.

52. Stacy BA, Wellehan JF, Foley AM, et al. Two herpesviruses associated with disease in wild Atlantic loggerhead sea turtles (Caretta caretta). Vet Microbiol 2008;126:63–73.

53. Pence DB, Wright SD. Chelonacarus elongatus n. gen., n. sp. (Acari: Cloacaridae) from the cloaca of the green turtle Chelonia mydas (Cheloniidae). J Parasitol 1998;84:835–9.

54. Santoro M, Morales JA, Rodríguez-Ortíz B. Spirorchiidiosis (Digenea: Spirorchiidae) and lesions associated with parasites in Caribbean green sea turtles (Chelonia mydas). Vet Rec 2007;161(14):482–6.

55. Frick MG, Williams KL, Bolten AB, et al. Diet and fecundity of Columbus crabs, Planes minutus, associated with oceanic-stage loggerhead sea turtles, Caretta caretta, and inanimate flotsam. J Crustacean Biol 2004;24(2):350–5.

56. Stacy BA, Santoro M, Morales JA, et al. Renal oxalosis in free-ranging green turtles Chelonia mydas. Dis Aquat Organ 2008;80(1):45–9.

57. Nutter FB, Lee DD, Stamper MA, et al. Hemiovanosalpingecomy in a loggerhead sea turtle (Caretta caretta). Vet Rec 2000;146(3):78–80.

58. Frutchey KP, Ehrhart LM, Pritchard PCH. Eversion and detachment of the oviduct in nesting loggerhead turtles (Caretta caretta). In: Proceedings 22th annual symposium on sea turtle biology and conservation. 2002. p. 184.

59. Crespo JL, García-Párraga D, Giménez I, et al. Two cases of pseudohermaphroditism in loggerhead sea turtles Caretta caretta. Dis Aquat Org 2013;105(3):183–91.

60. Rostal DC, Robeck TR, Owens DW, et al. Ultrasound imaging of ovaries and eggs in Kemp's ridley sea turtles (Lepidochelys kempi). J Zoo Wildl Med 1990;21:27–35.

61. Valente AL, Parga ML, Espada Y, et al. Ultrasonographic imaging of loggerhead sea turtles (Caretta caretta). Vet Rec 2007;161(7):226–32.

62. Pease A, Blanvillain G, Rostal D, et al. Ultrasound imaging of the inguinal region of adult male loggerhead sea turtles (Caretta caretta). J Zoo Wildl Med 2010;41(1):69–76.

63. Blanco GS, Morreale SJ, Velez E, et al. Reproductive output and ultrasonography of endangered population of East Pacific Green Turtles. J Wildl Manage 2011;76(4):841–6.

64. Di Bello A, Valastro C, Staffieri F. Surgical approach to the coelomic cavity through the axillary and inguinal regions in sea turtles. J Am Vet Med Assoc 2006;228(6):922–5.

65. Whittaker BR, Krum H. Medical management of sea turtles in aquaria. In: Fowler ME, Miller RE, editors. Zoo and wild animal medicine: current therapy. 4th Edition. Philadelphia: WB Saunders; 1999. p. 217–31.

66. Wyneken J, Mader DR. Medical care of sea turtles. In: Mader DR, editor. Reptile medicine and surgery. 2nd edition. Philadelphia: WB Saunders; 2006. p. 972–1007.

67. Erlacher-Reid CD, Norton TM, Harms CA, et al. Intestinal and cloacal strictures in free-ranging and aquarium-maintained green sea turtles (*Chelonia mydas*). J Zoo Wildl Med 2013;44(2):408–29.

68. Knotek Z, Morici M, Spadola F. The value of endoscopy in emergency and critical care for loggerhead sea turtles (*Caretta caretta*), in Proceedings. 2nd International Conference on Avian Herpetological and Exotic Mammal Medicine (ICARE). 2015. p. 361.

69. Spadola F, Insacco G. Endoscopy of cloaca in 51 *Emys trinacris* (Fritz et al., 2005): morphological and diagnostic study. Acta Herpetol 2009;4(1):73–81.

70. Witherington BE. Reducing threats to nesting habitat. In: Eckert KL, Bjorndal KA, Abreu-Grobois FA, et al, editors. Research and management techniques for the conservation of sea turtles. Washington, DC: IUCN/SSC Marine Turtle Specialist Group; 1999. p. 179–83. Publication No 4.

71. Choi GY, Eckert KL. Manual of best practices for safeguarding sea turtle nesting beaches. Ballwin (MO): Wider Caribbean Sea Turtle Conservation Network (WIDECAST); 2009. p. 86. Technical Report No. 9.

72. Johnson SA, Bjorndal KA, Bolten AB. Effects of organized turtle watches on loggerhead (*Caretta caretta*) nesting behaviour and hatchling production in Florida. Conserv Biol 1996;10(2):570–7.

73. Miller JD. Determining clutch size and hatchling success. In: Eckert KL, Bjorndal KA, Abreu-Grobois FA, et al, editors. Research and management techniques for the conservation of sea turtles. Washington, DC: IUCN/SSC Marine Turtle Specialist Group; 1999. p. 124–9. Publication No 4.

74. Margaritoulis D, Argano R, Baran I, et al. Loggerhead turtles in the Mediterranean sea: present knowledge and conservation perspectives. In: Bolten AB, Witherington BE, editors. Loggerhead sea turtles. Washington, DC: Smithsonian Books; 2003. p. 175–98.

75. Limpus CJ, Baker V, Miller JD. Movement-induced mortality of loggerhead eggs. Herpetologica 1979;35:335–8.

76. Boulon RH. Reducing threats to eggs and hatchlings: in situ protection. In: Eckert KL, Bjorndal KA, Abreu-Grobois FA, et al, editors. Research and management techniques for the conservation of sea turtles. Washington, DC: IUCN/SSC Marine Turtle Specialist Group; 1999. p. 169–74. Publication No 4.

77. Howard R, Bell I, Pike DA. Thermal tolerances of sea turtle embryos: current understanding and future directions. Endanger Species Res 2014;26:75–86.

78. Mrosovsky N. Pivotal temperatures for loggerhead turtles (*Caretta caretta*) from northern and southern nesting beaches. Can J Zool 1988;66:661–9.

79. Mclean K, Dutton P, Whitmore C, et al. A comparison of three methods for incubating turtle eggs. Mar Turtle Newsl 1983;26:7–9.

80. Mortimer JE. The influence of beach sand characteristics on the nesting behavior and clutch survival of green turtles (*Chelonia mydas*). Copeia 1990;3:802–17.

81. Limpus CJ, Reed P, Miller JD. Temperature dependent sex determination in Queensland sea turtles: intraspecific variation in *Caretta caretta*. In: Grigg G, Shine R, Ehmann H, editors. Biology of Australian frogs and reptiles. Sydney (Australia): Surrey Beatty and Sons; 1985. p. 343–51.

82. Mrosovsky N. Thermal biology of sea turtles. Am Zool 1980;20:531–47.

83. Wallace BP, Sotherland PR, Santidrian Tomillo P, et al. Egg components, egg size, and hatchling size in leatherback turtles. Comp Biochem Physiol A Mol Integr Physiol 2006;145(4):524–32.
84. Foti M, Giacopello C, Bottari T, et al. Antibiotic resistance of gram negatives isolates from loggerhead sea turtles (*Caretta caretta*) in the central Mediterranean Sea. Mar Pollut Bull 2009;58:1363–6.
85. Santoro M, Hernadez G, Caballero M, et al. Aerobic bacterial flora of nesting green turtles (*Chelonia mydas*) from Tortuguero National Park, Costa Rica. J Zoo Wildl Med 2006;37(4):549–52.
86. Santoro M, Orrego CM, Hernández Gómez G. Flora normal bacteriana nasal y cloacal de *Lepidochelys olivacea* (Testudines: Cheloniidae) en el Pacífico Norte de Costa Rica. Rev Biol Trop 2006;54(1):43–8.
87. Santoro M, Hernández G, Caballero M, et al. Potential bacterial pathogens carried by nesting leatherback turtles (*Dermochelys coriacea*) in Costa Rica. Chelonian Conserv Biol 2008;7(1):104–8.
88. Wyneken J, Burt TJ, Pederson DE. Egg failure in natural and relocated sea turtle nests. J Herpetol 1988;22(1):88–96.
89. Bézy VS, Valverde RA, Plante CJ. Olive ridley sea turtle hatching success as a function of the microbial abundance in nest sand at ostional, Costa Rica. PLoS One 2005;10(2):e0118579.
90. Solomon SE, Baird T. Effect of fungal penetration in the eggshell of the green turtle (*Chelonia mydas*). J Exp Mar Bio Ecol 1980;36:295–303.
91. Sarmiento-Ramírez JM, Abella E, Martín MP, et al. *Fusarium solani* is responsible for mass mortalities in nests of the loggerhead sea turtle, *Caretta caretta*, in Boavista, Cape Verde. FEMS Microbiol Lett 2010;312:192–200.
92. Craven KS, Awong-Taylor J, Griffiths L, et al. Identification of bacterial isolates from unhatched loggerhead (*Caretta caretta*) sea turtles eggs in Georgia, USA. Mar Turtle Newsl 2007;115:7–9.
93. Keene EL. Microorganisms from sand, cloacal fluid, and eggs of *Lepidochelys olivacea* and standard testing of cloacal fluid antimicrobial properties. 2012. Available at: http://opus.ipfw.edu/masters_theses/19.
94. Alberghina D, Panzera M, Maccarrone V, et al. Study of some blood parameters in *Caretta Caretta* during a recovery period. Comp Clin Path 2015;24(1):193–5.

Reproductive Medicine in Freshwater Turtles and Land Tortoises

Sean M. Perry, DVM*,
Mark A. Mitchell, DVM, MS, PhD, DECZM (Herpetology)

KEYWORDS

• Chelonian • Dystocia • Infertility • Reproduction • Surgery • Tortoise • Turtle

KEY POINTS

• As pressure continues to mount for wild populations of chelonians, the need for developing long-term and sustainable breeding programs will increase.
• Veterinarians can play an important role in ensuring the success of these programs for both institutions and individuals.
• It is important for veterinarians to develop a solid foundation of knowledge regarding the reproductive anatomy, physiology, and behaviors of these animals to differentiate normal from abnormal.
• Fortunately, most of the reproductive diseases seen in these animals are similar to those in other classes of animals and case management follows similar protocols.

INTRODUCTION

With the increased popularity of chelonians as pets, there is a need to establish successful captive breeding programs to ensure animals are available in the commercial trade without further affecting wild populations of animals. Chelonians are one of the most highly impacted groups of animals in the world because of demands on them for the pet trade, as sources of food, and for cultural/medicinal purposes. As with many other species commonly found in the pet trade, captive breeding programs are needed to ensure that these animals can be successfully raised and the necessary numbers to satiate the public are provided. In the United States and Europe, breeding programs are ongoing and have been, for many species, quite successful. However, herpetoculturists still have difficulty consistently reproducing some species, and for those that are successful, may still have some issues arise (eg, dystocia) that require

Disclosure Statement: The authors have nothing to disclose.
Department of Veterinary Clinical Sciences, Louisiana State University, School of Veterinary Medicine, Skip Bertman Drive, Baton Rouge, LA 70803, USA
* Corresponding author.
E-mail address: seanmperry87@gmail.com

Vet Clin Exot Anim 20 (2017) 371–389
http://dx.doi.org/10.1016/j.cvex.2016.11.004
1094-9194/17/© 2016 Elsevier Inc. All rights reserved.

intervention by a veterinarian. Because of these potential concerns or complications, it is important that veterinarians become familiar with the reproductive biology and potential diseases associated with the reproductive tracts of these animals to better serve their clients and chelonian patients. The purpose of this article is to review the reproductive anatomy of chelonians, discuss the diagnostic management of these types of cases, and review potential treatments.

CHELONIAN REPRODUCTIVE ANATOMY AND PHYSIOLOGY
Male Anatomy

Chelonians have paired testicles. The testicles are elongated and originate cranial to and course ventrally to the kidney; they are adhered loosely to the kidneys by the mesorchium. The color of the testicles can vary greatly based on species and age. In some species, melanin may be seen on the surface of the testes, but in most they are pink, white, tan, or yellow.[1–4] Sperm originates in the testicles and are transported though the epididymis to the ductus deferens, where they are deposited into the urodeum of the cloaca through an orifice at the neck of the bladder. Urinary excreta are deposited into the urodeum and flows retrograde into the bladder or are excreted from the cloaca. Semen samples collected by one of the authors (M.A.M.) using electroejaculation are commonly contaminated with urine as a result of their anatomy.[5] Just ventral to the opening of the ductus deferens, ureter, and bladder neck is the bulbous urethralis and the beginning of the penile corpus cavernosa. Compared with squamates, chelonians possess a single phallus that does not invert like hemipenes. The chelonian phallus is a single grooved organ arising from the ventral surface of the cloaca. The midline groove lies between 2 seminal ridges that run longitudinally along the phallus to the distal tip; these ridges are formed from coelomic canals and corpus cavernosa or corpus spongiosa. Erection occurs when the corpus cavernosa becomes engorged with blood from the internal iliac vessels, curling the seminal ridges dorsally and medially where they meet to form a tube called the seminal groove. Sperm is transported from the ductus deferens into the seminal groove and then down the phallus. The phallus contains corpora fibrosa, which supports the phallus ventrally and then cranially at full erection. Ventral to the corpora fibrosa is the muscularis retractor of the phallus, which when contracted replaces the phallus into the cloaca after the corpus cavernosa relaxes. The distal phallus consists of a spade-shaped glans penis with 3 distinct folds: the plica externa, plica media, and plica interna. This allows the male to successfully deposit the seminal fluid into the coprodeum of the female.[1–4]

Male Physiology

Spermatogenesis is a complex process in chelonians that is similar to other amniotes. Chelonians are considered postnuptial regarding spermatogenesis, and therefore, the process does not coincide with mating. Sperm is typically produced after the mating season and stored for extended periods of time in the male urogenital system. Spermatogenesis immediately before the breeding season has only been documented in sea turtles. Testosterone concentrations increase during spermatogenesis, and in some species, elevated testosterone concentrations have also been documented during peak mating activity. Two forms of gonadotropin-releasing hormone (GnRH) are present in chelonians: cGnRH-I and cGnRH-II.[6] Mammalian GnRH has no effect on plasma luteinizing hormone (LH) or steroid concentrations in male turtles. These GnRH-like hormones act at the level of the pituitary to promote production of follicle-stimulating hormone (FSH) and LH-like gonadotropins. Compared with mammals, the function of the FSH and LH-like gonadotropins in chelonians is poorly understood, although it is known that mammalian FSH can regulate steroidogenesis in chelonians.[7]

Female Anatomy

Female chelonians have paired ovaries in the dorsal, caudal coelomic cavity, cranial to the kidneys. Oviducts are caudal to the ovaries and suspended by the mesovarium. Ovarian size varies with the reproductive cycle. Mature reproductively active ovaries can occupy a significant area within the coelmic cavity, whereas juvenile ovaries are thin, elongated, and occasionally lobular. In many chelonian species, ovaries undergo a period of quiescence where ovarian size and activity are reduced. The oviduct can be histologically divided into 5 segments: the proximal segment with the ostium abdominale, the convoluted glandular segment or pars albuminifera, the isthmus where the shell membrane is formed, the uterus where the outer egg shell is deposited, and the short vagina or cervix that opens to the urodeum.[1-4]

Female Physiology

Oogenesis and folliculogenesis continue throughout the reproductive lifespan of a chelonian. In species that live in temperate climates, reproductive activity is typically restricted to the warmer months of the year when day length is longest. Females ovulate and are fertilized in spring, nest in late spring and summer, and begin folliculogenesis for the following year's eggs in late summer and fall. Comparatively, in tropical climates, temperature and day length fluctuations are minimal, and reproductive cycles are tied to changes in precipitation. Some species prefer to be reproductively active in the dry season, whereas others prefer to be active during peak rainfall.[7,8]

During the periovulatory period, a surge of both testosterone and progesterone occurs. After egg deposition, concentrations of estrogen, progesterone, and testosterone decrease. Other hormones may also assist in mediating ovulation; however, more research is needed to confirm this. Copulation is not thought to have an influence in ovulation, because solitary females can sometimes produce eggs in the absence of a male. Ovulation typically occurs over a 12- to 48-hour period, during which ova enter the oviduct. After ovulation, corpora lutea may be observed at ovulation sites. Follicles that did not ovulate may regress and undergo follicular atresia.

After ovulation, the ova enter the oviduct through the ostium. Fertilization occurs before the oviductal secretions envelop the ovum. The ovum passes through the glandular segment of the uterus, and albumin is secreted around the ova. Afterward, a fibrous egg or shell membrane is generated in the isthmus. The final segment of the uterus excretes calcium and forms the shell.[9] Finally, the egg is formed and passes to the short terminal portion of the uterus (vagina) before passing through the urodeum. Shelled eggs are held in the oviduct before oviposition for a variable amount of time depending on species. Some species will hold their eggs for as little as 9 days or as long as up to 4 to 6 months. Turtles can retain their eggs for extended periods of time if conditions are not suitable for egg laying.[7-9]

Sperm Storage in Females

Female chelonians can store semen for extended periods of time (eg, months to years). Semen storage is primarily associated with the uterus; however, in some turtle species, sperm storage has been demonstrated in the infundibulum. Female sperm storage has been documented in the families Emydidae, Kinosternidae, Chelydridae, Trionychidae, Cheloniidae, and Testudinidae.[7] Female chelonians can store sperm from several males simultaneously, which is why chelonian clutches commonly demonstrate multiple paternity.

SEXING CHELONIANS
External Sexual Characteristics

General guidelines used to externally differentiate male from female chelonians include tail length and plastron conformation (tortoises only). In males, the tail is longer and the vent more caudal (beyond carapacial rim) than in females. In addition, male tortoises tend to have a more concave plastron; however, this may be altered in animals with shell pyramiding because of abnormal shell growth. The plastron concavity and longer tail are evolutionary adaptations to help facilitate mating behaviors such as mounting and intromission (**Fig. 1**). Species-specific secondary sexual characteristics may also be useful for determining the sex of chelonians, including skin color, eye color, toenail length, scute size, and adult size. Examples of species-specific sexual dimorphism in chelonians include the following: the red iris color of male eastern box turtles (*Terrapene carolina carolina*) (**Fig. 2**), elongated toenails of the forelimb of male red-eared slider turtles (*Trachemys scripta elegans*), painted turtles (*Chrysemys picta*) and map turtles (*Graptemys* spp) (**Fig. 3**), and enlarged gular scutes of male sulcatta tortoises (*Centrochelys sulcata*). Body size may also help differentiate the sexes. For example, in diamondback terrapins (*Malaclemys terrapin*) and map turtles, females are generally larger; however, for desert tortoises (*Gopherus agassizii*), males are, on average, larger. It is important for veterinarians to learn these species-specific characteristics to assist their clients with sexing their mature animals.[2,4]

Chelonian Coelioscopy for Sex Identification

Coelisoscopy can be used to determine sex in juvenile animals or those without overt dimorphic characteristics (**Figs. 4** and **5**).[10–12] Ideally, endoscopic examination should be performed under general anesthesia, although the technique can be performed using local anesthetics. However, one study did observe higher pain scores in Chinese box turtles (*Cuora flavomarginata*) endoscopically sexed under local anesthetics versus general anesthesia.[13]

The prefemoral approach for coelioscopy includes the following:

- Develop appropriate plan for analgesia, anesthesia, and cardiorespiratory monitoring.
- Position chelonian in lateral or oblique recumbency.
- Extend the hindlimb caudally to expose the prefemoral fossa.

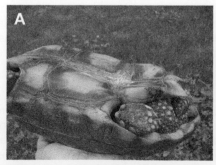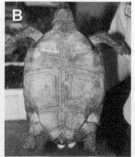

Fig. 1. (*A*) Male yellow-footed tortoise (*Chelonidis denticulata*). Note the concave plastron, which is characteristic in some male tortoise species. (*B*) Female gopher tortoise (*Gopherus polyphemus*). (*Courtesy of* Charlie Innis, VMD, DABVP(Reptile & Amphibian), Boston, MA.)

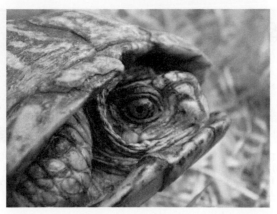

Fig. 2. Male eastern box turtle. Note the red iris color of male eastern box turtles (*T carolina carolina*). (*Courtesy of* Charlie Innis, VMD, DABVP(Reptile & Amphibian), Boston, MA.)

- Aseptically prepare prefemoral region and surrounding shell.
- Make small craniocaudal skin incision at the center of the prefemoral fossa.
- Dissect subcutaneous tissues and fat to expose aponeuroses of transverse and oblique muscles; aponeuroses and coelomic membrane are incised with a combination of blunt and sharp dissection.
- Insert endoscope and direct dorsally to visualize gonad.
- Closure is routine and can be done with absorbable suture.
- Skin closure can be done with suture or surgical glue.
- Aquatic turtles should be dry docked for 24 to 48 hours if using suture or glue, respectively.

Chelonian Cloacoscopy and Cystoscopy for Sex Identification

Endoscopic examination of gonads may also be attempted through the cloaca/urinary bladder.[14–16] One advantage of this technique is that it does not typically require surgical anesthesia. A disadvantage to this technique is that uric acid sediment can hinder visualization. In addition, the accessory vesicle can be highly vascularized and

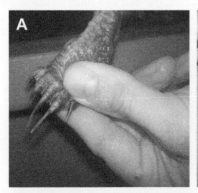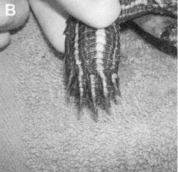

Fig. 3. (*A*) Elongated toenails of the forelimb of male red-eared slider (*T scripta elegans*). (*B*) Female red-eared sliders (*T scripta elegans*) show sexual dimorphism with shortened forelimb nails when compared with males. (*Courtesy of* Charlie Innis, VMD, DABVP(Reptile & Amphibian), Boston, MA.)

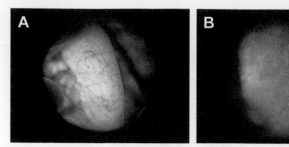

Fig. 4. (*A*) Endoscopic image of a testicle in a juvenile testicle of a Blanding's turtle (*Emydoidea blandingii*). (*B*) Endoscopic image of an immature ovary a Blanding's turtle (*E blandingii*). (*Courtesy of* Charlie Innis, VMD, DABVP(Reptile & Amphibian), Boston, MA.)

impede visualization. Unfortunately, the sensitivity of this method may not be high. One study attempted to identify sex in red-eared sliders by the presence of the phallus/clitoris; however, males were misdiagnosed as females (100%) and females as males (38%).[15] In addition, a recent study performed in 30 immature (36–90 g) red-eared sliders showed that only 10% (3/30) of the animals had their sex accurately identified by cystoscopy and 23% (7/30) of the animals experienced bladder or cloacal rupture.[15]

Measuring Hormone Concentrations for Sex for Identification

In juveniles, the measurement of plasma testosterone concentrations is also a useful method to determine sex. Rostral and colleagues[10] showed that animals that were endoscopically sexed to be male had a significantly higher plasma testosterone concentration compared with females. There was 98% agreement observed between the 2 methods. An FSH test has also been shown to be useful in confirming sex. FSH can be injected intracoelomically and blood drawn 4 hours later to measure plasma testosterone. Male concentrations will be >0.5 ng/mL, whereas females will be <0.2 mg/mL.[2]

Temperature Sex Determination

Most chelonians are considered to have temperature-dependent sex determination. Of the 149 species that have been karyotyped, genetic sex determination was only identified in 8 species distributed through the families Kinosternidae, Chelidae, Trionychidae, and Bataguridae. Incubation temperatures and specific-sex ratios are species

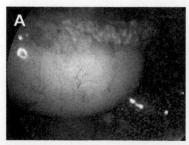
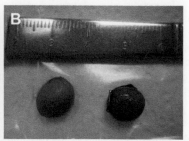

Fig. 5. (*A*) Endoscopic image of a testicle yellow-spotted river turtle (*Podocnemis unifilis*). (*B*) Testicles after endoscopic castration in a red-eared slider (*T scripta elegans*). (*Courtesy of* Charlie Innis, VMD, DABVP(Reptile & Amphibian), Boston, MA.)

specific. Recently, a candidate protein called cold-inducible RNA-binding protein was identified in the common snapping turtle (*Chelydra serpentina*) to mediate temperature effects on the developing gonads. Further research is needed on this candidate protein to determine if a genetic marker can be developed to accurately sex animals based on its expression.[17,18]

SEXUAL MATURITY AND REPRODUCTIVE LIFESPAN

Chelonians are long lived and are slow to mature. Although many species in the wild can produce large numbers of eggs, more often than not few hatchlings survive to sexual maturity. After achieving sexual maturity, chelonians can have a long reproductive life. Sexual maturity in chelonians is attributed to size (energy) rather than age. Captive specimens provided high levels of calories can become reproductive much sooner than their wild counterparts. For example, captive leopard tortoises (*Geochelone pardalis*) can reproduce within 4 to 6 years, whereas wild conspecifics can take 15 years to become sexually mature.[2]

Courtship and Mating Behavior

Most chelonians show some evidence of courtship behavior. Behaviors can be species specific due to natural history, evolution, and sexual selection. Examples of courting behavior include head bobbing, head swaying, falling forelimb movements, stroking females, nudging to gentle biting, trailing, and cloacal touching and sniffing. Intromission only occurs if the female is receptive. Courtship behaviors can last for several minutes (ie, claw vibration/titillation or head bobbing) to days (ie, trailing females) depending on the species; however, copulation and intromission only lasts for minutes at a time. Vocalization among male tortoises is common during copulation. Female chelonians may also display male-type reproductive behavior, such as mounting other females and ramming conspecifics. Clinicians should not determine chelonian sex based solely on courtship or mounting behaviors. These behaviors may occur secondary to the elevated testosterone concentrations noted during certain periods of the female reproductive cycle.

In chelonians, mate fidelity has not been demonstrated, although males have been shown to fertilize a given female repeatedly. Male-male combat also has been observed in chelonian species, and it is thought males who are successful in these battles have more reproductive success.

NATURAL HISTORY AND HUSBANDRY

In order to fully understand chelonian reproduction, it is vital to understand the natural history and husbandry requirements that are necessary for each species to flourish in captivity. Understanding their evolutionary history, home range, annual rainfall, temperatures, mating behaviors, reproductive capabilities, and nesting habits will allow the clinician to fully understand and create the optimal environment for them to reproduce. For example, some traits that vary significantly between species are clutch size, egg size, and nesting frequency. Pancake tortoises (*Malacochersus tornieri*), bowsprit tortoises (*Chersina angulate*), spider tortoises (*Pyxis arachnoides*), black-breasted leaf turtles (*Geoemyda spengleri*), Sulawesi forest turtles (*Leucocephalon yuwonoi*), and Central American wood turtles (*Rhinoclemmys* spp) generally produce only one (rarely 2 eggs) very large eggs per clutch, but may nest several times per year. In comparison, other species, such as sea turtles, snapping turtles, and soft shell turtles, produce dozens of eggs per clutch.

Husbandry, especially at the time of oviposition, can contribute significantly to reproductive health. Without appropriate husbandry and understanding of some of these life history traits, some animals may not nest. Although nesting behavior is conserved throughout chelonian species, some species nest in a different manner, such as the Burmese mountain tortoise (*Manouria emys*). The female constructs a nest by gathering sticks, dirt, and leaf litter into a pile and then guards the nest for several days to weeks after oviposition. This species demonstrates a level of maternal care not common in chelonians.[1,2,19]

MANAGING REPRODUCTIVE DISEASE IN CHELONIANS
Physical Examination and Diagnostics

When a chelonian is presented for a reproductive issue, it is important for the veterinarian to manage the patient as with any other case. Specifically focusing on the reproductive issue may misdirect the clinician managing the case, leading them to miss the primary disease/issue responsible for the development of the secondary reproductive disease/issue (eg, secondary nutritional hyperparathyroidism). Collecting a standard anamnesis focused on signalment, husbandry, the reproductive status of the patient, and duration of the presenting problem is the first step in directing the clinician toward a diagnosis. The physical examination should be thorough to ensure all systems are evaluated; this is key because with reproductive disease other systems (eg, endocrine, liver, skeletal) may also be affected. Once the anamnesis and examination are completed, the clinician should develop a problem list, identify all systems associated with the disease process, and develop a diagnostic plan. While this plan is being implemented, supportive care and initial treatments should be initiated.

REPRODUCTIVE TRACT DISORDERS IN CHELONIANS
Infertility

Infertility in males can occur for numerous reasons. A full evaluation of each animal that is intended for breeding should be performed. Individuals may exhibit or lack the drive or are unable to mate for several reasons. Husbandry-related causes of infertility are common in reptiles because of an incomplete understanding of life histories. Husbandry-related causes include no provision for brumation, insufficient humidity (precipitation), and incorrect sized animals or social structure. Cohabitation long term can suppress mating behaviors in certain animals; however, these animals may reproduce if separated and then reintroduced. Nonreproductive comorbidities can also lead to infertility; thus, it is important to rule out any comorbidities by performing a full workup. Finally, disease within the reproductive tract can also lead to infertility (eg, phallic infection or trauma).[4,20] To confirm infertility, evaluation of semen is necessary. Electroejaculation has been found to be successful in leopard tortoises and green turtles (*Chelonia mydas*) to evaluate semen[5,21,22] (**Fig. 6**). Gross abnormalities in sperm can be evaluated and confirmed microscopically. In addition, congenital testicular atresia or orchitis can be associated with infertility and can be diagnosed with endoscopy and testicular biopsy (see **Fig. 4**).

True fertility issues can also occur in females, although they are uncommonly reported. As with males, husbandry-related causes and comorbidities are common reasons female chelonians do not reproduce. In addition to those mentioned for males, inappropriate nesting material and poor nutrition are other contributors. Ultrasonography may be used to determine if folliculogenesis is occurring and to follow the progression of follicular development. In some cases, eggs are produced but fail to develop. This may suggest male infertility or improper egg management (eg, excessive

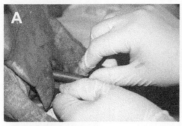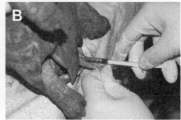

Fig. 6. (*A*) Electroejaculation probe inserted into an anesthetized leopard tortoise (*Stigmochelys pardalis*) cloaca for collections. (*B*) Collection of semen with a 1-mL syringe after electroejaculation.

handling, incorrect incubation parameters). It has been suggested that repeated radiography of free-ranging chelonians during sensitive stages of gamete and embryo development may cause damage to the germlines and/or embryos, increasing the risk of decreased fecundity; however, this has not been proven experimentally.[2] Although no evidence exists, it may be prudent to evaluate reproductively active individuals with ultrasound rather than radiography. Additional causes of infertility in females include salpingitis, cloacaitis, oophoritis, neoplasia, and follicular stasis. If suspected, these should be worked up using blood work, diagnostic imaging, endoscopy, and biopsy.

Dystocia/Egg Retention

Dystocia is defined as the failure to oviposit eggs within the appropriate time for a species; however, this is often referred to as egg retention. It is often difficult to differentiate between pathologic and normal egg retention because gravid females can retain eggs in the uterus for an extended period of time. Eggs have been documented to remain within the chelonian uterus well beyond the time they should normally be deposited without any pathologic consequence. Females can elect to not lay eggs when husbandry parameters and social factors are not appropriate. Failure to provide an appropriate nesting site/substrate and inappropriate temperature and humidity may lead to egg retention. Social factors such as competition for nest sites and intraspecific aggression can also lead to failure to oviposit in breeding colonies.[23–25] Chronically retained eggs can lead to infectious salpingitis, rupture of the oviduct with a resulting egg yolk coelomitis, and urinary/colonic obstruction. True egg retention is often incidental or determined based on the knowledge of the species and is not associated with any clinical signs. In many cases, these animals are past their due date. Individuals may pass part of a clutch or only 1 to 2 eggs, but not the entire clutch. These cases can be managed conservatively without any intervention or with suggestions to improve husbandry.[24,25] When making suggestions regarding nesting sites/substrates, a good rule of thumb is that it should be at least 1 to 2 times the length of the carapace, and loosening the substrate (eg, play sand) may be helpful[2] (**Fig. 7**).

Diagnosing a dystocia can be done based on the knowledge of the species normal egg-retention time, owner/institution's previous experience, and the clinical examination of the chelonian. Educating clients on how to maintain breeding records can be quite helpful in assessing these cases. Eggs can often be palpated in the prefemoral fossa, and radiographs can be used to help identify the number, position, shell quality, and integrity of the eggs; these images can also be used to help identify if obstructive causes of dystocia are present (eg, pelvic canal stenosis or fractures)[26] (**Fig. 8**). Large, misshaped eggs with thick walls typically indicate prolonged retention and a need to

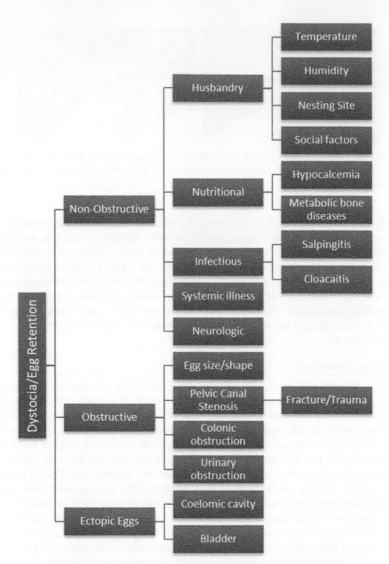

Fig. 7. Flow chart indicating different causes for Dystocia/Egg Retention.

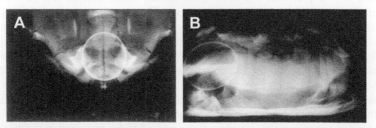

Fig. 8. An egg lodged in the cloaca of a desert tortoise (*G agassizii*). (*A, B*) Repeated oxytocin and calcium injections failed to induce oviposition, and the egg had to be broken down and removed through the cloaca. An egg in such a position is not accessible via plastron or inguinal coeliotomy. (*From* Innis CJ, Boyer TH. Chelonian reproductive disorders. Vet Clin North Am Exot Anim Pract 2002;5(3):568; with permission.)

pursue the case (**Fig. 9**). Ectopic eggs may be identified within the bladder or coelomic cavity from the radiographs or ultrasound.[26–29] Blood work should be performed to rule out underlying conditions such as infection or hypocalcemia (ionized calcium <1 mmol/L), which typically indicates a preexisting nutritional deficiency.

Treatment of dystocia in chelonians is rarely an emergency, unlike other reptiles. In chelonians, dystocia can often be resolved with conservative management/husbandry changes or medical therapy.[2,4,24,25,30] Healthy individuals with normal radiographically appearing eggs can often oviposit with an appropriate nest site and removal of any social stressors. Oviposition can be medically induced in chelonians with a combination of oxytocin, β-blockers, fluid therapy, and calcium supplementation. Patients that are clinically dehydrated should have their dehydration and electrolyte abnormalities corrected first because medical management will not be successful without correction. Parenteral fluids should be used to correct any deficits. Inducing oviposition in a dehydrated or unstable patient may lead to a worsening of a metabolic disorder or rupturing the oviduct.[31–34] In hypocalcemic animals, parenteral calcium supplementation is needed to assist in oviductal contractions; this can be done with either calcium glubionate or calcium gluconate (**Table 1**). Oxytocin can be administered intramuscularly or continuously through an intravenous or intraosseous catheter. In chelonians, the low end of the dose range is often effective (see **Table 1**). If the animal does not respond to the oxytocin, the dose can be repeated. Various recommendations exist for oxytocin treatment, including administering 3 doses at 90-minute intervals, and increasing the dose with each treatment. Another protocol recommends administering 50% to 100% of the original dose 1 to 12 hours later (**Box 1**).[24,25,34] Arginine vasotocin is reported to be more effective in reptiles than oxytocin; however, chelonians are one group of reptiles that respond well to oxytocin.[25] Adjunct therapies and medications may also be beneficial for dystocia cases in chelonians; however, they are not well studied. Prostaglandins are one such adjunct. A combination of oxytocin (7.5 U/kg) and prostaglandin $F_{2\alpha}$ (1.5 mg/kg subcutaneously) has been effective in inducing oviposition in red-eared sliders; however, this may be less effective in turtles weighing greater than 5 kg.[4] Topical application of prostaglandin E gel on the cloaca has been recommended by Innis and Boyer[2]; however, no adverse or beneficial effects have been reported. β-Blockers are thought to potentiate the effects of oxytocin in chelonians, and β-blockers that have been used include atenolol and propranolol (see **Table 1** and **Box 1**).[24] Propranolol has been successfully used in lizards and may

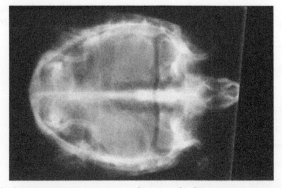

Fig. 9. Abnormally large eggs in an ornate box turtle (*Terrapene ornata*). The eggs were removed by bilateral prefemoral coeliotomy, aspiration of the egg contents, and salpingotomy. (*From* Innis CJ, Boyer TH. Chelonian reproductive disorders. Vet Clin North Am Exot Anim Pract 2002;5(3):567; with permission.)

Table 1
Reproductive assistive medications in chelonians

Medication	Dose	Route
Nutritional supplementation		
Calcium gluconate	50–100 mg/kg	IC, IM, SC
Calcium glubionate	23 mg/kg	PO
Hormones		
Oxytocin	1–20 IU/kg	IM, IO, as a CRI
Prostaglandin $F_{2\alpha}$	1.5 mg/kg	SC
Prostaglandin E gel	—	Topically to vent/cloaca
β-Blockers		
Atenolol	7 mg/kg	PO
Propranolol	1 mg/kg	IC

Abbreviations: CRI, constant rate infusion; IC, intracoelomically; IM, intramuscular; IO, intraosseous; PO, orally; SC, subcutaneous.

translate to chelonians.[23] When conservative management fails, more aggressive therapies are indicated; this is especially true for animals showing signs of debilitation, tenesmus, or abnormally shaped/sized eggs on radiographs. Salpingotomy can be performed via a plastronotomy or a prefemoral approach. A plastronotomy is the preferred approach when a large field of vision is required; however, the prefemoral approach is less invasive. These procedures are both well described in the literature.[35–38] A coelioscopy-assisted approach for ovariectomy and salpingectomy has also been described for species with a small prefemoral area.[39–41] This technique can also be used to approach a cystotomy to extract eggs found in the urinary bladder. Ovocentesis can be performed via the cloaca on eggs that can be visualized or palpated. A speculum aids in visualization, and a large-gauge needle should be used to aspirate the contents. Eggs tend to fracture after aspiration, but fragments usually pass on their own or can be removed carefully with forceps.[2,25] A technique exists for punctured eggs that do not pass. The tip of a Foley catheter is cut so the balloon is at the end of the catheter; the amount of air needed to inflate the balloon to the appropriate size for the egg to be removed is determined, and the infusion port is filled with water and placed in the freezer to improve the rigidity of the catheter. The catheter is then placed into the egg via the centesis hole; the balloon is inflated, and traction is applied to remove the egg. Care must be taken not to overinflate the

Box 1
McArthur chelonian dystocia protocol

1. Rehydrate
2. Lubricate cloaca
3. Provide nesting area, heat, and humidity
4. Calcium supplementation if needed
5. In evening atenolol (7 mg/kg PO)
6. Oxytocin 1 to 3 IU/kg the following morning
7. Continue this protocol daily if eggs continue to be produced

* Discontinue protocol when oviposition discontinues.

balloon or tear the oviduct during this process.[4,34] The authors recommend irrigating the cloaca and oviduct after the procedure. McArthur additionally recommends continuing oxytocin and β-blockers to assist in expulsion of the egg remnants. When eggs are adhered to the uterus, a salpingotomy/salpingectomy may be required.

Follicular Stasis

Follicular stasis (ie, preovulatory egg-binding or retained follicles) is commonly reported in lizards; however, it also occurs in chelonians. Inappropriate nutrition and environmental conditions are common causes of follicular stasis. Follicles that neither ovulate nor regress can become inspissated or necrotic, rupture, and lead to egg yolk coelomitis. These follicles may remain static for months. Affected chelonians often present for anorexia and lethargy. Clinical pathologic findings in affected animals include elevated concentrations of calcium, albumin, total protein, and alkaline phosphatase, with anemia, leukopenia, and heteropenia.[42,43] A diagnosis is typically made using ultrasound to show the presence of persistent nonovulated follicles. Ovariectomy is the preferred treatment. A technique for coelioscopy-assisted ovariectomy has been described and used successfully to treat follicular stasis in chelonians.[40] Briefly, an endoscope is inserted through a prefemoral incision to visualize and gently grasp and retract the ovary out of the prefemoral incision. Oocentesis can be done on larger follicles to facilitate further exteriorization of the ovary and the ovarian vessels ligated to complete the ovariectomy[44] (**Fig. 10**).

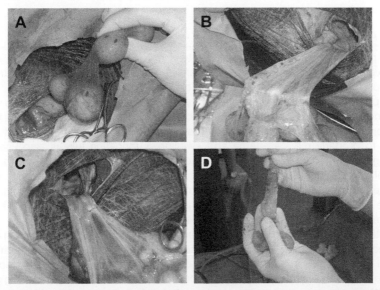

Fig. 10. Prefemoral approach to the coelmic cavity in a hybrid Galapagos tortoises (*Geochelone nigra*) undergoing an endoscopic-assisted oophorectomy. These photographs were taken after exposure and externalization of the ovary and oviduct. (*A*) Ova within the oviduct are exteriorized after the prefemoral approach. (*B*) Full exteriorization of the oviduct to visualize the ovary for removal (*C*) Hemal clips are placed on the vasculature within the mesovarium. (*D*) Ovary after successful removal. (*Courtesy of* S.J. Divers, BVetMed, DZooMed, DECZM(Herp), DECZM(ZHM), DACZM, FRCVS, Athens, GA, J.P. Flanagan, DVM, Houston, TX and S. Rivera, DVM, MS, DABVP(Avian), DACZM, DECZM(Zoo), Atlanta, GA.)

Egg Yolk Coelomitis

Egg yolk coelomitis can occur secondary to retained follicles, oophoritis, salpingitis, or dystocia. Inflammation, degenerative changes, and infection can all affect the ovaries of chelonians. Follicular stasis and dystocia often predispose chelonians to developing egg yolk coelomitis.[25,42,43] During a stasis event, retained follicles undergo follicular necrosis, which can lead to the coelomitis. In a dystocia, rupture of the oviduct can lead to egg contents spilling into the coelomic cavity. Clinical signs are often nonspecific, including anorexia, lethargy, inactivity, diarrhea, and/or decreased fecal/urate production. Clinical pathologic findings include hypercalcemia, hyperproteinemia, and anemia. Many of these animals develop multiorgan dysfunction syndrome. Ultrasonography and radiography can be used to assist in identifying follicular stasis or dystocia. Ultrasound can also be used to confirm the presence of free fluid within the coelomic cavity and aid with coelomocentesis. Endoscopy is the definitive method of diagnosing egg yolk coelomitis because the clinician can visualize degenerative, hyperemic, brown or purple follicles and see free fluid or adhesions within the coelom. Chelonians with retained eggs and a ruptured oviduct must be diagnosed quickly because they tend to decline rapidly. The source of the egg material should always be removed as well as strong consideration given toward performing an ovariectomy and salpingectomy to permanently correct the issue.[42,43,45] Samples collected during surgery should be submitted for histopathology and both bacterial and fungal cultures. The coelomic cavity should be flushed thoroughly with warmed saline to remove all possible yolk material. Postoperative care should include supportive care (eg, fluid therapy, enteric nutrition), analgesics, anti-inflammatories, and antimicrobials. Egg-yolk coelomitis in chelonians carries a grave prognosis.

Phallus Prolapse

Phallus prolapse may occur due to a variety of causes, including debilitation, neurologic dysfunction, excessive libido, urogenital or gastrointestinal disease, trauma, tenesmus, constipation, gastrointestinal foreign bodies, and cystic calculi.[2,4,46] A normal phallus should only be exposed for a few minutes. A prolapsed phallus should be cleaned with warmed saline and returned to the cloaca if the tissue appears viable. Hypertonic solution, such as 50% dextrose, should be immediately applied to the phallus to properly reduce edema and swelling. Lubricating jelly is also useful for reducing the prolapse. In some cases, sedation is required to limit straining. Once the phallus is reduced, a purse-string suture or simple continuous sutures should be placed in the vent to maintain the reduction. It is important that the clinician evaluate the sutures to ensure they are loose enough to allow the chelonian to urinate and defecate. Sutures should remain for 7 to 14 days.

If the tissue is not viable, a phallus amputation is indicated. An appreciation of chelonian phallus anatomy is required to successfully perform a proper amputation. A detailed review of this anatomy is described earlier in this article. In small chelonians, the base of the phallus may be ligated without clamping and by using encircling or vertical mattress sutures. Absorbable suture material should be used for this procedure. In larger chelonians, the surgical procedure is more complicated, and a description can be found in the following list[2,4,47] (Fig. 11):

- Surgical area is draped and aseptically prepared.
- Phallus is retracted caudally.
- Blood supply to each longitudinal ridge is identified and double ligated using absorbable sutures.

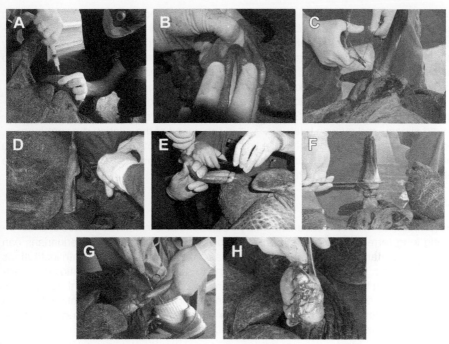

Fig. 11. Phallus amputation in a hybrid Galapagos tortoise (*G nigra*). (*A*) Intrathecal injection for local anesthesia/analgesia. (*B*) Exteriorization of the phallus from the cloaca. (*C*) Placement of a transfixation ligature. (*D*) Movement of the phallus can allow for better exposure for ligature placement. (*E*) Placement of another transfixation ligature. (*F*) Clamp placed distally to ligatures before transection. (*G*) Phallus is transected for removal. (*H*) Cloacal tissue remaining after dissection can then be closed over the stump of the phallus in a simple continuous pattern. (*Courtesy of* S.J. Divers, BVetMed, DZooMed, DECZM(Herp), DECZM(ZHM), DACZM, FRCVS, Athens, GA, J.P. Flanagan, DVM, and S. Rivera, DVM, MS, DABVP(Avian), DACZM, DECZM(Zoo), Houston, TX.)

- The main body of each longitudinal ridge, the corpus cavernosa, is separately clamped and double ligated.
- The phallus can then be dissected free of the cloaca and transected.
- Cloacal tissue remaining after dissection can then be closed over the stump of the phallus in a simple continuous pattern.
- Postoperative antibiotic and analgesic medications should be provided.
- Confirm underlying cause of prolapse.

Neoplasia of the Reproductive System

Reproductive cancer in chelonians is rare. A retrospective study evaluating 3500 reptile necropsies from a zoo over a period of 100 years found a prevalence of cancer of 2.3% for all reptiles and 1.2% in chelonians.[48] An additional study compiling the results from more than 5000 biopsy specimens submitted to a laboratory found a prevalence of cancer of 9.8% for all reptiles and 2.7% in chelonians.[49,50] Neither report listed reproductive tract tumors in chelonians. Case reports in male chelonians include a testicular interstitial cell adenoma and a seminoma. In the interstitial cell adenoma case report, the testes were grossly unremarkable and rafts of tumor cells were found within the testicular blood vessels; this testicle did not produce any viable sperm within the seminiferous tubules. The seminoma was reported in a 13-year-old male spur-thighed tortoise (*Testudo graeca*) that presented for anorexia, apathy, and prolapse of penile tissue. An antemortem diagnosis was made with ultrasonography and MRI, because the appearance and signal intensities were similar to those reported in testicular neoplasms, specifically seminomas in humans. A definitive diagnosis was confirmed on necropsy based on histopathological findings.[51]

Reports of cancer in female chelonians are also limited and include oviductal leiomyoma in a desert tortoise (*G agassizii*), ovarian dysgerminomas in 2 unrelated red-eared sliders, and ovarian teratoma.[52–54] In the cases of the ovarian dysgerminomas, each ovary was effaced by soft white tissue masses, one of which was large enough to prevent the turtle from retracting her head and neck into the shell. Cloacal polyps have also been reported in a box turtle.[53]

SUMMARY

As pressure continues to mount for wild populations of chelonians, the need for developing long-term and sustainable breeding programs will increase. Veterinarians can play an important role in ensuring the success of these programs for both institutions and individuals. It is important for veterinarians to develop a solid foundation of knowledge regarding the reproductive anatomy, physiology, and behaviors of these animals to differentiate normal from abnormal. Fortunately, most of the reproductive diseases seen in these animals are similar to those in other classes of animals and case management follows similar protocols.

REFERENCES

1. Kuchling G. The reproductive biology of the chelonia. Berlin: Springer; 1999. Available at: http://catalog.hathitrust.org/api/volumes/oclc/39368593.html. Accessed July 25, 2016.
2. Innis CJ, Boyer TH. Chelonian reproductive disorders. Vet Clin North Am Exot Anim Pract 2002;5(3):555–78.
3. Innis CJ. Endoscopy and endosurgery of the chelonian reproductive tract. Vet Clin North Am Exot Anim Pract 2010;13(2):243–54.
4. Sykes JM. Updates and practical approaches to reproductive disorders in reptiles. Vet Clin North Am Exot Anim Pract 2010;13(3):349–73.
5. Mitchell MA, Zimmerman D, Heggem B. Collection and characterization of semen from leopard tortoises. In: Proceedings of the Association of Reptilian and Amphibian Veterinarians. Milwaukee (WI): 2009. p. 166.
6. Kumar S, Roy B, Rai U. Hormonal regulation of testicular function. In: Norris DO, Lopez KH, editors. Hormones and reproduction of vertebrates reptiles volume 3. London: Elsevier; 2011. p. p.63–84.
7. Hormones and reproductive cycles in turtles. In: Norris DO, Lopez KH, editors. Hormones and reproduction of vertebrates reptiles volume 3. London: Elsevier; 2011. p. 277–99.
8. Hormonal regulation of ovarian function. In: Norris DO, Lopez KH, editors. Hormones and reproduction of vertebrates reptiles volume 3. London: Elsevier; 2011. p. 89–109.
9. DeNardo D. Reproductive biology. In: Mader D, editor. Reptile medicine and surgery. 1st edition. St Louis (MO): Elsevier; 1994. p. 214.
10. Rostal D, Grumbles J, Lance V, et al. Non-lethal sexing techniques for hatchling and immature desert tortoises (Gopherus agassizii). Herpetol Monogr 1994;8: 83–7.

11. Mitchell MA, Thompson D, Burgdorf A, et al. Coelioscopy as an antemortem method for confirming temperature dependent sex determination in Blanding's turtles (Emydoidea blandingii). In: Proceedings of the Association of Reptilian and Amphibian Veterinarians. Milwaukee (WI): 2009. p. 136.
12. Perpinan D, Costa T, Bargallo, et al. Correlation between gonad histology and endoscopic sex determination in juvenile red-eared turtles (Trachemys scripta elegans). In: Proceedings of International Conference on Avian, Herpetological and Exotic Animal Medicine (ICARE). Wiesbaden (Germany): 2013. p. 126–7.
13. Hernandez-Divers SJ, Stahl SJ, Farrell R. An endoscopic method for identifying sex of hatchling Chinese box turtles and comparison of general versus local anesthesia for coelioscopy. J Am Vet Med Assoc 2009;234(6):800–4.
14. Martínez-Silvestre A, Bargalló F, Grífols J. Gender identification by cloacoscopy and cystoscopy in juvenile chelonians. Vet Clin North Am Exot Anim Pract 2015;18(3):527–39.
15. Proenc a L. Comparison between coelioscopy versus cloacoscopy for gender identification in immature turtles (Trachemys scripta). In: Proceedings of International Conference on Avian, Herpetological and Exotic Animal Medicine (ICARE). Paris (France): 2015. p. 142–3.
16. Selleri P, Di Girolamo N, Melidone R. Cytoscopic sex identification of posthatchling chelonians. J Am Vet Med Assoc 2013;242:1744–50.
17. Madge D. Temperature and sex determination in reptiles with reference to chelonians. BCG Testudo 1994;2(3):9–14.
18. Schroeder AL, Metzger KJ, Miller A, et al. A novel candidate gene for temperature-dependent sex determination in the common snapping turtle. Genetics 2016;203(1):557–71.
19. Ernst CH, Barbour RW. Turtles of the world. Washington, DC: Smithsonian Press; 1998.
20. Innis C. Infertility and embryonic death. In: McArthur S, Wilkinson R, Meyer J, editors. Medicine and surgery of tortoises and turtles. Oxford (United Kingdom): Blackwell Publishing; 2004. p. 63–8.
21. Wood F, Platz C, Critchley K, et al. Semen collection by electroejaculation of the green turtle, Chelonia mydas. Br J Herpetol 1982;6:200–2.
22. Platz CC, Mengden BS, Quinn H, et al. Semen collection, evaluation and freezing in the green sea turtle, Galapagos tortoise, and red-eared pond turtle. In: Proceedings of the American Association of Zoo Veterinarians. 1980. p. 47–54.
23. Gross T, Guillette LJ, Gross DA, et al. Control of oviposition in reptiles and amphibians. In: Proceedings of the American Association of Zoo Veterinarians. 1992. p. 143–50.
24. McArthur S. Dystocia. In: McArthur S, Wilkinson R, Meyer J, editors. Medicine and surgery of tortoises and turtles. Oxford (United Kingdom): Blackwell Publishing; 2004. p. 316–8.
25. DeNardo D. Dystocias. In: Mader D, editor. Reptile medicine and surgery. 2nd edition. St Louis (MO): Elsevier Inc; 2006. p. 787–92.
26. Cheng Y, Chen T, Yu P, et al. Observations on the female reproductive cycles of captive Asian yellow pond turtles (Mauremys mutica) with radiography and ultrasonography. Zoo Biol 2009;28:1–9.
27. Stetter M. Ultrasonography. In: Mader D, editor. Reptile medicine and surgery. 2nd edition. St Louis (MO): Elsevier Inc; 2006. p. 665–74.
28. Knotek Z, Jekl V, Knotkova Z, et al. Eggs in chelonian urinary bladder: is coeliotomy necessary? In: Proceedings of the Association of Reptilian and Amphibian Veterinarians. 2009. p. 118–21.

29. Thomas HL, Willer CJ, Wosat MA, et al. Egg-retention in the urinary bladder of a Florida cooter turtle, Pseudemys floridana floridana. J Herp Med Surg 2001;11(4): 4–6.

30. Johnson R. Dystocia in an injured common eastern long-necked turtle (Chelodina longicollis). Vet Clin North Am Exot Anim Pract 2006;9:575–81.

31. Tucker JK, Thomas DL, Rose J. Oxytocin dosage in turtles. Chelonian Conserv Biol 2007;6(2):321–4.

32. Feldman ML. Some options to induce oviposition in turtles. Chelonian Conserv Biol 2007;6(2):313–20.

33. Innis CJ. Innovative approaches to chelonian obstetrics. In: Proceedings of the Association of Reptilian and Amphibian Veterinarians. Naples (Italy): 2004. p. 1–5.

34. McArthur S. Reproductive system. In: McArthur S, Wilkinson R, Meyer J, editors. Medicine and surgery of tortoises and turtles. Oxford (United Kingdom): Blackwell Publishing; 2004. p. 57–63.

35. Mader DR, Bennett RA, Funk RS, et al. Surgery. In: Mader D, editor. Reptile medicine and surgery. 2nd edition. St Louis (MO): Elsevier Inc; 2006. p. 581–630.

36. McArthur S, Hernandez-Divers S. Surgery. In: McArthur S, Wilkinson R, Meyer J, editors. Medicine and surgery of tortoises and turtles. Oxford (United Kingdom): Blackwell Publishing; 2004. p. 403–59.

37. Minter LJ, Landry MM, Lewbart GA. Prophylactic ovariosalpingectomy using a prefemoral approach in eastern box turtles (Terrapene carolina carolina). Vet Rec 2008;163(16):487–8.

38. Nutter FB, Lee DD, Stamper MA, et al. Hemiovariosalpingectomy in a loggerhead sea turtle (Caretta caretta). Vet Rec 2000;146:78–80.

39. Innis CJ, Feinsod R, Hanlon J, et al. Coelioscopic orchiectomy can be effectively and safely accomplished in chelonians. Vet Rec 2013;172(20):526.

40. Innis CJ, Hernandez-Divers S, Martinez-Jimenez D. Coelioscopic-assisted prefemoral oophorectomy in chelonians. J Am Vet Med Assoc 2007;230(7):1049–52.

41. Proença LM, Divers SJ. Coelioscopic and endoscope-assisted sterilization of chelonians. Vet Clin North Am Exot Anim Pract 2015;18(3):555–70.

42. McArthur S. Follicular stasis in captive chelonian, Testudo spp. In: Proceedings of the Association of Reptilian and Amphibian Veterinarians. Eighth Annual Conference. Orlando (FL): 2001. p. 75–86.

43. McArthur S. Follicular stasis. In: McArthur S, Wilkinson R, Meyer J, editors. Medicine and surgery of tortoises and turtles. Oxford (United Kingdom): Blackwell Publishing; 2004. p. 325–9.

44. Knafo SE, Divers SJ, Rivera S, et al. Sterilisation of hybrid Galapagos tortoises (Geochelone nigra) for island restoration. Part 1: endoscopic oophorectomy of females under ketamine-medetomidine anaesthesia. Vet Rec 2011;168(2):47.

45. Mans C, Sladky KK. Diagnosis and management of oviductal disease in three red-eared slider turtles (Trachemys scripta elegans). J Small Anim Pract 2012; 53(4):234–9.

46. Barten SL. Penile prolapse. In: Mader D, editor. Reptile medicine and surgery. 2nd edition. St Louis (MO): Elsevier Inc; 2006. p. 862–4.

47. Rivera S, Divers SJ, Knafo SE, et al. Sterilisation of hybrid Galapagos tortoises (Geochelone nigra) for island restoration. Part 2: phallectomy of males under intrathecal anaesthesia with lidocaine. Vet Rec 2011;168(3):78.

48. Sykes JM, Trupkiewicz JG. Reptile Neoplasia at the Philadelphia Zoological Garden, 1901–2002. J Zoo Wildl Med 2006;37:11–9.

49. Garner MM, Hernandez-Divers SM, Raymond JT. Reptile neoplasia: a retrospective study of case submissions to a specialty diagnostic service. Vet Clin North Am Exot Anim Pract 2004;7:653–71.

50. Hernandez-Divers SM, Garner MM. Neoplasia of reptiles with an emphasis on lizards. Vet Clin North Am Exot Anim Pract 2003;6:251–73.

51. Pees M, Ludewig E, Plenz B, et al. Imaging diagnosis- Seminoma causing liver compression in a spur-thighed tortoise (Testudo gracea): seminoma in a Tortoise. Vet Radiol Ultrasound 2015;56(2):E21–4.

52. Frye FL, Dybdal NO, Harshberger JC. Testicular interstitial cell tumor in a desert tortoise (Gopherus agassizii). J Zoo Anim Med 1988;19(1–2):55–8.

53. Frye FL. The diagnosis and surgical treatment of reptilian neoplasms with a compilation of cases 1966–1993. In Vivo 1994;8:885–92.

54. Newman SJ, Brown CJ, Patnaik AK. Malignant ovarian teratoma in a red-eared slider (Trachemys scripta elegans). J Vet Diagn Invest 2003;15(1):77–81.

Reproductive Disorders in Snakes

Nicola Di Girolamo, DMV, MSc(EBHC), PhD, DECZM(Herpetology),
Paolo Selleri, DMV, PhD, DECZM(Herpetology &Small Mammals)*

KEYWORDS

- Ophidians • Surgery • Reptiles • Squamate • Dystocia

KEY POINTS

- Snake species are oviparous and viviparous; knowledge of biology and physiology of each species is fundamental to properly treat a snake with reproductive disorders.
- Several factors, including body condition, temperature, humidity, light cycle, and presence of conspecifics, need to be considered when approaching a snake with reproductive disorders.
- Ultrasonographic visualization of ovaries, testes, or hemipenes may assist correct snake sex identification in certain instances.
- Diagnostic imaging is fundamental during dystocia to identify obstructive and nonobstructive cases.
- In cases of egg dystocia, the goal of surgery is usually to preserve reproductive function. In such cases the eggs may be removed from the oviducts via salpingotomy.

 Video content accompanies this article at http://www.vetexotic.theclinics.com.

INTRODUCTION

Reproduction of snakes is a complex aspect of herpetologic medicine. To breed snakes, several factors need to be considered. The clinician needs to be aware of such factors to assist amateur and professional breeders. Because of the complexity of reproduction, several disorders may present before, during, or after this process. Most of infertility problems can be resolved by knowing appropriate reproductive management techniques. Disorders during gestation or egg deposition are extremely common (**Fig. 1**) and may result in death of the snake and loss of the eggs/fetuses (**Fig. 2**). Disorders following mating or oviposition (eg, prolapses, infections) are less common but may preclude future ability to reproduce the snake.

The authors have nothing to disclose.
Clinica per Animali Esotici, Centro Veterinario Specialistico, Via Sandro Giovannini 53, Rome 00137, Italy
* Corresponding author.
E-mail address: paolsell@gmail.com

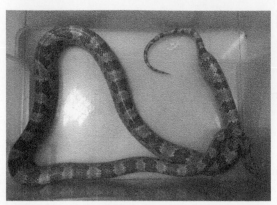

Fig. 1. Clinical presentation of a corn snake (*Panterophis guttatus*) with retention of an egg in the cloaca. (*Courtesy of* Paolo Selleri, DMV and Nicola Di Girolamo, DMV, Rome, Italy.)

REPRODUCTIVE PHYSIOLOGY

Snake species are classified as oviparous (egg layers) and viviparous. Some viviparous snakes (placental viviparous) have a placenta (eg, boa constrictors, green anacondas), whereas other viviparous snakes (eg, most vipers) do not have placental connection and develop eggs that hatch before parturition (previously defined as ovoviviparous). One blind snake species (*Ramphotyphlops braminus*) is obligate parthenogenetic (ie, offspring are produced by females without the genetic contribution of a male),[1] and facultative parthenogenesis has been rarely observed in other snakes.[2] Male snakes achieve internal fertilization by inserting one of the two hemipenes, the copulatory organs, into the female's cloaca (**Fig. 3**). The sperm is delivered through ductus deferens from the testes located in the coelomic cavity to the hemipenes. At the end of mating, the pair separate. Depending on the species, females may store the semen for multiple reproductive seasons.

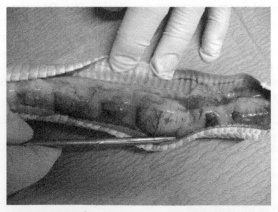

Fig. 2. Postmortem examination of a western hognose snake (*Heterodon nasicus*) deceased during gestation. (*Courtesy of* Francesco De Filippo, DMV Naples, Italy.)

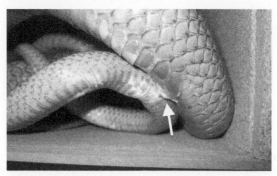

Fig. 3. Mating of Baron's green racer (*Philodryas baroni*) by insertion of one of the hemipenes in the female's cloaca (*arrow*). (*Courtesy of* Marcello Devincenzi, DVM, Mantova, Italy.)

REPRODUCTIVE TRACT ANATOMY
Ovaries and Oviducts

The reproductive tract of female snakes is generally composed of two ovaries and two oviducts,[3] although in few species (eg, *Tantilla* sp) the left oviduct is vestigial or absent.[4,5] Ovaries are elongated and present numerous variably sized, whitish to yellowish, follicles (**Fig. 4**). They are suspended by a mesovarium and exhibit seasonal changes, with the greatest size reached during the breeding season, before ovulation. In snakes, the right ovary is usually bigger and localized anteriorly than the left one.[3] Oviducts run from the ovaries to the urodeum, where they open through the urogenital papillae. Gonadal arteries, originating from the dorsal aorta, vascularize the ovaries and oviducts. Ovarian veins drain into the postcaval veins.[6]

Testes and Hemipenes

In most snake species, testes are elongated, cylindrical, yellowish white organs, attached dorsally to the body wall by the mesorchium in the caudal third of the body cranial to the kidneys (**Fig. 5**). They are vascularized by spermatic arteries and

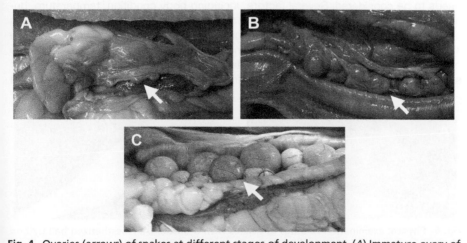

Fig. 4. Ovaries (*arrows*) of snakes at different stages of development. (*A*) Immature ovary of a boa constrictor (*Boa constrictor*). (*B*) Mature ovary of a boa constrictor. (*C*) Preovulatory follicles of a Burmese python (*Python bivittatus*). (*Courtesy of* Nicola Di Girolamo, DMV and Paolo Selleri, DMV, Rome, Italy.)

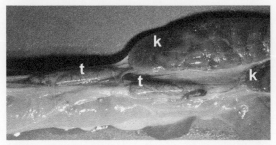

Fig. 5. Gross appearance of testes (t) and their anatomic relationship with respective kidneys (k) in snakes. (*Courtesy of* Nicola Di Girolamo, DMV and Paolo Selleri, DMV Rome, Italy.)

veins and their size may vary depending on the season with larger testes during spermatogenesis. One ductus deferens per each testis is present.[6] Male snakes have paired hemipenes, which lie in respective sacs caudal to the cloaca in the ventral part of the tail.

Cloaca

Compared with other reptiles the cloacal divisions in snakes are simple, with minimal to no separation and often poor delineation between each other.[6] The coprodeum is the area where the terminal colon and rectum end. Caudal to the coprodeum, the urodeum is where the urinary tract and the reproductive tracts terminate. Snakes have no urinary bladder, therefore in this area the ureters empty. The proctodeum, which is, the most caudal division of the cloaca, is associated with the vent. Material leaving the cloaca passes through the vent, where musk glands empty.

CLINICAL APPROACH TO DISORDERS OF REPRODUCTION
Physical Examination

To approach a snake with reproductive problems, the normal biology of the species needs to be considered. Several factors, including body condition, temperature, humidity, light cycle, or introduction of a male, are thought to trigger folliculogenesis and ovulation in snakes.[7,8] During physical examination the body condition of the snake need to be assessed because female snakes may not reproduce if they do not have enough fat stores. In case of gestation, eggs are visible as multiple coelomic swellings, especially in colubrids (**Fig. 6**). In larger snakes, palpation may be required

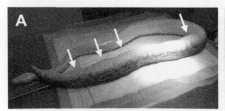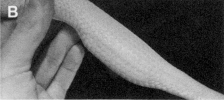

Fig. 6. Physical examination findings in snakes with dystocia. (*A*) Anesthetized ball python (*Python regius*) in dorsal recumbency. Notice that eggs are evident as multiple coelomic swellings (*arrows*). (*B*) Single coelomic swelling in an albino radiated ratsnake (*Coelognathus radiatus*) with one dystocic egg. (*Courtesy of* Nicola Di Girolamo, DMV and Paolo Selleri, DMV, Rome, Italy.)

to detect eggs or fetuses. Palpation should be gentle, because the practitioner may be responsible for rupture of structures associated with the reproductive tract (eg, cysts, follicles) with subsequent death of the snake.[9]

Sex Determination

Most snakes lack definitive secondary sexual characteristics even in adulthood. Sometimes individuals have been sexed when young by breeders and then maintained by inexperienced owners. Therefore, owners may not be aware of the real sex of the animal. Depending on the species, there are certain sexing techniques that are more indicated than others, including:

- Evaluation of secondary sexual characteristics
- Probing (**Fig. 7**)
- Manual hemipenile eversion (ie, popping) (**Fig. 8**)
- Hydrostatic hemipenile eversion
- Contrast radiography[10]
- Ultrasonography (USG)

Secondary sexual characteristics (eg, cloacal spurs in boids) are not reliable indicators because they may be influenced by management and growth. Probing consists of the insertion of cylindrical, atraumatic probes at the base of the tail just caudal and lateral to the cloaca, where hemipenile sacs are located in males. A deep ingress of the probes indicates a male, whereas superficial ingress of the probes indicates a female. The deepness of the access of the probes is then compared with reference values for each species (**Table 1**). However, when a snake is referred for a reproductive disorder, it is always advisable to not completely rely only on such techniques. Probing may be flawed by iatrogenic lesions of the hemipenile sacs (ie, lesions in the vestigial hemipenile sacs in female snakes caused by probing make them seem like hemipenile sacs and therefore males).

Ultrasonographic visualization of ovaries, testes, or hemipenes is a more definite sex identification technique. However, there is conflicting evidence on the diagnostic accuracy of ultrasound to visualize hemipenes, with one study reporting accuracy of

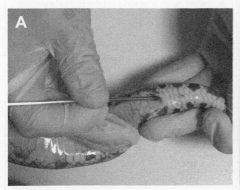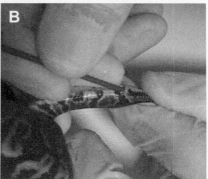

Fig. 7. Sexing of adult (*A*) and posthatchling (*B*) ball pythons (*Python regius*) by probing. The technique consists of insertion of cylindrical, atraumatic probes at the base of the tail just caudal and lateral to the cloaca, where hemipenile sacs are located in males. The deepness of the access of the probes is then compared with reference values for each species. A deep ingress of the probes indicates a male, whereas a superficial ingress of the probes indicates a female.

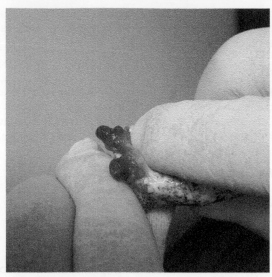

Fig. 8. Manual eversion of the hemipenes in a ball python (*Pyton regius*). This sexing technique is referred by breeders as "popping" and may potentially lead to spinal trauma if performed in young individuals. (*Courtesy of* Francesco De Filippo, DMV, Naples, Italy.)

100% (17 out of 17 male snakes identified) and one study reporting accuracy of 48% (10 out of 21 male snakes identified).[10,11]

Diagnostic Imaging

Radiography
Radiography may be a useful tool to evaluate a snake with breeding problems. Before reproduction, radiology allows visualization of eggs or fetuses retained from the

Table 1
Number of subcaudal scales that are generally accessed with a sexing probe in male versus female in selected snake species

Species	Male	Female
Acrantophis sp	10–12	4–5
Aspidites sp	10–12	3–4
Boa constrictor	9–12	2–4
Corallus caninus	14–15	3
Epicrates cenchria cenchria	11	3
Eunectes murinus	19	2–3
Morelia sp	9–10	2–5
Python molurus bivittatus	10–16	3–5
Python molurus molurus	10–12	3–5
Python regius	10	3
Python reticulatus	9–10	2–3
Sanzinia madagascariensis	8–10	3

Modified from Ross RA, Marzec G. The reproductive husbandry of pythons and boas. Stanford (CT): Institute for Herpetologic Research; 1990.

previous season and to assess presence of celomic fat. In snakes with dystocia, radiography usually provides a rough estimate on the number of eggs present, even if the exact number is better determined with USG.

Radiographic technique Ideally, a dorsoventral and a lateral view are obtained. Radiographs in snakes are commonly obtained by placing conscious snakes in radiotransparent plastic bags, plastic containers, or plastic tubes. Placement of snakes in containers that make them assume a curled position is discouraged by the authors. The radiograph would not easily allow identification of the eggs (**Fig. 9**). There is some evidence that lung fields would not be properly evaluated in a curled recumbence as opposite to a straight recumbence.[12] Dorsoventral and lateral radiographs may be obtained in sedated snakes or in conscious snakes by manual restraint or by use of plastic tubes.

Radiographic findings Because of the limited calcification of eggs in most snakes, radiography is limited. However, radiography is useful to have a general image of the snake and in the specific to:

- Evaluate the presence of eggs or in some instances large follicles
- Estimate the number of eggs (before treatment confirm with ultrasound)
- Evaluate the morphology of the eggs (**Fig. 10**)
- Evaluate additional problems that may be associated with or responsible for reproductive disorders

Ultrasonography
USG is one of the more useful tools to assist snake reproduction and to cope with reproductive disease of snakes. Indications for USG include the following:

- Definitive sex determination by identification of ovaries or testes. Active ovaries are easily visualized even by inexperienced operators.
- Monitoring of the follicular development and elect optimal reproduction time.[13]
- Estimate of viable clutch size (**Fig. 11**).[14]
- Monitoring of viability of fetuses.

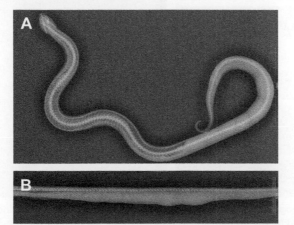

Fig. 9. Comparison of radiographs obtained unrestrained in dorsoventral projection (*A*) and manually restrained in lateral projection (*B*) in a conscious western hognose snake (*Heterodon nasicus*). Notice that the profile of the eggs is clearer in the lateral projection. (*Courtesy of* Paolo Selleri, DMV and Nicola Di Girolamo, DMV, Rome, Italy.)

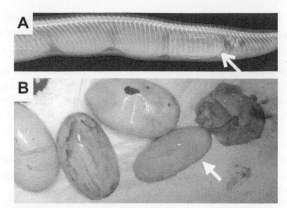

Fig. 10. Role of radiography during dystocia. (*A*) Lateral radiographic projection in a ball python (*Python regius*). (*B*). Eggs retrieved from the same individual. A solidified egg (*arrow*) was the cause of dystocia in the ball python. The radiographic appearance of the altered egg (*empty arrow*) was diagnostic. (*Courtesy of* Nicola Di Girolamo, DMV and Paolo Selleri, DMV, Rome, Italy.)

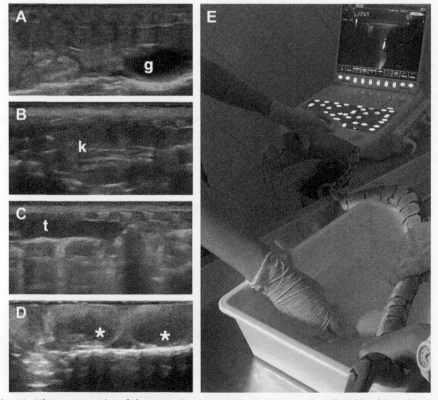

Fig. 11. Ultrasonography of the reproductive tract in snakes. (*A, B*) Gallbladder (g) and kidney (k) are, respectively, the cranial and caudal anatomic landmarks for the identification of ovaries and testes. (*C*) Testis (t) during inactive season in a ball python (*Python regius*). (*D*) Visualization of multiple eggs (*asterisks*) in a western hognose snake (*Heterodon nasicus*). (*E*) Placement of the snake in warm water may reduce the artifacts because of entrapment of air through the scales. (*Courtesy of* Nicola Di Girolamo, DMV and Paolo Selleri, DMV, Rome, Italy.)

Ultrasonography technique Understanding of snake topographic anatomy is mandatory to properly perform a USG examination. Linear array transducers of medium-high frequencies (6–18 MHz) are used depending on the size of the snake. To reduce the artifacts generated by the scale, USG may be performed placing the snake and the transducer in warm water.

Ultrasonographic findings Ovaries may be identified cranial to the corresponding kidney, or at the same level of the kidneys if the snake is ovulating, with the right ovary being cranial to the left one. Usually visualization of the ovarian parenchyma is impossible and follicles are identified as a landmark of the ovaries. Size of the follicles varies with season and age of the snake. The follicles appear as multiple round anechoic structures surrounded by a capsule with an echoic inner layer and an anechoic outer layer.[11]

Oviducts in nongravid snakes are small tubular structures with a hyperechoic wall, usually difficult to visualize. They are visible medial to the kidneys and run lateral to the ureters.[11]

Testes are visualized as elongated structures (longitudinal scan) and oval-round structures (transverse scan) slightly less echogenic than fat bodies cranial to the cranial pole of the kidneys. Color flow Doppler USG may be used to differentiate the renal vein (flow present) from the deferent duct (no flow).[11]

Scent glands are identifiable in male and female snakes as paired circular structures, with a rough and nonhomogeneous echotexture and a poor echogenicity. In male snakes, scent glands are dorsal to hemipenes. In females, the scent glands are more prominent and occupy most of the cranial portion of the tail.[11]

The hemipenes are better identified in longitudinal scans than in transverse scans.[11] In longitudinal scan, the hemipenes appear as two echoic lines within two parallel anechoic lines, whereas in transverse scan they appear as two echoic circular structures positioned ventrally or laterally to the scent glands.

Endoscopy
Cloacoscopy is a useful diagnostic tool to evaluate cloacal pathology associated with reproduction in snake patients including prolapses and dystocia.[15]

Endoscopic equipment Cloacoscopy in small-to-medium size snakes has been successfully performed with a 2.7-mm diameter, 18 cm in length, 30° viewing rigid endoscope housed within a 3.5-mm protective sheath (Storz, Karl Storz GmbH & Co KG, Tuttligen, Germany) or a 14.5F catheter instrumented sheath system containing multiple ports (Storz, Karl Storz GmbH & Co KG) and/or with a 9.5F catheter, 14 cm in length, 30° viewing operating telescope (Storz, Karl Storz GmbH & Co KG). In very small snakes the use of smaller equipment, such as 1.9-mm rigid endoscope, should be considered. In large snakes the use of flexible endoscopes should be considered.

Patient preparation and technique The snake patient is anesthetized and is placed in either ventral or dorsal recumbency. Recumbency is gently inverted during the procedure to allow a more complete evaluation of the cloaca. The endoscope is inserted in the vent and directed cranially. Warm (30°C) fluids are infused (one drop every 3–4 seconds) to allow distention of the cloacal opening. To allow appropriate distention of the cloaca, the lips of the vent may initially be gently held closed while warm saline water is infused. The investigation of the cloaca is performed easily once it is properly dilated.

The urodeum and associated structures can also be thoroughly examined, including the oviducts of females and ureteral openings. Maintaining a gentle pressure and with fluid being infused the access to the interested areas is possible. Cloacoscopy during dystocia often permits visualization of the most caudal egg. The irrigation of sterile saline dilates the oviduct, facilitating the passage of the egg when manually manipulated. Endoscopy of the cloaca also permits visualization, video recording, and biopsy of lesions found in the cloaca or in the oviducts.

REPRODUCTIVE TRACT SURGICAL TECHNIQUES
Ovariectomy and Ovariosalpingectomy

Reproductive tract disorders may require surgical intervention in female snakes. Ovariectomy and ovariosalpingectomy are rarely indicated in snakes, the most common clinical indication for these surgeries being neoplastic disorders. Rarely, other disorders of the oviduct may require partial or complete salpingectomy.[16] Ovariectomy may be performed as an elective surgery for preventive care in female snakes with recurrent reproductive disorders and in severe cases of preovulatory stasis. To relieve dystocic eggs, salpingotomy is often preferred to ovariosalpingectomy.

Standard access to the coelom is performed.[17] In case of ovariosalpingectomy, a large coelomic incision is needed. If the snake is immature or ovulation has already occurred (ie, the oviducts contain postovulatory follicles or eggs), the ovaries are small. If ovulation has not occurred (ie, preovulatory stasis), the ovaries may be large and present several yellow-to-orange follicles and should be gently exteriorized. Size of the follicles may significantly affect the surgical anatomy and techniques. Once identified, the ovaries should be elevated to expose the mesovarium with its vessels. Microsurgical instruments, ligation clips, and radiosurgical and electrosurgical devices are required to facilitate and accelerate the removal of the entire ovaries (**Fig. 12**). If the oviduct needs to be removed, the oviductal vessels are carefully ligated using radiosurgery or ligatures and the oviduct is ligated at its base.

Salpingotomy

In cases of postovulatory stasis (ie, egg dystocia), the goal of surgery is usually to preserve reproductive function. In such cases the eggs may be removed from the oviducts (ie, cesarean section, salpingotomy) (**Fig. 13**). Alternatively, if only one oviduct is dystocic, a unilateral ovariosalpingectomy preserves the breeding function. If an

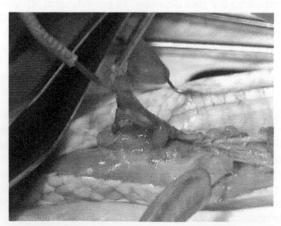

Fig. 12. Removal of inactive ovary in a corn snake (*Panterophis guttatus*) using radiosurgical device. (*Courtesy of* Paolo Selleri, DMV, Rome, Italy.)

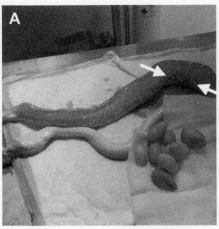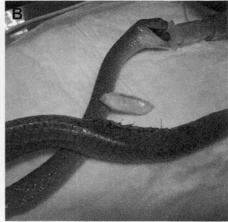

Fig. 13. Outcomes of salpingotomy in a green three python (*Morelia viridis*) (*A*) and in a green cat snake (*Boiga cyanea*) (*B*). Notice the large number of nonviable eggs retrieved from a relatively small incision (*arrow*). (*Courtesy of* Paolo Selleri, DMV and Nicola Di Girolamo, DMV, Rome, Italy.)

oviduct is removed also the respective ovary should be removed. Inadvertent remnants of ovarian tissue may provoke future ovulation into the coelomic cavity and yolk coelomitis, ovarian neoplasia, or ovarian cysts.[18]

The number of eggs and their exact location is determined by ultrasound and marked on the body of the snake. Depending on the size and the species of the snake and the number of dystocic eggs, several celiotomy accesses may be required to remove all the eggs. As a rule, from an incision approximately the size of the egg, the egg right after the incision and the preceding and following eggs may be removed without exerting too much pressure on the oviduct (**Fig. 14**A). Access to both oviducts is possible from a single coelomic incision (**Fig. 14**B). Furthermore, eggs often adhere to the oviduct and removal from a single oviductal incision may be difficult (**Fig. 14**C, D).[19] Once the eggs are removed, the incisions are closed with absorbable monofilament suture (eg, polydioxanone or polyglyconate, 3-0 to 5-0) in an inverting or apposing pattern (**Fig. 14**E, F). The oviducts are generally fragile in small snakes and the rims may invert, making closure of the incisions difficult.

Orchiectomy

Orchiectomy (orchidectomy) in male snakes has been performed to treat testicular tumors and for physiologic research.[20,21] Because of the intracoelomic location of the testicles, orchiectomy is a more invasive procedure in snakes as compared with most mammals. Identification with ultrasound and labeling the location of the testicles before surgery is suggested. After standard coeliotomy, the testicles are identified. Testicles are elongated and friable and must be handled carefully. The testicle may be gently elevated from the coelomic cavity by placing a suture or a needle through them as in lizards.[22,23] In general, full exteriorization is difficult because of the intimate relationship between the testis and major blood vessels. Therefore, ligation of the testicular vessels is facilitated by use of ligation clips or radiosurgical or electrosurgical equipment. While removing the testicles, care should be used to avoid damaging the vena cava that is contiguous to them. The vascular pedicles are checked for hemorrhage and the coelom is routinely closed.

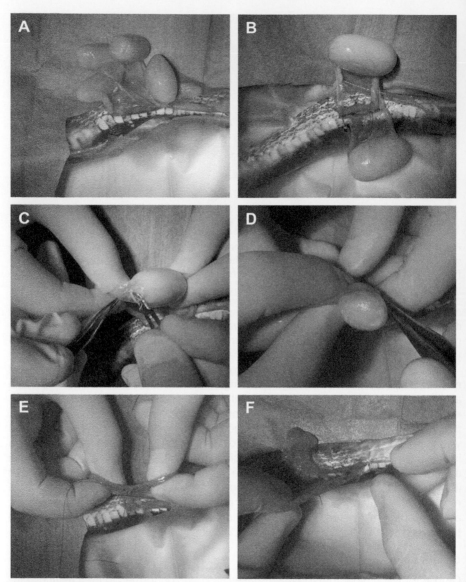

Fig. 14. Salpingotomy for egg retrieval in a western hognose snake (*Heterodon nasicus*). (*A*) From a cutaneous incision slightly larger than a single egg, several eggs may be retrieved. (*B*) The two oviducts may be manipulated from a single incision. (*C*) The oviduct is incised at the apex of the egg, paying care to avoid lesioning the egg. (*D*) The egg is gently exteriorized from the incision. It is difficult to retrieve multiple eggs from a single oviductal incision. (*E, F*) Oviductal incision is sutured with monofilament absorbable suture. (*Courtesy of Nicola Di Girolamo, DMV and Paolo Selleri, DMV, Rome, Italy.*)

Hemipenectomy

Hemipeneal amputation (hemipenectomy) is indicated in case of recurring or chronic hemipeneal prolapse (**Fig. 15**). Amputation can be performed *in toto*, because hemipenes do not contain the urethra. Amputation of a single hemipene in snakes does

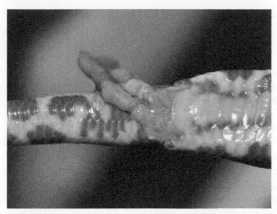

Fig. 15. Chronically prolapsed and necrotic hemipenes in a boa constrictor (*Boa constrictor*). (*Courtesy of* Paolo Selleri, DMV and Nicola Di Girolamo, DMV, Rome, Italy.)

not preclude reproduction. The snake is anesthetized and positioned in dorsal recumbency and the hemipene is surgically prepared. Depending on the size of the snake, one or two transfixing ligatures are placed at the base of the hemipene. The tissue is excised distal to the ligatures.

SPECIFIC DISORDERS
Dystocia

Dystocia is probably the most common disorder of reproduction in snakes.[24–26] Typically, oviparous snakes are presented with single or multiple abdominal bulgings. It is not always straightforward to diagnose a dystocia in snakes. Gestational duration, clutch size, egg size, egg type, and even placentation vary among species of snakes. An in-depth understanding of each species reproductive cycle is required. Even knowing that, it is not easy to understand when a snake is suffering egg retention. Untreated dystocia may result in oviductal prolapse and death (**Fig. 16**).

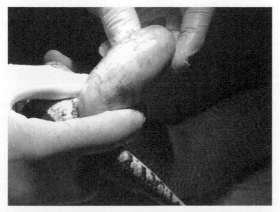

Fig. 16. Oviductal prolapse in a ball python (*Python regius*) with dystocic eggs. (*Courtesy of* Nicola Di Girolamo, DMV and Paolo Selleri, DMV, Rome, Italy.)

Dystocia is diagnosed when the snake laid part of her clutch and retained one or more eggs (or fetus in case of viviparous species), there is evidence of a mechanical impediment of oviposition (eg, strictures, cloacal calculi), or there is evidence of abnormally long clutch retention with presence of one or more abnormal eggs (eg, solidified, broken, extremely large) (see **Fig. 10**). Dystocia should be suspected when despite proper care, the gravid female suddenly becomes anorectic and lethargic, or there is evidence that the clutch has been retained for an abnormally long period.

Obstructive versus nonobstructive dystocia

Cases in which there is evidence that lack of egg-laying is secondary to abnormal reproductive canal, or abnormal eggs or fetuses are defined as obstructive dystocias. These cases usually require surgical treatment. Often there is no evidence of an obstruction in the female reproductive canal and eggs (or fetuses) are of normal size and morphology (ie, nonobstructive dystocias). Often, nonobstructive dystocias are secondary to poor reproduction planning and management, including poor physical condition of the female, improper nesting site, improper temperature, malnutrition, and dehydration. In nonobstructive dystocias medical treatment may be successful.

Diagnostics

Radiography is useful to obtain a preliminary clinical picture, but is limited by lack of calcification of eggs in snakes. USG permits visualization and counts of the number of eggs. Cloacoscopy permits visualization of the distal oviducts. Computed tomography and MRI have been rarely reported as a tool for assisting dystocic snakes, but may be useful in specific cases.

Treatment

Medical treatment When obstructive causes have been discarded, a preliminary medical approach consists of fluid therapy, calcium support, and eventually oxytocin. Is uncommon for snakes that have retained eggs for several days to respond to oxytocin. Usually oxytocin is effective when treating snakes 2 to 3 days after the start of nesting behavior.[15] Dosages used in snakes range from 0.4 to 10 IU/kg.[25] Anecdotally, increasing dosages of 5 to 20 IU/kg intramuscularly have been used in snakes with a 6- to 12-hour interval. There is no scientific evidence of the safety of this treatment.

Manual voiding In some cases, manual voiding is feasible with minimal pressure (Video 1). When eggs are retained for a consistent period of time, there is formation of a layer of fibrin that creates adherence with the oviduct. In such case manual voiding is difficult, and even if the eggs are in the cloaca, surgical removal may be needed (**Fig. 17**).

Endoscopic-assisted voiding Endoscopic-assisted voiding consists of visualization of the eggs by means of an endoscope before manual voiding (**Fig. 18**). Endoscopic-assisted voiding has two advantages over manual voiding: it allows visualization and opening of the cervix, and it permits instillation of fluids in the oviduct, which diminish the attrition.

Percutaneous ovocentesis Percutaneous ovocentesis should be limited to those cases of obstructive dystocia in which there is one very large egg occluding the oviduct. Percutaneous ovocentesis is ineffective in cases in which there is solidification of the egg (see **Fig. 10**).

To perform percutaneous ovocentesis the snake needs to be properly sedated. Usually the needle is inserted between the first and second line of lateral scutes to

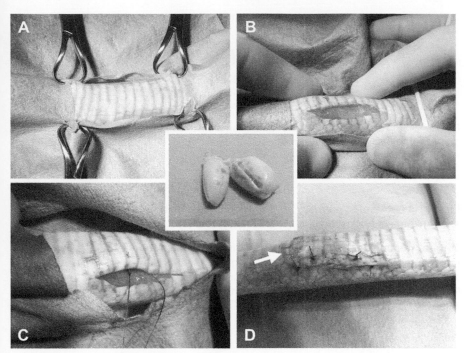

Fig. 17. Cloacotomy for egg retrieval in an albino corn snake (*Panterophis guttatus*). Even if the eggs were inside the cloaca (*arrow*), their adherence to surrounding tissue impeded manual or endoscopic voiding. (*A*) Surgical field. (*B*) Exposure of the muscles around the cloaca by incision of the skin between the lateral and ventral scale (alternatively skin is incised between the first and second rows of lateral scales). (*C, D*). Closure of the incision on a double layer, muscles and skin. *Inset*: Cloacal eggs retrieved. (*Courtesy of* Nicola Di Girolamo, DMV and Paolo Selleri, DMV, Rome, Italy.)

avoid damage to vessels or internal organs. The site elected for needle insertion is scrubbed. A large, 20-to-22-gauge needle is inserted in the egg and the material is aspirated (**Fig. 19**). After ovocentesis, if the problem was only related to the size of the egg, the snake should be able to eject the shell in the following days. In case

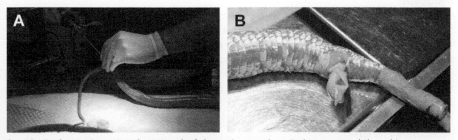

Fig. 18. Endoscopic-assisted retrieval of dystocic eggs in a *Boiga cyanea* (*A*) and in a western hognose snake (*Heterodon nasicus*) (*B*). Often as shown in (*B*), after the first egg is retrieved the other eggs are easily voided. (*Courtesy of* Paolo Selleri, DMV and Nicola Di Girolamo, DMV, Rome, Italy.)

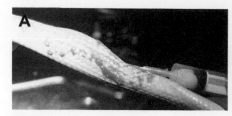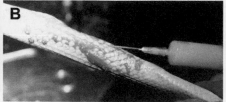

Fig. 19. (*A, B*) Transcutaneous ovocentesis in an albino radiated ratsnake (*Coelognathus radiatus*) with one dystocic egg from **Fig. 6**. The reddish foam on the scales is povidone-iodine solution. (*Courtesy of* Nicola Di Girolamo, DMV and Paolo Selleri, DMV, Rome, Italy.)

the egg is not ejected normally, other procedures should be used to retrieve the egg shell (manual or endoscopic voiding, surgery).

Surgical treatment Surgical treatment includes salpingotomy and ovariosalpingectomy. Immediately after removal of the eggs, all the viable eggs should be incubated as soon as possible. Often professional snake breeders take care of future hatchlings more than the mother snake. Egg management is reported elsewhere in this issue.

Follicular Stasis

Follicular stasis or preovulatory stasis is a condition in which follicles neither ovulate nor regress over time and are associated with clinical signs (eg, lethargy and/or anorexia). Depending on snake size and species the follicles may be evident as a swelling of the middle to caudal third of the snake. This condition is difficult to diagnose with certainty mainly because of the interspecific differences in follicular size and development time.

Diagnostics

Ultrasound allows identification of the follicles and evaluation of their echogenicity. Recent follicles generally have homogenous echogenicity, whereas old follicles have a hypoechoic to anechoic center. When follicular stasis is suspected, multiple USG examinations should be carried out over a period of time to monitor follicle size. A characteristic of follicular stasis is the presence of large follicles over an abnormal period of time (generally several weeks).

Treatment

Anecdotally, calcium administration has been used to treat follicular stasis[27] because it is thought that this is a consequence of the lack of available calcium. However, there is no scientific evidence of the cause of this disorder, or of effectiveness or the safety of this treatment. In case of persisting follicles associated with anorexia and in the absence of other evident disorders, ovariectomy should be considered. Other medical alternatives, including hormonal treatments, need proper scientific assessment before implementation in clinical practice.

Hemipenile Prolapse

Cloacal prolapses are less common in snakes than in other reptiles, with hemipenile prolapse being identified in 0.16% of snakes (1 of 628, both sexes) examined in a single institution.[28]

Diagnostics

A hemipenile prolapse should be considered as a primary disease only when occurring during or after copulation. Most often hemipenile prolapse is an unspecific sign of illness and diagnostics should be carried out as appropriate.

Treatment

If the snake has been presented soon after prolapse, and the tissue is viable, the hemipene can be gently repositioned. Soaking the hemipene in a hypertonic solution may reduce the swelling and facilitate prolapse reduction. A temporary suture of the hemipenile sac after reduction may avoid recurrence of the prolapse. Often, the owner notices the hemipenile prolapse late after occurrence. If the tissue is already necrotic, amputation is required.

Neoplasia of the Reproductive Tract

Neoplasia of the reproductive tract is among the most common tumors in snakes, with hemangiomas, carcinomas, fibromas, and granulosa cell tumor affecting the ovary, and leyomiosarcomas the oviduct.[29] In males, germ cell (ie, seminoma)[20] and gonadal stromal tumors (ie, Sertoli cell tumor, Leydig cell tumor)[29] may occur. Typically, snakes are presented with enlargement between their middle and caudal third.

Diagnostics

Radiography, ultrasound, and computed tomography scan provide important clinical information, including size and anatomic relationship with contiguous structures of the mass. Fine-needle aspiration or percutaneous biopsies allows identification of the tissue of origin and differentiation of the neoplasia.

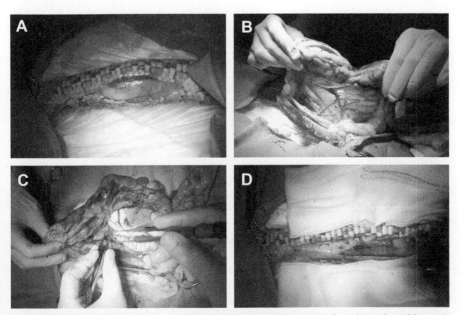

Fig. 20. Ovariosalpingectomy in a corn snake (*Panterophis guttatus*) with oviductal leyomiosarcoma. (*A, B*). Exposure of the oviduct. (*C*) Closure of oviductal vessels with radiosurgical equipment. (*D*) Appearance of the surgical site after removal of the neoplasia. (*Courtesy of* Nicola Di Girolamo, DMV and Paolo Selleri, DMV, Rome, Italy.)

Treatment

Depending on the type, dissemination, and aggressiveness of the neoplasia different treatments should be considered. In case of localized lesions ovariectomy, ovariosalpingectomy, or orchidectomy may be performed as appropriate (**Fig. 20**).[20]

SUPPLEMENTARY DATA

Supplementary video related to this article can be found online at http://dx.doi.org/10. 1016/j.cvex.2016.11.007.

REFERENCES

1. Nussbaum RA. The brahminy blind snake (*Ramphotyphlops braminus*) in the Seychelles Archipelago: distribution, variation, and further evidence for parthenogenesis. Herpetologica 1980;36:215–21.
2. Booth W, Smith CF, Eskridge PH, et al. Facultative parthenogenesis discovered in wild vertebrates. Biol Lett 2012;8:983–5.
3. Blackburn DG. Structure, function, and evolution of the oviducts of squamate reptiles, with special reference to viviparity and placentation. J Exp Zool 1998;282: 560–617.
4. Greer AE. On the adaptive significance of the loss of an oviduct in reptiles. Proc Lin Soc NWS 1976;101:242–9.
5. Clark DR. Loss of the left oviduct in the colubrid snake genus *Tantilla*. Herpetologica 1970;26:130–3.
6. Fox A. The urinogenital system of reptiles. In: Gans C, Parsons TS, editors. Biology of the reptilia. Volume 6, Morphology E. London: Academic Press; 1977. p. 1–157.
7. Bonnet X, Naulleau G, Mauget R. The influence of body condition on 17-beta estradiol levels in relation to vitellogenesis in female *Vipera aspis* (Reptilia, Viperidae). Gen Comp Endocrinol 1994;93:424–37.
8. DeNardo DF, Autumn K. Effect of male presence on reproductive activity in captive female blood pythons, *Python curtus*. Copeia 2001;4:1138–41.
9. Michaels SJ, Sanecki R. Undifferentiated carcinoma in the ovary of a boa constrictor (*Boa constrictor ortoni*). J Zoo Wildl Med 1988;19:237–40.
10. Gnudi G, Volta A, Di Ianni F, et al. Use of ultrasonography and contrast radiography for snake gender determination. Vet Radiol Ultrasound 2009;50:309–11.
11. Banzato T, Russo E, Finotti L, et al. Ultrasonographic anatomy of the coelomic organs of boid snakes (*Boa constrictor imperator, Python regius, Python molurus molurus*, and *Python curtus*). Am J Vet Res 2012;73:634–45.
12. Hedley J, Eatwell K, Schwarz T. Computed tomography of ball pythons (*Python regius*) in curled recumbency. Vet Radiol Ultrasound 2014;55:380–6.
13. Nielsen E. Evaluation of the follicular cycle in Ball Pythons (*Python regius*). In: Proceedings of the Annual Conference Association of Reptilian and Amphibian Veterinarians. Houston (TX), August 29-September 2, 2015. p. 475.
14. Taylor EN, DeNardo DF. Reproductive ecology of Western Diamond-Backed Rattlesnakes (*Crotalus atrox*) in the Sonoran Desert. Copeia 2005;2005:152–8.
15. Stahl SJ. Introduction to cloacoscopy in snakes. Proceedings of the North American Veterinary Conference. Orlando (FL), January 7-11, 2006. p. 1684–1685.
16. Zwart P, Kik MJ, Das AH. Dysfunction of the oviducts and salpingectomy in a boa (*C. constrictor*). Description of a case. Tijdschr Diergeneeskd 1988;113:494–7 [in Dutch].

17. Di Girolamo N, Mans C. Reptile soft tissue surgery. Vet Clin North Am Exot Anim Pract 2016;19:97–131.
18. Cruz Cardona JA, Conley KJ, Wellehan JF, et al. Incomplete ovariosalpingectomy and subsequent malignant granulosa cell tumor in a female green iguana (*Iguana iguana*). J Am Vet Med Assoc 2011;239:237–42.
19. Stahl SJ. Clinical approach to dystocia in snakes. In: Proceedings of the Annual Conference Association of Reptilian and Amphibian Veterinarians. Baltimore (MD); 2006. p. 105–109.
20. Willuhn J, Hetzel U, Preuss D, et al. Seminoma in a Brown Housesnake (*Lamprophis fuliginosus fuliginosus*). Tierärztliche Praxis 2003;3:176–9.
21. Parker MR, Mason RT. A novel mechanism regulating a sexual signal: the testosterone-based inhibition of female sex pheromone expression in garter snakes. Horm Behav 2014;66:509–16.
22. Mader DR, Bennett RA. Surgery: soft tissue, orthopedics and fracture repair. In: Mader DR, editor. Reptile medicine and surgery. 2nd edition. St Louis (MO): Saunders Elsevier; 2006. p. 581–612.
23. Alworth LC, Hernandez SM, Divers SJ. Laboratory reptile surgery: principles and techniques. J Am Assoc Lab Anim Sci 2011;50:11–26.
24. Grain E Jr, Evans JE Jr. Egg retention in four snakes. J Am Vet Med Assoc 1984; 185:679–81.
25. Millichamp NJ, Lawrence K, Jacobson ER, et al. Egg retention in snakes. J Am Vet Med Assoc 1983;183:1213–8.
26. Patterson RW, Smith A. Surgical intervention to relieve dystocia in a python. Vet Rec 1979;104:551–2.
27. Stahl SJ. Reptile obstetrics. Proceedings of the North American Veterinary Conference. Orlando (FL), January 7–11, 2006. p. 1680–1683.
28. Hedley J, Eatwell K. Cloacal prolapses in reptiles: a retrospective study of 56 cases. J Small Anim Pract 2014;55:265–8.
29. Mauldin GN, Done LB. Oncology. In: Mader DR, editor. Reptile medicine and surgery. 2nd edition. St Louis (MO): Saunders Elsevier; 2006. p. 299–322.

Reproductive Medicine in Lizards

Zdenek Knotek, DVM, PhD, DECZM (Herpetology)*, Eva Cermakova, DVM,
Matteo Oliveri, DVM

KEYWORDS

- Lizards • GnRH • Hemipenile prolapse • Dystocia • Ovarian follicles • Salpingotomy
- Salpingectomy • Ovariectomy

KEY POINTS

- Sexual dimorphism is present in many lizard species. In clinical practice, the most feasible method for sex determination in lizards is probing with lubricated or wet stainless steel rod with blunt ends.
- The most common reproductive problems in captive male lizards are hemipenile plugs and prolapsed hemipene.
- Female lizards suffer from preovulatory follicular stasis (POFS) and dystocia. It is important for the veterinarian to be able to differentiate between these reproductive disorders because the course of treatment differs.
- Mating, physical contact, or even the visual contact between male and female lizards should stimulate the ovulation and prevent the problem of POFS.
- Surgical intervention is usually required for causes of dystocia or retained ovarian follicles.

INTRODUCTION

Knowledge in the reproductive biology of lizards is essential for veterinarians in accurate and effective diagnosis and treatment of lizard patients.[1] In many lizard (eg, iguanas) species sex is determined by presence of sex chromosomes (genotypic sex determination); however, temperature-dependent sex determination exists in some lizards (*Agama agama*, *Pogona vitticeps*, *Eublepharis macularius*). Females can develop at low incubation temperatures; or females develop at either the low or high incubation temperatures, whereas males develop in at midrange temperatures.[1] Sexual maturity in lizards is determined primarily by size, with age possibly playing a less significant role. Although standard ages of sexual maturity can be found in the

This project was partially supported by the Internal Grant of the Faculty of Veterinary Medicine, University of Veterinary and Pharmaceutical Sciences Brno (IGA FVL 130/2016).
Avian and Exotic Animal Clinic, Faculty of Veterinary Medicine, University of Veterinary and Pharmaceutical Sciences Brno, 1946/1 Palackeho Street, Brno 612 42, Czech Republic
* Corresponding author.
E-mail address: knotekz@vfu.cz

Vet Clin Exot Anim 20 (2017) 411–438
http://dx.doi.org/10.1016/j.cvex.2016.11.006
1094-9194/17/© 2016 Elsevier Inc. All rights reserved.

vetexotic.theclinics.com

literature, these numbers are usually based on free-ranging animals in which all individuals in a population have similar environmental influences. However, in captivity, care and, more importantly, diet can vary dramatically; therefore, captive lizards may sexually mature at dramatically different ages.[1] Parthenogenesis, or asexual reproduction, has been reported in lizards, including monitor lizards (Komodo dragon) and lizards of the family Teiidae (more than 30% of the genus *Cnemidophorus* are parthenogenetic species). Clutch size is extremely variable in lizards with ranges from 1 to 2 (anoles, leopard gecko), 40 to 90 (oviparous species: iguanas, oviparous chameleons, veiled chameleon), 1 (some skinks), and 10 to 50 (viviparous species: slow worm *Anguis fragilis*, Jackson's chameleon).

MALE REPRODUCTIVE ANATOMY

The reptile testis is an ovoid mass of seminiferous tubules, interstitial cells, and blood vessels encased in a connective tissue sheath.[1–4] The testes are located dorsomedially within the coelomic cavity but may vary in location depending on species. The right testis is located cranial to the left. The copulatory organs are paired hemipene located laterally in the cloaca and inverting into the base of the tail. The hemipene are maintained in the tail base by a retractor muscle.[1–4]

FEMALE REPRODUCTIVE ANATOMY

The ovaries are similarly located as the testes and consist of epithelial cells, connective tissue, nerves, blood vessels, and germinal cell beds encased in an elastic tunic. The variable gross appearance depends on the stage of oogenesis, ranging from small and granular in an inactive ovary to a large lobular sac (**Fig. 1**) filled with spherical vitellogenic follicles in an active ovary.[1–4] The oviducts have both an albumin-secreting and shell-secreting function (**Fig. 2**), and no true uterus exists. The oviducts empty directly into the cloaca through genital papillae (**Fig. 3**).

Once ovulation occurs, usually little transfer of nutrients occurs between the female and the ova (in oviparous reptile species). The ovum becomes an egg when albumin and a shell are added in the oviduct. The degree of shell calcification varies between lizard species, ranging from pliable (most lizards) to rigid (geckos).[1–4] Although most lizard species lay eggs, some bear live young. Besides providing gas and possibly nutrient exchange to the developing offspring, viviparity provides some protection to the developing embryos and permits a female to easily adjust the developmental temperature.[1,4] By retaining the developing fetuses within the body for an extended period of time, the female lizard is limited to a limited number of clutches per year.

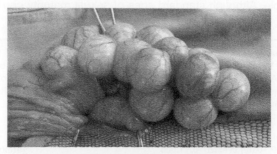

Fig. 1. Vitellogenic follicles in an active ovary (*Iguana iguana*).

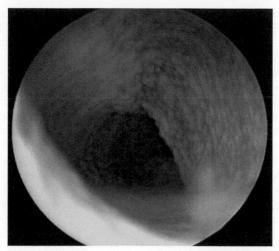

Fig. 2. Cloacoscopy. Endoscopic view of the oviducts in an adult female green iguana (*Iguana iguana*).

In addition, the space occupied by the fetuses limits the function of the gastrointestinal tract; therefore, reptiles usually limit or cease feeding during the latter stages of pregnancy.[4]

In captivity, however, extensive postpartum feeding may allow for naturally biannual breeding species to produce annually. Oviparous species may also suspend feeding during the later stages of egg development; however, the length of time during which feeding is reduced is much shorter (some weeks) and has a less significant effect.[1]

A major step in the maturation of the reptilian follicle is the accumulation of yolk, or vitellogenesis. Estrogen stimulates the liver to convert lipid from the body's fat stores and to synthetize the precursor of the lipoproteins and phosphoproteins

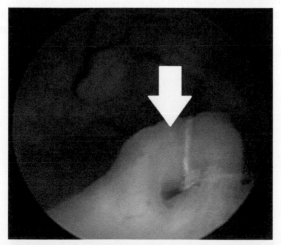

Fig. 3. Cloacoscopy. Endoscopic view of the urodeum with the papilla (*arrow*) in an adult female green iguana (*Iguana iguana*).

(vitellogenin). During this time, the liver enlarges dramatically and takes on a yellowish color. The vitellogenin is selectively absorbed from the bloodstream by the follicles. The mature ovum is 10-fold to 100-fold larger than its previtellogenic size.[1,4] In most lizards, calcium is predominantly supplied to the offspring in the yolk. Therefore, plasma calcium levels are extremely high during vitellogenesis.[5,6] In oviparous species of female lizards, 3 main reproductive stages were identified, including the previtellogenic stage (with the absence of visible follicular structures), the vitellogenic stage (with the presence of round follicular structures), and the gravid stage (with the presence of eggs in oviducts).[7] The follicles selectively absorb the vitellogenin from the bloodstream, plumping the follicle with yolk. Before ovulation, the mature follicles will appear as a cluster of grapes and are of soft-tissue opacity on radiographs. Once the ovum has ovulated, it will have albumen and the shell added in the oviduct, and it becomes an egg (**Figs. 4** and **5**) visible on radiographs due to its calcification (**Fig. 6**). Clinical problems associated with reproducing captive lizards are relatively common.

The important prerequisite for any study focused on successful hormonal management of reptile reproduction in captivity is to understand of how gonadal activity in reptiles is regulated by the hypothalamus-pituitary-gonadal axis and other hormones.[8] In female veiled chameleons, the difference between ovulatory and anovulatory cycles appears to be associated with plasma progesterone concentration (P_4). In ovulatory cycles, a marked increase in P_4 was noted when plasma estrogen concentration (E_2) was declining and plasma testosterone concentration (T) was increasing; whereas, in anovulatory cycles, P_4 peak maximum values were significantly lower than in ovulatory cycles.[9] In a group of captive chameleon females, E_2 rose during the vitellogenesis stage and peaked in the late vitellogenesis period, and P_4 rose during the late vitellogenic stage, peaked in mid-gravidity, and fell to baseline values at oviposition. T levels varied during the previtellogenic and vitellogenic stages, then mirrored P_4 with a distinct peak during the time of ovulation and gravidity.[7] Ovulation did occur with the decreasing estrogen: progesterone ratio. The influence of the first anovulatory ovarian cycle on the outcome of the subsequent cycle in female veiled chameleons is supposed. Several females underwent an ovulatory cycle after 1 or even 2 anovulatory cycles. It was observed that approximately 50% female veiled chameleons that did not lay eggs through the normal reproductive period contained large masses of ovarian follicles at the time of necropsy or ovariectomy, some of which were atretic based on histopathologic examination (**Fig. 7**).[9]

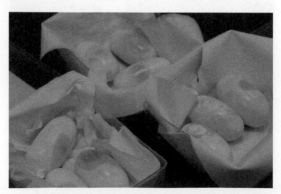

Fig. 4. Fertilized eggs with the presence of pink spots (*Iguana iguana*).

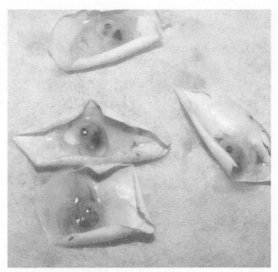

Fig. 5. The inside view of the fertilized eggs with embryos (*Iguana iguana*).

SEXING

Sexual dimorphism of adult animals is present in many lizard species (**Figs. 8–10**).[1–4] Some species are dimorphic from hatching (presence of heel spurs on the rear limbs in male veiled chameleons). Femoral, preanal, or anal pores are enlarged in mature males and smaller or absent in females (**Fig. 11**). In clinical practice, probing is the most feasible method for sex determination in medium to large species of lizards. Probing the inverted hemipenis is done with a gentle narrow sexing-probe (stainless steel rod with blunt ends, fine catheter). A lubricated or wet probe is gently inserted in the external opening of the hemipenial sac and directed slowly toward the tail tip (**Fig. 12**). In male lizards, the probe will pass to the depth of one-quarter to one-third of the tail length, whereas the probe will only pass to a depth of 2 to 6 scales in female lizards.[1,2] Ultrasonography and endoscopy (coelioscopy, cloacoscopy) may be used for gender determination (**Fig. 13**) in monomorphic lizard species (skink, monitor lizard, Gila monster, and bearded lizard) and in juvenile lizards.[10–15]

COMMON REPRODUCTIVE DISEASES IN MALE LIZARDS

The most common reproductive problems in captive male lizards are the presence of caseous mass with desquamated cornified epithelial cells (hemipenile plugs) in hemipenial sac, testicular cyst (**Fig. 14**), and unilateral or bilateral hemipenile prolapse.[1–3,16]

Hemipenile Plugs

The tips of plugs are dried and hardened, plugs become large and cause discomfort in animal (**Fig. 15**). The plug can be grasped with a fine forceps and pulled in a cranial direction. Additional manual assistance, by pushing the caudal end of the plug forward, or the surgical treatment of the retained hemipenile plug, may be necessary in some cases.[2]

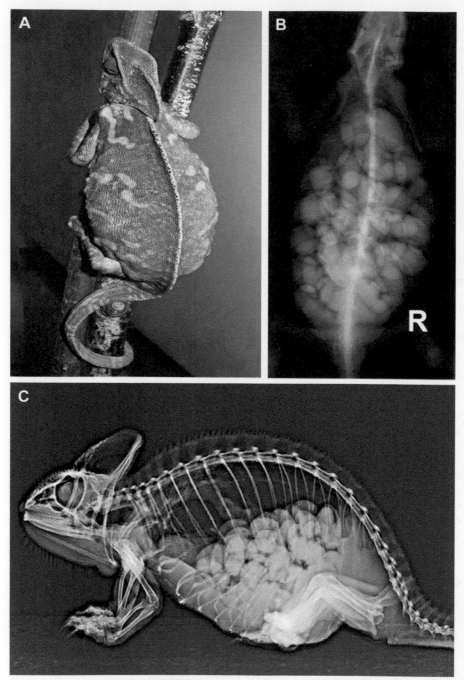

Fig. 6. Gravid female veiled chameleon (*Chamaeleo calyptratus*). The typical color pattern of the skin and shape of the body (*A*). The eggs are visible on dorsal (*B*) and lateral (*C*) radiographs due to their calcification.

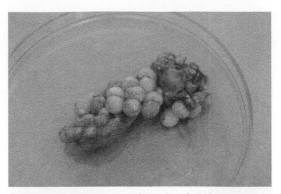

Fig. 7. Chronic oophoritis with large mass of ovarian follicles and necrotic ovary in veiled chameleon (*Chamaeleo calyptratus*).

Hemipenile Prolapse

Hemipenile prolapse is a common condition of male lizards (**Fig. 16**). Prolapse occurs as a result of trauma while the hemipenis is everted for copulation. Severely trauma-tized tissue is highly vascularized and quickly swells, making hemipenile retraction difficult or impossible.[1–3,16] Therapy in uncomplicated (acute) cases is by reposition of cleaned and moistened hemipenis after reduction of the edema and pain with cold compresses, topical (EMLA cream), and/or systemic (meloxicam, 0.3–1 mg/kg, every 24 hours, intramuscularly) administration of analgesics. In more complicated cases, short anesthesia, with propofol or alfaxalone, is necessary before the reposition of prolapsed hemipenis. The sac is filled with an antibiotic ointment and the opening of the sac is sutured with monofilament absorbable material to prevent recurrence for 3 to 5 days.

In chronic cases, the exposed swollen tissue is subjected to further trauma with bleeding. Because of the extensive desiccation and necrosis, prolapsed hemipenis must be amputated (phallectomy).[1–3,16–21] Before the hemipenis amputation, the

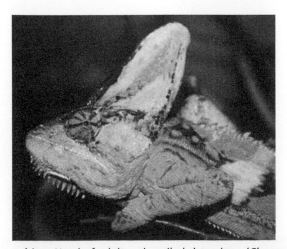

Fig. 8. Sexual dimorphism. Head of adult male veiled chameleon (*Chamaeleo calyptratus*).

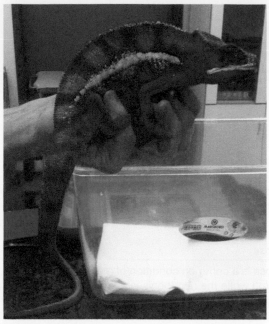

Fig. 9. Sexual dimorphism. Typical color pattern of the skin in adult male panther chameleon (*Furcifer pardalis*).

base of hemipenis is ligated with 2 or 3 absorbable transfixing sutures. The hemipenis is excised distal to the ligatures. Short anesthesia (propofol or alfaxalone) and analgesia (EMLA cream, meloxicam) are necessary before the hemipenile amputation.

Cloacal Prolapse

Cloacal prolapse, as the possible consequence of the reproductive tract disease, is very uncommon in male lizards.

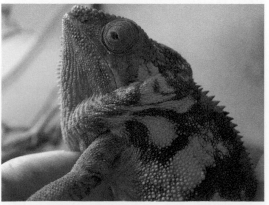

Fig. 10. Sexual dimorphism. Typical shape of the head and color pattern of the skin in adult female panther chameleon (*Furcifer pardalis*).

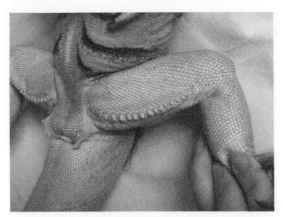

Fig. 11. Sexual dimorphism. Enlarged femoral pores in adult male green iguana (*Iguana iguana*).

Therapeutic and Preventive Orchiectomy

Therapeutic orchiectomy may be performed in male lizards as a treatment of testicular disease.[12,16–19] The effectiveness of preventive castration (**Fig. 17**) to reduce male behavioral problems in robust reptile species (iguanas, monitor lizards) is still not clear and is controversial with principles of animal welfare (anesthesia and surgery that are not necessary for the wellbeing of the animal). Due to short mesorchium with testicular artery and veins, and position of adrenal gland, vascular clips are recommended for ligation the testicle-associated vessels before dissection, rather than use of suture material.[12,19] The most challenging step in orchiectomy is to prevent

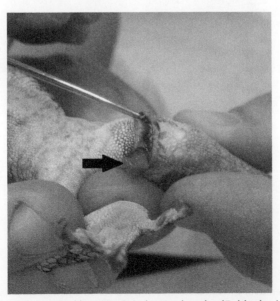

Fig. 12. Probing the left inverted hemipenis in leopard gecko (*Eublepharis macularius*) with lubricated narrow stainless steel rod. The right hemipenis (*arrow*) is everted.

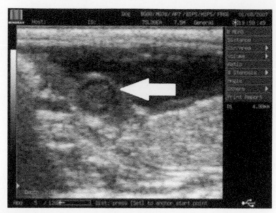

Fig. 13. Ultrasonography used for gender determination in monomorphic lizard Gila monster (*Heloderma suspectum*). The follicle (*arrow*) is present on ovary.

any trauma on the left adrenal gland and left renal vein. Endoscopic orchiectomy is recommended.[12,13]

COMMON REPRODUCTIVE DISEASES IN FEMALE LIZARDS

Reproductive diseases are important causes of morbidity in captive female reptiles. It is difficult to determine whether a female reptile is undergoing a physiologic or a pathologic reproductive cycle. Gestational duration, clutch size, or number of

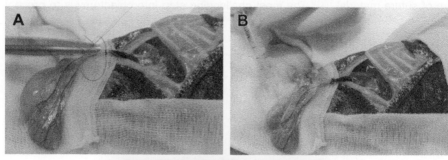

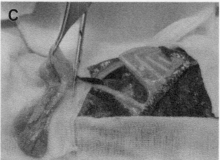

Fig. 14. Surgical removal of testicular cyst in male veiled chameleon (*Chamaeleo calyptratus*). Ligature of the vessel connection (*A*), aspiration of the fluid from the cyst (*B*), and excision of the cyst distal to the ligature (*C*).

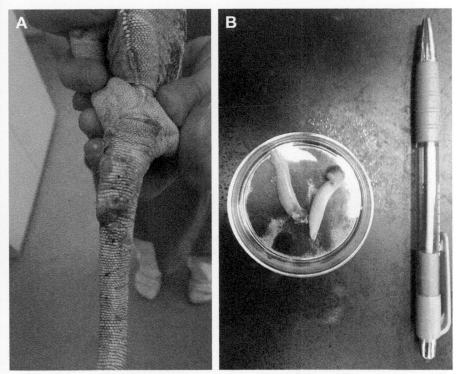

Fig. 15. The chronic inflammation of the right hemipenial sac due to the presence of hemipenile plugs in male veiled chameleon (*Chamaeleo calyptratus*). The left hemipenis is partially everted (*A*). Hemipenile plugs (*B*).

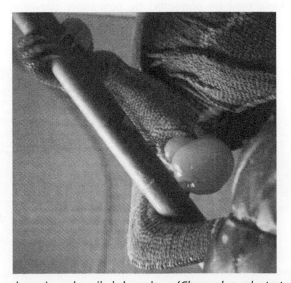

Fig. 16. Cloacal prolapse in male veiled chameleon (*Chamaeleo calyptratus*).

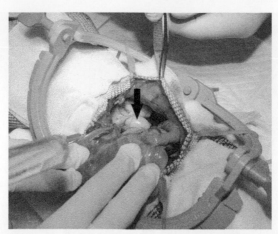

Fig. 17. Preventive castration (orchiectomy) in male green iguana (*Iguana iguana*). The oval-shaped white testicle (*black arrow*) is located in the center of the surgical field.

neonates (in viviparous lizard species) varies among species of lizards.[1,4] Female lizards (veiled chameleons, bearded dragons, and green iguanas) kept under low-quality husbandry practices (suboptimal temperature, limited exposure to ultraviolet radiation, small terrariums with crowding and stress, insufficient feeding regime) suffer from retained ovarian follicles (preovulatory follicular stasis [POFS]) and dystocia (egg binding, postovulatory egg stasis [POES]).[1–3,5–7,22–24] Cloacal prolapse or prolapse of the oviduct can be present in female lizard as a complication of chronic dystocia (**Fig. 18**).

It is very important for the veterinarian to be able to differentiate between 2 major reproductive disorders, POFS and POES, because the course of treatment differs. Mating, physical contact, or even the visual contact between male and female lizards should stimulate the ovulation and prevent the problem of POFS. Simple non-obstructive dystocia may be corrected by husbandry providing an appropriate nesting area.

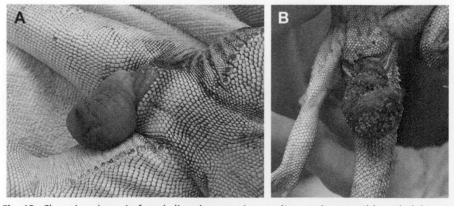

Fig. 18. Cloacal prolapse in female lizards: green iguana (*Iguana iguana; A*) bearded dragon (*Pogona vitticeps; B*).

Preovulatory Follicular Stasis

During the normal ovarian cycle, after ovulation, the postovulatory follicles are transformed into corpora lutea.[4] Under abnormal environment, preovulatory follicles persist for weeks (**Fig. 19**). Follicles enlarge and are filled with yellowish vitelline. POFS occurs in healthy young female lizards kept alone without any contact with males or females. Clinical signs of POFS can be very varied (**Fig. 20**) and female lizards may remain in a reasonable state for weeks. Manipulation of the animal (palpation of the coelom) may cause rupture of the follicles and subsequent inflammation of the ovary. Vitelline is highly irritating and can cause severe coelomitis (vitelline yolk pleuroperitonitis).[1–3,5,6,18]

Dystocia

Many conditions can lead to dystocia in female lizards. It can be caused by obstructive anatomic or nonobstructive physiologic abnormalities.[1–3,22,25] Anatomic abnormalities leading to obstructive dystocia in lizards include abnormally shaped eggs, necrotic masses, oviductal stricture, granulomas, and neoplasia. Nonobstructive conditions leading to dystocia in lizards may result from obesity, disease of the endocrine system, hypocalcaemia, infection of the oviduct, and inappropriate husbandry conditions.[1,22,25] Eggs become adherent to the walls of oviducts if they are not

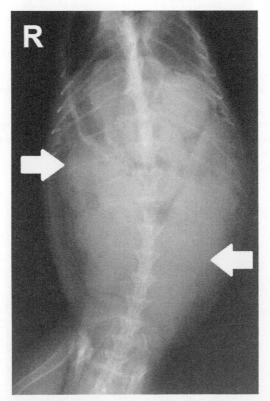

Fig. 19. Radiography, dorsal view. The presence of ovarian follicles (*arrows*) in coelom of female green iguana (*Iguana iguana*).

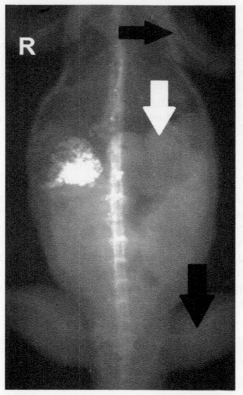

Fig. 20. Radiography, dorsal view. The presence of ovarian follicles (*white arrow*) and long bone fractures (*black arrows*) in female green iguana (*Iguana iguana*) suffering from POFS.

passed at the appropriate time. Clinical signs of dystocia can be very varied and lizards may remain in a reasonable state for weeks or months after the end of the gestation period before coming ill.[1–3,22,25] The female lizards may be either restless or subdued (**Figs. 21–23**).

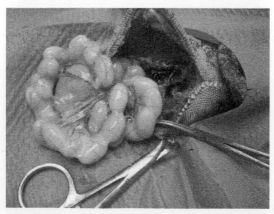

Fig. 21. Dystocia with salpingitis in veiled chameleon (*Chamaeleo calyptratus*).

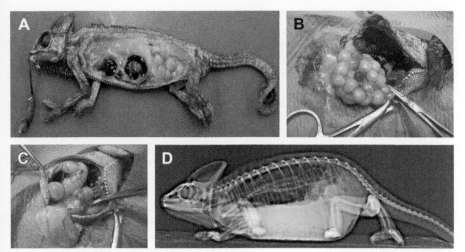

Fig. 22. Coelomitis (vitelline yolk pleuroperitonitis) in veiled chameleon (*Chamaeleo calyptratus*) (*A, B*). Egg yolk is present in coelom and oviduct (*C*). Lateral radiographic view of the female with chronic pleuroperitonitis (*D*).

Pharmacologic treatment options for dystocia

The efficacy of medical treatment varies depending on how long retained eggs or follicles persist. Calcium gluconate (100 mg/kg) is administered intramuscularly or subcutaneously twice in 6 hour intervals and oxytocin (5–10 IU) could be then administered intramuscularly. The problem of effective treatment the nonobstructive dystocia in lizards (the most common type of dystocia in these reptiles) is that conservative treatment with oxytocin and some other methods of conservative therapy are rarely effective.[1] It is also not common that gentle manipulation of eggs caudally with the coelom and cloacal massage are effective in removing retained eggs from female lizards, and the method of percutaneous aspiration of yolk (ovocentesis) that would "help to collapse the egg in female snakes"[3] proved to be dangerous for the female lizards in clinical practice.

Cloacal Prolapse, Prolapse of the Oviduct

Prolapse of cloaca and/or oviduct are common in female lizards.[1–3,22,25,26] Minor, uncomplicated, cloacal prolapse can be gently replaced after the mucosa has been cleaned and moistened (EMLA cream). Simple interrupted sutures, placed near the

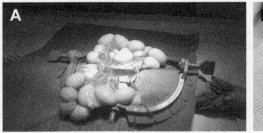
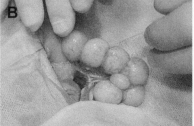

Fig. 23. Female green iguana (*Iguana iguana*). Patient with POE (*A*). Patient with POFS (*B*).

edges of cloaca, prevent recurrence. Severe prolapse is treated by transcutaneous cloacopexy or cloacal resection.[1-3,17,19,26] In full accordance with Hernandez-Divers,[17] the author (ZK) considers that cloacal or oviduct prolapses are often treated inappropriately by replacement of the prolapsed organ (mucosa) without proper investigation of the underlying case with the standard diagnostic protocol and methods (plasma chemistry, radiography, ultrasonography, coelioscopy). Therefore, in case of oviduct prolapse, even if the prolapsed tissue is viable, a coeliotomy with salpingotomy or salpingectomy is recommended.[17]

Concurrently with the continual development of modern minimally invasive surgical methods, advanced nonsurgical techniques for management of reproduction in captive lizards have been also performed (to stimulate or to suppress effectively sexual activity, to improve a quality of semen for artificial insemination, to decrease a percentage of embryonic or fetal mortality).[27-29]

Recent studies focused on the clinical use of gonadotropin releasing hormone (GnRH) implants (deslorelin) in young female green iguanas and veiled chameleons. In the experimental groups, implants did effectively suppress the reproductive activity of female green iguanas but did not suppress the reproductive activity of female veiled chameleons kept in groups.[24,28]

Therefore, surgical intervention (ovariectomy, salpingotomy, salpingectomy, or salpingectomy with ovariectomy) is usually required for causes of dystocia or preovulatory follicles especially in female lizards.

PREOPERATIVE CARE

Fluid support (20 mL/kg every 24 hours) via a subcutaneous route helps maintain hydration and protect function of the kidney. Keeping the patient warm with an electric heating pad during and after surgery is very important.

ANESTHESIA, ANALGESIA

The standard protocol of anesthesia in the author's (ZK) practice is based on the use of inhalation anesthesia after induction with short-acting anesthetics, propofol, or alfaxalone.[30-32] Anesthesia starts with combination of analgesics butorphanol (0.3–2 mg/kg, intramuscularly) and meloxicam (0.3–1.0 mg/kg, intramuscularly), followed after 30 to 45 minutes by alfaxalone (5 mg/kg, intravenously) or propofol (5 mg/kg, intravenously).

An endotracheal tube is inserted within 1 to 2 minutes and the patient is kept under inhalation anesthesia with isoflurane and oxygen. An intravenous plastic catheter is most often used as an endotracheal tube. Tracheal tube insertion is easy in iguanas and agamid lizards; however, in chameleons it is a difficult procedure that must be done with patience and delicacy. It is challenging due to a narrow and deep oral cavity and large tongue and, particularly, to an unusually sigmoid trachea and very small glottis. Vital functions of the lizard during anesthesia and surgery can be monitored by various devices. A Doppler heart rate monitor proved to be the most useful and available method of noninvasive monitoring in clinical practice. Reflexes (toe-pinch, tail-pinch, palpebral, righting, tongue-pinch) and reaction to external stimuli are gently evaluated at regular intervals before and after the surgery.[30,31]

SURGICAL TREATMENT OPTIONS

For ovariectomy, salpingectomy, or salpingotomy, most female lizards, iguanas, agamid lizards, and geckos are placed in dorsal recumbence.[17-19,22] Female chameleons are placed in lateral recumbence (left or right side) and lateral (flank) coeliotomy is performed.[17–19,22,30] The female is placed on a heating pad in the dorsal position (lateral position in chameleons) and the head and hind legs are secured with tape and fixed to the drape. Skin is prepared for a surgery by the standard protocol (disinfection with chlorhexidine). In female green iguanas and robust agamid lizards the paramedian approach or the midline approach with craniocaudal incision of the ventral abdominal skin is provided with a small scalpel blade or with scissors. The advantage of the paramedian approach is the safe preservation of the abdominal vein, which is easily seen laterally to the incision line. The advantage of the midline approach is the easy accessibility, equal to both sides, of the left and right ovaria and oviducts in the coelom (**Fig. 24**). In the paramedian approach, the incision is made sagittally. In small lizard species, such as leopard geckos or anoles, the paramedian approach is the best choice and is preferred over the median approach to avoid the ventral abdominal vein. The distance of the incision from the midline depends on the size of the lizard (less than 1 cm in very small lizards, more than 2 cm in large lizards). At the moment of complete loss of reactions, wet sterile drapes are placed around the surgical wound. The skin is delicately separated from the muscle layer. The abdominal musculature and pleuroperitoneum are thin and can be easily incised by laser or radiosurgery.[17–19] Sharp dissection of the muscles is avoided to minimize bleeding and to optimize healing. The author (ZK) prefers the method of blunt dissection using the small hemostat and fingers of the surgeon. Abdominal retractors are useful to achieve appropriate exposure of coelom organs (**Fig. 25**). With gentle care, the paired fat bodies are partially exteriorized and placed on the wet sterile drapes (**Fig. 26**).

With POFS, the best choice is to remove both large ovaries to prevent future problems. The avascular area of ovarian interfollicular connective tissue is selected for placement of finger or the grasping forceps (**Fig. 27**), taking care to avoid rupture of ovarian follicles.[17–19,22,30] Gentle traction is applied and the ovary is cautiously retracted toward the coelom incision. Exteriorization is continued until all follicles are visible and clear cranial and caudal borders of the mesovarium are visible (**Fig. 28**). The ovarium-associated vessels in mesovarium are ligated with absorbable suture material (or vascular clips) and the mesovarium is transected distal to the ligatures (**Fig. 29**). Examination of the ligation sites is performed

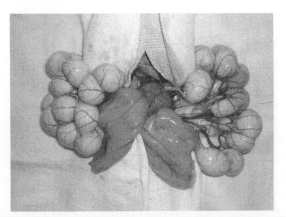

Fig. 24. The midline approach with easy accessibility of the left and right oviducts in the coelom in female green iguana (*Iguana iguana*).

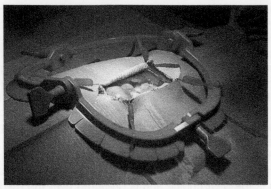

Fig. 25. Lone star retractor is useful tool for appropriate exposure of coelom and female reproductive organs.

to verify hemostasis and to confirm complete excision of all ovarian tissue. If any small follicles (smaller than a pinhead) are overlooked (**Fig. 30**), they can dramatically enlarge within few weeks or months and the patient must be operated on again.

Ovariectomy is generally recommended to prevent POFS in solitary female pet lizards. Based on the author's (ZK) experience, the optimum time for standard ovariectomy is when active ovaries are maximally enlarged and easily grasped and elevated on entering the female lizard's coelom. Preventive ovariectomy in female with inactive (small) ovaries is more difficult and is best provided by minimally invasive surgery (endosurgery).[12–14,17]

In dystocia (POES), the eggs (salpingotomy) or eggs with oviducts (salpingectomy) must be removed (**Fig. 31**). The oviduct must be gently exteriorized and placed on wet sterile drapes (**Fig. 32**). The oviduct is incised and the eggs are removed (salpingotomy). The oviduct is then gently sutured using absorbable monofilament material in a single layer. The presence of eggs just in front of the cloaca can complicate surgery. If they cannot be easily exteriorized via the cloaca, they should be carefully pushed

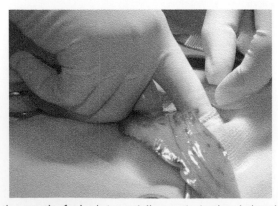

Fig. 26. With gentle care, the fat body is partially exteriorized and placed on the wet sterile drape in female bearded dragon (*Pogona vitticeps*).

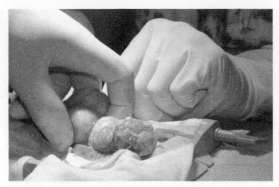

Fig. 27. Remove large ovaries with follicles by grasping the avascular area of ovarian inter-follicular connective tissue in female green iguana (*Iguana iguana*).

proximally through the cloaca so they can be removed via the incision in the oviduct wall.

In many cases the whole oviduct must be removed. Before the salpingectomy, the distal end of the oviduct (close to its insertion with cloaca) is closed with 2 transfixing ligatures and all of the oviduct-associated vessels in the mesosalpinx must be ligated with absorbable sutures (or vascular clips). The oviduct with eggs is removed after transection between the oviduct and the ligatures (**Fig. 33**).[17–19,22]

In female chameleons, the skin is incised along the curvature of the ribs.[17–19,30] Here, the surgeon must be very careful not to damage the small veins located close to the caudal margin of the ribs. Before entering the coelom, inhalation anesthesia should be adequately adjusted to stop breathing for 15 to 30 seconds. If this is not done, air sacs may sharply protrude into the surgical wound, which will make the operation in chameleons difficult. The muscle layer and pleuroperitoneum are transected with small scissors. Once the coelom cavity is entered, the fat body and the ipsilateral ovarium with follicles (or the oviducts with eggs) are gently exteriorized (**Fig. 34**). Forceps or the fingers of the surgeon are passed gently into the coelom to facilitate manipulation of follicles or oviducts. In female chameleons, the contralateral ovary can often be exteriorized and resected in the same way as the

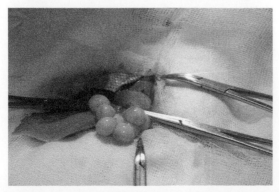

Fig. 28. Gentle exteriorization of the ovary in female bearded dragon (*Pogona vitticeps*). Ovarian follicles and cranial and caudal borders of the mesovarium are visible.

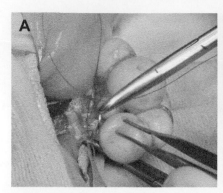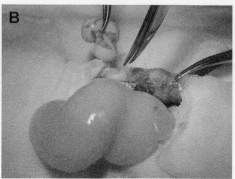

Fig. 29. Ovariectomy in female green iguana (*Iguana iguana*) (*A*) and Chinese water dragon (*Physignathus cocincinus*) (*B*). The ligation of ovarium-associated vessels in mesovarium (*A*) and the trans-section between the ovary and the ligatures (*B*).

ipsilateral. It means that bilateral ovariectomy or salpingectomy may be achieved via a unilateral incision. If needed, a contralateral incision can be made for additional access.

It is generally accepted that if oviducts have to be removed, then the ovaries also should be removed to prevent future ovulation. The problem is that ovaries in this situation (POES) are small, they are deeply situated, and it is technically difficult to provide the ovariectomy. Endoscopic ovariectomy can be an option or the reptile owner can be asked to control the animal's health condition and behavior within the next weeks or months. In the author's (ZK) clinical practice, the system of 2 surgeries (ovariectomy some weeks or months after previous salpingectomy) proved to be good solution of the problem, especially in female chameleons.

Once the procedure (ovariectomy, salpingotomy, or salpingectomy) has been completed, the fat bodies are gently returned back to coelom. The muscle layer and pleuroperitoneum are closed (usually together in small lizard species) with 4-0 absorbable monofilament material in a simple continuous pattern. The skin must be closed

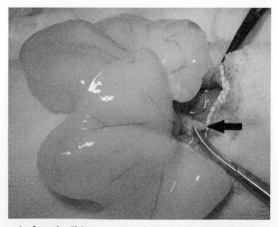

Fig. 30. Ovariectomy in female Chinese water dragon (*Physignathus cocincinus*). Exteriorization of small pinhead-shaped follicles (*arrow*).

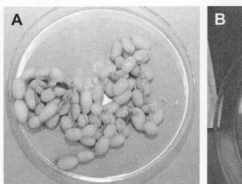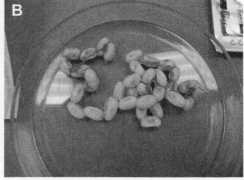

Fig. 31. Salpingectomy in female veiled chameleon (*Chamaeleo calyptratus*). Fresh eggs (*A*) and old eggs (*B*) are present in the oviduct.

using an everting suture pattern, the horizontal mattress, with appropriate size nonabsorbable suture, or absorbable suture (4-0, 3-0).

POSTOPERATIVE CARE

In the moment of restoration of reflexes (tail-pinch, toe-pinch, palpebral, tongue withdrawal), the female patient is extubated and placed back in a heated terrarium. Postoperative care may include administration of antibiotics for 8 days. For at least 10 to 14 days postoperatively, the patient should remain in a warm and clean environment. Fluid therapy (amino acids, minerals, vitamins, and glucose) may be necessary to prevent dehydration after surgery. If the patient is anorectic, it may require force-feeding with a critical care diet for exotic animals to prevent weight loss and nutritional deficiencies. Skin sutures should be removed in approximately 6 weeks after the surgery.

REPRODUCTIVE ULTRASONOGRAPHY

Ultrasonography can be used to distinguish the general stages of follicle development, including gonadal inactivity, early previtellogenic follicle growth, vitellogenesis, ovulation, and either shelling or fetal development (**Fig. 35**). Birth can be predicted with

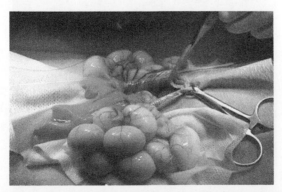

Fig. 32. Gentle exteriorized oviduct is placed on wet sterile drapes. Green iguana (*Iguana iguana*).

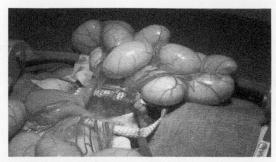

Fig. 33. Salpingectomy in female green iguana (*Iguana iguana*). Ligated oviduct-associated vessels in mesosalpinx before the transection between the oviduct and the ligatures.

monitoring of the loss of yolk by the use of ultrasonography. Birth usually occurs about a week after yolk is no longer detectable.[1,33]

REPRODUCTIVE ENDOSCOPY

Coelioscopy and cloacoscopy are valuable diagnostic techniques that can be used in reproductive medicine in lizards. Performing endoscopy requires an in-depth knowledge of the anatomy of lizards. The methods of reproductive endoscopy need practical training and good clinical experience because any kind of technical mistake during the endoscopy would be dangerous for the animal.

Indications or Contraindications

Indications and contraindications include the following:

- Coelioscopy is indicated for the evaluation of lizards with clinical signs of reproductive disease, including oophoritis and salpingitis (**Fig. 36**).
- Coelioscopy is also used for treatment as a minimally invasive surgical procedure (reproductive endosurgery) in lizards.
- Cloacoscopy allows minimally-invasive, yet detailed, visual examination of the mucosa of cloaca, urinary bladder, distal colon, ovaries, and oviduct (**Fig. 37**).

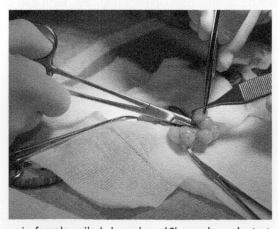

Fig. 34. Ovariectomy in female veiled chameleon (*Chamaeleo calyptratus*).

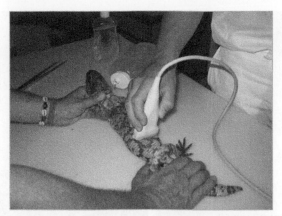

Fig. 35. The practical use of ultrasonography in monitoring the ovarian activity in a Gila monster (*Heloderma suspectum*).

- Both methods are safe, no changes in the general health of lizards have been observed following cloacoscopy.
- The only known contraindication is associated with anesthesia.

Coelioscopy

The coelom of lizard is examined with rigid endoscopes of various diameters, depending on the size of the animal.[11–15] The Hopkins Documentation Forward-Oblique Telescope (30°, ø 2.7 mm, 18 cm) and the Hopkins Slender Telescope (30°, ø 1.9–2.1 mm, 18 cm) can be used with or without operating sheaths, depending on the size of the animal. Lizards are positioned in dorsal or lateral recumbence (lateral recumbence in chameleons). There is no significant difference in visualization of reproductive organs in male or female lizards from either the left or the right approach.[11–15] However, the left

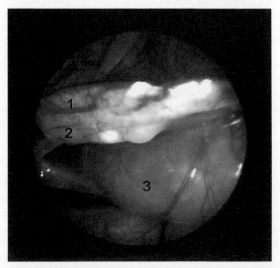

Fig. 36. Coelioscopy in young female green iguana (*Iguana iguana*). Adrenal gland (*1*), ovarium (*2*), colon (*3*).

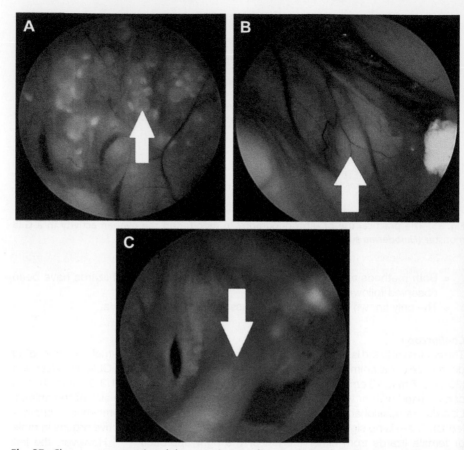

Fig. 37. Cloaca cystoscopy in adult green iguana (*Iguana iguana*). Endoscopic indirect view of the ovarian surface (*white dots, arrow*) through the semitransparent wall of the urinary bladder (*A*). Endoscopic indirect control of eggs presence (*arrow*) through the semitransparent wall of the urinary bladder (*B*). Urodeum with the septum (*arrow*) between the distal colon and the urogenital tract (*C*).

approach is generally preferred for coelioscopy in lizards. The entry area is bordered by ribs, the spine, and the left hind limb. A small skin incision is made in the center of this area. The rigid endoscope is inserted into coelom through the operating sheath and pneumocoelom is created with carbon dioxide insufflation.[11–15] Testes are ovoid and smooth, the ovaries appear as clusters of follicles. The size of gonads varies with season (**Fig. 38**).

Cloacoscopy
The lizard's cloaca is examined with the standard instrumentation as for coelioscopy. The following clinical implications exist for cloacoscopy in lizards: cloacal examination of the reptile patient, presence of discharges from oviduct (can be observed and sampled if necessary). The standard cloacoscopy is recommended for clinical practice with lizards for visualization of the proctodeum, urodeum, and coprodeum. The method is safe and allows a detailed evaluation of the distal colon, urogenital papillae, and urinary bladder. Short-time anesthesia can be performed with propofol or alfaxalone administered intravenously. The cloacoscopy technique relies on

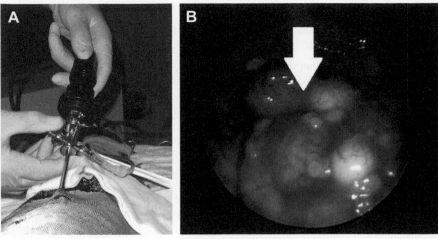

Fig. 38. Coelioscopy in green iguana (*Iguana iguana*). The rigid endoscope with endoscopy camera inserted into coelom through the operating sheath (*A*). Clusters of follicles (*arrow*) in different stadia of maturation (*B*).

directing and supporting the end of the telescope with the left hand while supporting the scope and camera with the right hand. Irrigation with sterile saline solution is used as the feasible method for distension of the cloaca. Moreover, flushing the cloaca with the sterile fluid is optimal for cleaning the mucosa and removal of the small pieces of tissue, urine, or feces from the tip of endoscope. A bag of sterile saline is suspended above the examination table and an intravenous giving set is used to connect the bag to 1 of the ports of the working sheath. A second giving set is connected from the other sheath port to a collecting bowl under the examination table. By controlling both inflow and outflow, the operator can infuse and aspirate saline, thereby providing a clean view of the cloaca and distal colon. The cloacal opening must be held shut around the scope to keep the cloaca distended[11] (**Fig. 39**).

Fluid irrigation and gently insertion the endoscope deep into the cloaca help to dilate the urodeum of cloaca and visualize the opening of colon and the opening of urinary bladder. The surgeon must check (with continuous fluid irrigation that enables opening the sphincters and distension the space) the oviducts, urinary bladder, and colon.

The author (ZK) did not record any negative health consequences associated with short-term cloacoscopy in the lizards (green iguana, bearded dragon) examined.

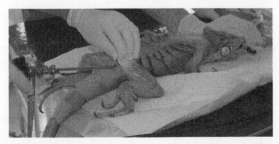

Fig. 39. Cloacoscopy in adult male green iguana (*Iguana iguana*). The cloacal opening is held shut around the scope to keep the cloaca distended with sterile saline irrigation.

SUMMARY

The results of clinical studies of reproductive medicine in female veiled chameleons, green iguanas, and bearded dragons indicate that

- High temperatures, long days, and high energy diet can initiate the breeding activity earlier and maintain it for longer than environmental conditions permit in the wild.
- Stress and social conditions, including unwanted sexual composition of the group (absence of a male in the same terrarium with a female during the heat season, presence of a male in the same terrarium with gravid female), would influence ovarian activity in captive females.
- Female are commonly presented to veterinarians for a variety of reproductive problems and, often, these problems require surgical intervention.
- Performing the diagnostics necessary to ascertain whether the reproductive problem is preovulatory or postovulatory is very important because the medical and surgical treatment varies according to which condition the female lizard is suffering from.
- Nonsurgical treatment of POFS is based on the presence of adult healthy male, which presence and active sexual behavior stimulate the female to ovulate.
- In captive females, surgical ovariectomy is recommended and commonly used to treat POFS.
- GnRH implant (deslorelin) did not suppress effectively the reproductive activity of female veiled chameleons kept in groups.[24,30]
- GnRH implant (deslorelin) may suppress effectively the reproductive activity of female green iguanas for at least 1 year.[28]

The results of clinical studies of reproductive medicine in female leopard geckos indicate

- Female leopard geckos are commonly presented to veterinarians with dystocia (POES), which usually requires surgical intervention.
- In female leopard geckos, salpingotomy is recommended and commonly used to treat POES.
- GnRH implants did not suppress effectively the reproductive activity of female leopard geckos.

REFERENCES

1. DeNardo D. Reproductive biology. In: Mader DR, editor. Reptile medicine and surgery. 2nd edition. St Louis (MO): Elsevier Saunders; 2006. p. 376–90.

2. Zwart P. Urogenital system. In: Beynon PH, Lawton MPC, Cooper J, editors. BSAVA manual of reptiles. 1st edition. Cheltenham (United Kingdom): BSAVA; 1992. p. 117–27.

3. Johnson JD. Urogenital system. In: Girling SJ, Raiti P, editors. BSAVA manual of reptiles. 2nd edition. Quedgeley (United Kingdom): BSAVA; 2004. p. 261–72.

4. Fox A. The urogenital system of reptiles. In: Gans C, Parsons TS, editors. Biology of the Reptilia, vol. 6. London: Academic Press; 1977. p. 1–157.

5. Knotkova Z, Pelrilova S, Knotek Z. Haemogram and plasma chemistry in female green iguana with POOS versus POFS syndrome. Proceedings of the Annual Conference European Association of Zoo and Wildlife Veterinarians. Ebeltoft, May 19–23, 2004. p. 287–9.

6. Knotek Z, Dorrestein GM, Knotkova Z, et al. Haematology and plasma chemistry in female veiled chameleons (Chamaeleo calyptratus) suffering from preovulatory follicle stasis (POFS). Proceedings of the Annual Conference European Association of Zoo and Wildlife Veterinarians. Leipzig, April 30–May 3, 2008. p. 189–95.

7. Kummrow MS, Smith DA, Crawshaw G, et al. Characterization of fecal hormone patterns associated with the reproductive cycle in female veiled chameleons (*Chamaeleo calyptratus*). Gen Comp Endocrinol 2010;168:340–8.

8. Phillips JA, Frye F, Bercovitz A, et al. Exogenous GnRh overrides the endogenous annual reproductive rhythm in green iguanas, *Iguana iguana*. J Exp Zool 1987; 241:227–36.

9. Kummrow MS, Mastromonaco GF, Crawshaw G, et al. Fecal hormone patterns during non-ovulatory reproductive cycles in female veiled chameleons (*Chamaeleo calyptratus*). Gen Comp Endocrinol 2010;168:349–55.

10. Schildger BJ, Wicker R. Sex determination and clinical examination in reptiles using endoscopy. Herpetol Rev 1989;20:9–10.

11. Schildger B. Endoscopic examination of the urogenital tract in reptiles. Proceedings of the Annual Conference Association Reptilian and Amphibian Veterinarians. Pittsburgh, October 22–24, 1994. p. 60–1.

12. Divers SJ. Lizard endoscopic techniques with particular regard to the green iguana (*Iguana iguana*). Semin Avian Exot Pet Med 1999;8:122–9.

13. Hernandez-Divers SJ. Diagnostic and surgical endoscopy. In: Girling SJ, Raiti P, editors. BSAVA manual of reptiles. 2nd edition. Quedgeley (United Kingdom): BSAVA; 2004. p. 103–14.

14. Divers SJ. Reptile diagnostic endoscopy and endo-surgery. Vet Clin North Am Exot Anim Pract 2010;13(2):217–42.

15. Divers SJ. Diagnostic endoscopy. In: Mader DR, Divers SJ, editors. Current therapy in reptile medicine and surgery. St Louis (MO): Elsevier Saunders; 2014. p. 154–78.

16. Barten SL. Penile prolapse. In: Mader DR, editor. Reptile medicine and surgery. 2nd edition. St Louis (MO): Elsevier Saunders; 2006. p. 862–4.

17. Hernandez-Divers SJ. Surgery: principles and techniques. In: Girling SJ, Raiti P, editors. BSAVA manual of reptiles. 2nd edition. Quedgeley (United Kingdom): British Small Animal Veterinary Association; 2004. p. 147–67.

18. Mader DR, Bennet RA. Surgery. In: Mader DR, editor. Reptile medicine and surgery. 2nd edition. St Louis (MO): Elsevier Saunders; 2006. p. 581–612.

19. Di Girolamo N, Mans C. Reptile soft tissue surgery. Vet Clin North Am Exot Anim Pract 2016;19:97–131.

20. Biron K, Heckers K. Removal of a testicular tumor from a veiled chameleon (*Chamaeleo calyptratus*). Proceedings of the Annual Conference Association Reptilian and Amphibian Veterinarians. South Padre Island (TX), 2010. p. 77–8.

21. Knotek Z, Barazorda Romero S, Knotkova Z, et al. Surgical removal of cyst in the testis of Yemen chameleon (in Czech). Veterinarni klinika 2013;10:153–7.

22. Funk RS. Lizard reproductive medicine and surgery. Vet Clin North Am Exot Anim Pract 2002;5:579–613.

23. Knotek Z, Knotkova Z, Möstl E, et al. Reproductive endocrinology in reptiles. Proceedings of the Conference Amphibian and Reptilian Veterinarians. Cremona, May 13–15, 2012, p. 44–7.

24. Knotek Z. Reproductive strategies in captive female veiled chameleons. Proceedings of the UPAV/AAVAC/ARAV Conference. Cairns, April 22–24, 2014. p. 127–30.

25. DeNardo D. Dystocias. In: Mader DR, editor. Reptile medicine and surgery. 2nd edition. St Louis (MO): Elsevier Saunders; 2006. p. 787–92.

26. Bennet RA, Mader DR. Cloacal prolapse. In: Mader DR, editor. Reptile medicine and surgery. 2nd edition. St Louis (MO): Elsevier Saunders; 2006. p. 751–5.
27. Kirchgesser M, Mitchell M, Domenzain L, et al. Evaluating the effect of leuprolide acetate on testosterone levels in captive male green iguanas (*Iguana iguana*). J Herpetol Med Surg 2009;19:128–31.
28. Kneidinger N. GnRH implant in green iguana (*Iguana iguana*) [Thesis]. Vienna (Austria): University of Veterinary Medicine; 2009. p. 29.
29. Johnson JG. Therapeutic review: deslorelin acetate subcutaneous implant. J Exot Pet Med 2013;22:82–4.
30. Knotek Z. Surgery in chameleons. Proceedings of the UPAV/AAVAC/ARAV Conference. Cairns, April 22–24, 2014. p. 212–21.
31. Knotek Z, Hrda A, Knotkova Z, et al. Alfaxalone anaesthesia in the green iguana (Iguana iguana). Acta Vet 2013;82:109–14.
32. Knotek Z, Hrda A, Kley N, et al. Alfaxalone anaesthesia in veiled chameleon (*Chamaeleo calyptratus*). Proceedings of the Annual Conference Association Reptilian and Amphibian Veterinarians. Seattle, August 6–12, 2011. p. 179–81.
33. Hochleithner C, Holland M. Ultrasonography. In: Mader DR, Divers SJ, editors. Current therapy in reptile medicine and surgery. St Louis (MO): Elsevier Saunders; 2014. p. 107–27.

Reptile Perinatology

Krista A. Keller, DVM, DACZM

KEYWORDS

- Reptile • Perinatology • Amniotic egg • Hatchling

KEY POINTS

- In oviparous species, the amniotic egg includes the shell, albumen, yolk and yolk sac, and extraembryonic membranes; each structure serves physiologic function(s) to support the developing embryo.
- Artificial incubation of reptile eggs should mirror natural incubation conditions in terms of temperature and moisture and requires construction of an appropriate incubation chamber or use of a commercially available incubator.
- Egg viability can be determined through visual assessment, candling, or auscultation of the embryo heart rate.
- Manual pipping should be reserved for cases of viability of the embryo in question and requires sterile technique and magnification.
- Neonates/hatchlings are at risk for suffering from the same illnesses noted in adults, including husbandry-related and infectious processes; yolk-associated illness often requires veterinary surgical intervention.

INTRODUCTION

Reptile perinatology is the time period surrounding hatching in oviparous species and surrounding birth in viviparous species. For the purposes of this review, the term perinatology includes applicable information regarding the egg, incubation period, and hatching (relevant for oviparous species) as well as hatchling/neonatal care and medicine.

THE REPTILIAN (AMNIOTIC) EGG

The reptilian egg at oviposition is composed of the egg shell, albumen (or whites), and the yolk. Each structure is involved in some support mechanism for the developing embryo (**Table 1**). Unlike avian eggs, reptilian eggs do not have an air cell or chalazae.

The author has nothing to disclose.
Vida Veterinary Care, Denver, CO 80126, USA
E-mail address: krista.keller@live.com

Vet Clin Exot Anim 20 (2017) 439–454
http://dx.doi.org/10.1016/j.cvex.2016.11.005
1094-9194/17/© 2016 Elsevier Inc. All rights reserved.

Table 1
Structures of the reptile egg at oviposition and their physiologic functions to support the developing embryo

Structure	Function (s)	Additional Notes
Shell	• Barrier between the external environment and the embryo • Porous nature allows for gas and water vapor exchange • Calcium source for the developing embryo	• Can be either soft/leathery or hard in nature • Hard-shelled eggs laid by species that naturally incubate in arid environments • Soft-shelled eggs laid by species that naturally incubate in moist environment
Albumen	• Physical support for the embryo1 • Water storage • Antimicrobial peptides protect the developing embryo	• Created by specialized glands in the material oviduct
Yolk and yolk sac	• Primary energy source for embryo and hatchling • Storage site for retinal, hormones, fatty acids, proteins, minerals •Maternal transfer of antibodies	• Can be a source of maternally derived toxins

As incubation progresses, there is development of the embryo and the extraembryonic membranes within the egg. The extraembryonic membranes are composed of the amnion, allantois, and chorion and each has a physiologic function:

• The amnion is the membrane that directly surrounds the embryo. Contraction of smooth muscles in the amnion during hatching causes retraction and is ultimately responsible for the internalization of the yolk.[1,2]
• The allantois originates at the umbilicus and is a continuation of the embryo urachus. The allantoic cavity is the major storage site for urea excretion.[3]
• The chorion is the outermost membrane that encloses the embryo, amnion, allantois, yolk, and yolk sacs.

The yolk and its yolk sac attach to the developing embryo at the umbilicus and continue as the vitelline duct (also referred to as the omphalomesenteric duct) that allows direct transfer of nutrients from the yolk to the developing embryo intestines. During incubation and embryonic development, as the yolk contents traverse the vitelline duct, the yolk size decreases while the embryo size increases.[3]

ARTIFICIAL INCUBATION
Collection of Eggs

During collection of eggs, care should be taken not to change the spatial orientation of the egg during transport or when placed into the substrate of the incubator. Turning seems to be fatal once performed after embryo attachment.[4,5] Because the exact times of embryo attachment postoviposition are not elucidated for all species, the author recommends taking care to not change the spatial orientation of the egg during transport.

Incubator

Incubators can either be constructed or purchased. There are several commercially available reptile and avian incubators. Constructed incubators should be designed with a double-chamber principle (**Fig. 1**). The eggs and substrate are within the inner chamber

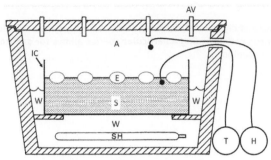

Fig. 1. Diagram of appropriate reptile incubator using an inner chamber and outer chamber design. A, air; AV, air vent; E, egg; H, hygrometer; IC, inner chamber; S, substrate; SH, submersible heater; T, thermometer; W, water.

that is suspended within a larger chamber. Either air or water can be present between the 2 chambers; when water is used, evaporation helps maintain the necessary high humidity within the incubation chamber. Buffering the heat through an air or water medium has the advantage of reducing incidence of hot spots that may reduce hatchability. When constructing an incubator, a waterproof container, such as a plastic storage bin, works well for the inner chamber whereas a larger plastic or polystyrene foam ice chest is appropriate for the outer chamber. Air flow through multiple vents should be ensured.

The incubator, whether purchased or constructed, should be set up and operational several days before the arrival of the eggs to allow for equilibration of temperature and humidity within the system. Once the ambient temperature within the incubator is established, frequent opening of the unit should be avoided. A window in the top of the incubator is standard in most commercial incubators and allows for monitoring the eggs and observation of the hatching process (**Fig. 2**).

Substrate

Within the inner chamber, various substrates are used (**Box 1**). Substrates are recommended to be moist but not wet. Use of tap water may introduce chlorine, chloramine,

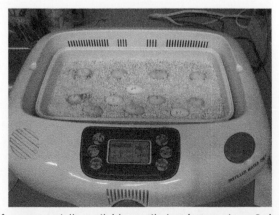

Fig. 2. Example of a commercially available reptile incubator using a 2-chamber design. The eggs or multiple species are being incubated at the same time using perlite as substrate. This incubator has a clear lid (removed in this photo) that allows for direct observation of the incubation process.

> **Box 1**
> **Substrates used successfully for artificial incubation of reptilian eggs. Consultation with an individual experienced with breeding a particular species allows for determination of the most ideal substrate medium**
>
> Vermiculite
>
> Sterilized potting soil
>
> Sand
>
> Sphagnum moss
>
> Shredded paper
>
> Coconut coir

and other potential toxins. Use of backyard-derived substrates may introduce toxins, such as pesticides. Prior to incubation, discussion with an experienced individual (breeder or zookeeper) enables more precise information regarding successful substrate types used for the species in question. Typically, the eggs are half buried in the substrate (**Fig. 3**).

Heat and Temperature Monitoring

Species-specific incubation temperatures should be followed, whenever available (**Table 2**). Abnormal incubation temperatures may lead to hatchling deficits, reduced growth and immunity, and latent effects on growth after hatching.[6–9] When kept within the species-specific temperature ranges, an inverse relationship exists between temperature and incubation length. For example, In the common wall lizard (*Podarcis muralis*), eggs incubated at a higher temperature (32°C) hatched more than 5 weeks earlier than those eggs incubated at a lower temperature (24°C).[10]

Outside of appropriate embryonic development, temperature manipulation is used to control the sex of the developing embryo(s). Many reptiles exhibit temperature-based sex determination (TSD). Unlike genotypic sex determination (GSD), where

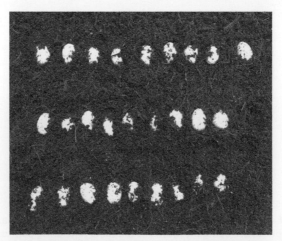

Fig. 3. Incubating panther chameleon (*Furcifer pardalis*) eggs. The substrate used is a moistened coconut coir product. Note that the eggs are half buried within the substrate.

Table 2
Clutch characteristics and recommended incubator settings for common companion reptile species

	Species	Typical Clutch Size	Humidity (%)	Temperature (°F)	Expected Hatch Time (d)[a]
Lizards	Bearded dragon (*Pogona vitticeps*)	16–24	70–80	82–86	50–80
	Leopard gecko (*Eublepharis macularius*)	1–2	80–90	80–90	35–89
	Crested gecko (*Correlophus ciliates*)	1–2	70–80	72–80	60–120
Chelonians	Red-eared slider (*Trachemys scripta elegans*)	4–25	75–85	81–86 (27.2–30)	60–80
	Eastern box turtle (*Terrapene carolina carolina*)	3–8	80–90	72–90	70–120
	Greek tortoise (*Testudo graeca*)	2–7	50–80	82–90	60–80
	Russian tortoise (*Agrionemys horsfieldii*)	1–5	50–80	84–90	80–120
Snakes	Corn snake (*Pantherophis guttatus*)	10–30	75–90	78–88	60–80
	Ball python (*Python regius*)	4–9	90–100	86–92	52–65

[a] Lower temperatures require longer incubation times whereas higher temperatures produce shorter hatch times.

sex phenotype is determined secondary to genes passed from the parents, in TSD sex phenotype is determined due to specific temperature ranges during incubation.[11] Most chelonian species studied exhibit TSD; notable exceptions include all species studied of the family Chelidae (suborder Pleurodira).[12] Of the crocodilian and Sphenodontia species studied to date, all follow a TSD pattern.[13,14] Lizards exhibit mixed patterns of sex determination, even within taxonomic families and genus. The leopard gecko (*Eublepharis macularius*) is a classically described TSD whereas the bearded dragon (*Pogona vitticeps*) exhibits GSD.[15]

Various heat sources are used to maintain incubator temperatures. Heating coils, strips, pads, and submersible aquarium heaters are commercially available. Ideally, heaters with adjustable capacities are used to maintain accurate incubation temperatures within the inner chamber. Reliable thermometers, ideally digital, should be used that allow external evaluation of the temperature in the inner chamber because repeated opening of the incubator allows loss of heat and moisture. Daily monitoring and recording of the temperature is recommended.

Moisture

If conditions are too dry, the eggs lose water mass to the environment and begin to crinkle or collapse (in cases of soft-shelled eggs). Intervention with additional moisture at this stage may be able to save an egg and its developing embryo.[3,16] At the other extreme, if an egg is surrounded by too much water, oxygen may be excluded from diffusing into the developing embryo and it may die from drowning.[16] Eggs from hard-shelled egg–laying species do not allow such impressive water diffusion; however, lack of moisture during incubation has been shown to influence hatchling size and performance in some species.[6,17] Common examples of reptile species with hard-shelled and soft-shelled eggs are presented in **Box 2**.

Moisture sources for the humidity required during incubation should come from the substrate and potentially from the water bath used between the inner and outer chamber based on incubation design. Daily misting of the substrate may help increase humidity levels but requires opening the incubator, which leads to loss of heat and moisture; thus, self-regulation of the humidity with a more closed incubator design is preferable. If misting is performed, the misting bottle should be kept at the same ambient temperature as the internal incubation temperatures. Reliable hygrometers should be used in the same fashion as thermometers that allow external evaluation of the humidity of the inner chamber with daily monitoring of humidity concentrations. Species-specific humidity recommendations are presented in **Table 2**.

DETERMINATION OF EGG VIABILITY

There are several ways to evaluate egg viability: evaluation of the external appearance, candling, and noninvasive heart rate monitoring.

- Daily monitoring of the appearance of the eggs should be performed and recorded. A healthy, viable egg should stay a consistent in color, although slight mottling to the surface of the egg may not be significant. Marked changes in color or texture or growth of fuzzy mold (**Fig. 4**) usually indicates that the embryo has either died or was nonfertile. Wrinkling and shrinking of the eggs do not always indicate embryo death but that moisture levels are too low and the egg is dehydrating (**Fig. 5**). Moistening of the surrounding substrate and checking humidity levels may be effective at rehydrating the egg, although severe dehydration may lead to embryo death.
- Candling can be performed with a high-intensity light source, such as an ophthalmic transilluminator or a commercially available egg candler. The light should be placed in direct contact with the far side of the egg in a darkened room. Candled viable eggs have a diffuse developing vascular pattern or the presence of an embryo. Nonviable eggs lack a vascular pattern and have a homogenous diffuse yellow-white appearance (**Fig. 6**). Care should be taken that the candling process is not prolonged, because heat from some light sources can damage the developing embryo and its membranes.

Box 2
Common companion reptile species categorized as laying either soft-shelled or hard-shelled eggs

Soft-Shelled (Leathery) Eggs	Hard-Shelled Eggs
Bearded dragon (*Pogona vitticeps*)	Greek tortoise (*Testudo graeca*)
Leopard gecko (*Eublepharis macularius*)	Russian tortoise (*Agrionemys horsfieldii*)
Crested gecko (*Correlophus ciliates*)	
Red-eared slider (*Trachemys scripta elegans*)	
Eastern box turtle (*Terrapene carolina carolina*)	
Corn snake (*Pantherophis guttatus*)	
Ball python (*Python regius*)	

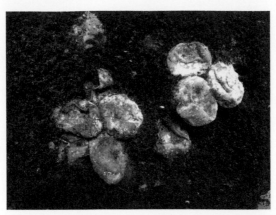

Fig. 4. Fuzzy growth on eggs during incubation often indicates a fungal or bacterial infection. The advanced state of decomposition paired with the fuzzy growth on these eggs of unknown species indicates lack of egg viability.

- Embryo heart rate monitoring can be performed for soft-shelled eggs. A standard high-frequency (7.5–10 MHz) ultrasound transducer can be used to evaluate the heart rate of the developing embryo. Water-soluble ultrasound gel can be used as an interface; however, because it may clog pores of the shell and prevent oxygen exchange, minimal gel should be used. In addition, a noninvasive commercially available infrared digital heart rate monitor (Buddy system, Avian Biotech International, Tallahassee, Florida) can be used on both hard-shelled and soft-shelled eggs. Because an infrared light is used, it can be a source of heat that may cause harm to the developing embryo if used for a prolonged amount of time.[18]

It is recommended that nonviable eggs or eggs that have an embryo that has died should be removed from the incubator, because they commonly become infected with opportunistic pathogens that can spread to other eggs in the clutch.[19] Necropsy of the removed egg and collection of samples for histopathologic and potentially bacteriologic and/or toxicologic examinations can be vital components of developing a successful incubation and hatching program. Assessment of records of daily temperatures and humidity is the most important first step in evaluation of causes of embryo death. Standard avian egg necropsy practices should be followed.

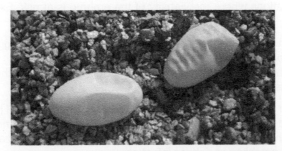

Fig. 5. Leopard gecko (*Eublepharis macularius*) eggs with a wrinkled appearance that indicates dehydration. Additional humidity to the environment often corrects this degree of dehydration. (*Courtesy of* Claire Vergneau-Grosset, méd. Vét., IPSAV (Médecine zoologique), DACZM, Universite de Montreal, Saint-Hyacinth, QC, Canada.)

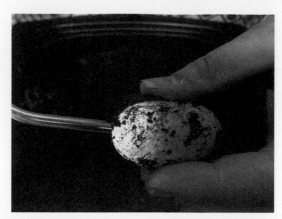

Fig. 6. Candling a box turtle (*Terrapene carolina*) egg using a high-intensity light source. This egg is nonviable based on the lack of developing vessels and/or a fetus at 60 days through incubation.

HATCHING AND MANUAL PIPPING

In the natural hatching process, immediately prior to hatching, the yolk sac is internalized into the coelomic cavity of the hatchling. After successful yolk internalization, the body wall closes around the navel. From this point, gas exchange can no longer take place through the membranes and the embryo must initiate gas exchange through its lungs. It is hypothesized that hypoxic conditions in the embryo during yolk internalization cause contraction of muscles in the neck of the hatchling, leading to pipping.[1] Pipping occurs when the egg tooth, or caruncle, is forced through the egg shell. Once the egg shell is broken, the process of emergence of the hatchling from the shell can take 24 hours to 48 hours.[1]

Hatching is expected to occur based on calculated species-specific hatch times that are additionally influenced by incubation temperatures (see **Table 2**). In many instances, the specific hatch time is not known and constant observation should be performed to investigate when the process should be expected. In some species of crocodilians, embryos begin vocalizing from within the egg prior to pipping.[20] Most eggs from the same clutch are expected to hatch within a few days of each other.

Manual pipping and intervention in the natural events of hatching should be reserved for situations where the viability of the embryo is at risk. Examples include the following:

- Vocalization was previously heard within an egg and other eggs in the clutch have been pipping, but this particular egg has not yet pipped.
- Hatchling has pipped but not progressed to full emergence in the same amount of time as its hatch mates.

The process of full emergence from the shell takes 24 hours to 48 hours[1] and prematurely initiated emergence can lead to rupture of membranes and bleeding or a hatchling emerging from the shell that has not completely internalized the yolk sac, thus placing that hatchling at risk for infection.

In cases of manual pipping indicated, sterile technique should be used with magnification. A small wedge incision is made in the top of the egg with sharp scissors. Care should be taken to avoid incising any internal vessels of the extraembryonic membranes. When performed properly, the extraembryonic membranes are left intact. If the extraembryonic membranes appear dry and tacky, rehydration can be performed with judicious use of a few drops of isotonic saline. After manual pipping is performed, the neonate should be allowed to emerge from the egg on its own.

NEONATAL/HATCHLING CARE AND MEDICINE
Husbandry

Reptile neonates are born precocious and find food, feed themselves, and perform normal functions as an adult. The housing and husbandry requirements of neonates mirror those of adults, although temperature and humidity requirements tend to be higher. Most breeders keep the neonates in an incubator for the first few days after hatching at the incubation temperatures with a humidity of 90% to 100%. Neonates do well on a simple substrate of moistened paper towels that are easy to keep clean and monitor fecal and urinary outputs. Group housing should only be pursued if appropriate for the species, and care should be taken to ensure that all individuals are eating. Cannibalism can be prevented by reducing stocking density and ensuring the neonates housed together are of similar sizes.

When considering feeding of a neonate, it is not uncommon for a neonatal reptile to not eat for the first few days to few weeks of life. During this time period, the internalized yolk is providing nutrition to the neonate. The time period that the yolk can sustain the neonate is species specific, with some snake species delaying the first meal after the first hibernation.[21] Inappropriately intervening with nutritional support during this physiologic period of fasting induces stress on the developing neonate.

In general, neonates should be fed items that mirror what adults eat, although smaller, with some exceptions. In the bearded dragon, adults tend toward herbivory whereas juveniles tend toward insectivory. Smaller versions of the adult diet should be offered, which may require breeding of insects to obtain the smallest insect size for insectivores or finely chopped vegetation in cases of herbivorous species. Because neonates are fast growing and have high nutrient demands, supplementation of foods with calcium supplement daily and a reptile-specific multivitamin weekly, whether dusted, gut loaded, or both, is recommended.

Techniques for stimulating slow-to-eat neonates are species specific or diet specific. As an example, frog-eating snakes may have little interest in the rodent prey easily fed in captivity. Individuals have had success scenting rodent prey with amphibian mucus to induce an appetite in these species. Other appetite-inducing techniques may include slap feeding in snakes, warming of food items, or placing food in a neonate's mouth. In cases were true assist or force feeding must be performed, care should be taken to carefully calculate stomach volume (typically 1%–3% of body weight) and to gently use a soft pliable tube, such as a 3.5-French or 5-French red rubber tube with water-based lubrication so as not to harm the delicate tissues.

Diagnostics

In many cases, diagnostics used for adults can be similarly used in neonatal patients.

- Complete blood cell count and plasma biochemical references intervals for neonates have not been evaluated for any companion reptile species known to the author; however, intervals for adults can be extrapolated to juvenile specimens judiciously. In several species of sea turtles, articles are available that report complete blood cell count and plasma biochemical reference intervals for juveniles and compare juvenile and adult blood parameters.[22,23] Many neonates are of a size that precludes or severely limits the volume of blood that can be obtained. Venipuncture sites available mirror those in the adult (**Fig. 7**).

- Radiographs may be used, and dentistry radiographic units may be most appropriate for the small size of hatchlings.
- Sex determination of hatchlings is an important topic, and there are many resources outlining endoscopic methods of sex identification in a variety of chelonian species.[24–26]
- Necropsy of deceased neonates is advisable and standard techniques similar to those used for adults are recommended.

Diseases

Yolk sac diseases

In most cases, the yolk sac is absorbed into the coelomic cavity before hatching.[1] If the sac is not internalized when the hatchling emerges, the neonate is at risk for yolk sac rupture, strangulation, and/or infection. If the yolk is mostly internalized (**Fig. 8**), the natural progression of internalization may progress on its own if the neonate is closely monitored and maintained on a clean damp surface. In cases of the umbilicus pendulously attached to the neonate, it is advisable to ligate and transect the yolk sac as proximal to the neonate as possible to reduce incidence of infection. After transection, if the body wall is open, surgical closure should be performed.

Yolk sac infection may occur even if the yolk was internalized prior to complete emergence. Infection of the yolk sac causes closure of the vitelline duct, cutting off nutritional sources to the neonate, and may lead to generalized coelomitis and toxic metabolite production. Affected neonates may have a palpable structure in the coelom and show clinical signs of lethargy, anorexia, and general malaise. Exploratory surgery with collection of bacteriologic samples after surgical removal of the yolk sac is indicated. Postoperatively, broad-spectrum antibiotics should be administered.

Infectious diseases

In general, any infectious disease that can affect an adult can also affect a neonate, although with their small size and incomplete immune function, neonates have higher morbidity and mortality when exposed to these same pathogens. For example, the common snake mite (*Ophionyssus natricis*) may cause subclinical infections in adult

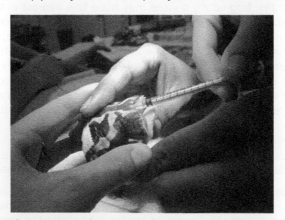

Fig. 7. Subcarapacial venipuncture in a neonatal spider tortoise (*Pyxis arachnoides*) using an insulin syringe and needle to reduce tissue trauma and allow precise measurement of blood volume collected. (*Courtesy of* Olivia Petritz, DVM, DACZM, ACCESS Speciality Animal Hospital, Culver City, CA, USA.)

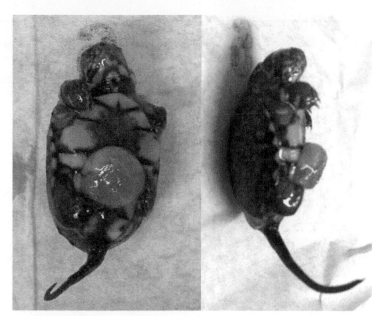

Fig. 8. Ventral (*left*) and lateral (*right*) views of a postmortem neonatal western pond turtle (*Emys marmorata*) that had fully internalized a retained yolk sac shortly after hatching but failed to close the umbilicus and was found dead the following morning.

saurians but this hematophagous mite can overwhelm and exsanguinate neonates in a short amount of time. Some classic species-specific pathogens in neonatal and juvenile reptiles are listed in **Table 3**.

The topic of salmonellosis should be discussed in more detail, because it is a common zoonosis. Despite a long-standing federal ban in the United States on the sale of turtles with a carapace length of less than 4 inches, continued multistate outbreaks of turtle-associated salmonellosis occur.[27] Most reptile-associated salmonellosis in humans is linked with turtle contact; a variety of species are implicated in infections, including bearded dragons, corn snakes (*Patherophis guttatus*), veiled chameleons (*Chamaeleo calyptratus*), and a variety of *Python* spp, among others.[28,29] Hatchlings are infected once they pip and are in the environment that is contaminated by *Salmonella* spp.[30] Basic hygiene and awareness when dealing with neonatal reptiles is appropriate to reduce chances of outbreaks in reptile and human patients. Salmonellosis in humans can be associated with a variety of risk factors and isolates should be serotyped to prove infection is from a reptile source.

Husbandry-associated diseases
In general, any husbandry-related disease that can affect an adult can also affect a neonate, although with rapid metabolism and growth, neonates have higher morbidity and mortality when husbandry deficiencies are present. Common husbandry-related diseases that affect neonates include the following:

- Nutritional secondary hyperparathyroidism occurs when diets low in calcium and lack of vitamin D (dietary, UV-B, or both) occur (**Fig. 9**A).
- Sand/substrate impaction occurs in individuals fed on particulate substrate. Even when fed on nonparticulate substrate, animals may ingest substrate (**Fig. 9**B).
- Predation by cage mates is often due to inappropriate pairings or high stocking densities and may lead to missing toes, tail tips, or death (**Fig. 9**C).

Table 3
Common infectious diseases and associated clinical signs in neonatal and hatchling reptiles

Taxonomic Group	Etiologic Agent	Species	Clinical Signs	Confirmatory Diagnostics to Perform
Saurians	*Cryptosporidium saurophilum/varanii*	Any lizard species, especially prevalent in the leopard gecko (*Eublepharis macularius*)	Poor body condition score, diarrhea, anorexia, failure to thrive	• *Cryptosporidium* spp PCR on gastric wash, feces
	Agamid adenovirus 1	Bearded dragon (*Pogona vitticeps*)	Diarrhea, weight loss, anorexia, central nervous system dysfunction	• Agamid adenovirus 1 PCR
	Chrysosporium sp	Most lizard species	Crusting/ulcerative dermatologic lesions. Lesions often yellow in color in bearded dragons	• Histopathology • Fungal culture • Cytology
	Ophionyssus spp	Snakes and lizards	Increased shedding frequency, visible ectoparasites, increased soaking, anorexia	• Direct observation of the mite
Chelonians	Testudid herpesvirus	Chelonians, especially Russian tortoises (*Agrionemys horsfieldii*)	Oronasal discharge, ocular discharge, fibrinous/necrotizing stomatitis	• Testudid herpesvirus PCR (nasal flush) • Testudid herpesvirus antibody titers
	Mycoplasma sp	Chelonians	Conjunctivitis and ocular discharge, nasal discharge/bubbling, choanal inflammation	• *Mycoplasma* spp PCR (nasal flush) • *Mycoplasma* spp antibody titers (maternal interactions for up to 1 y of age)

Abbreviation: PCR, polymerase chain reaction.

Congenital diseases

Many congenital diseases are reported in neonatal reptiles and may have a genetic or inappropriate incubation root cause. Recently reported congenital lesions include patent urachus in a prehensile-tailed skink (*Corucia zebrata*), ankyloblepharon in a leopard gecko, amelia in Morelet's crocodile (*Crocodylus moreletii*), and dicephaly in a Greek tortoise (*Testudo graeca ibera*).[31–34] A recent large-scale study in neotropical viperids found that spinal abnormalities were the most common malformations noted,

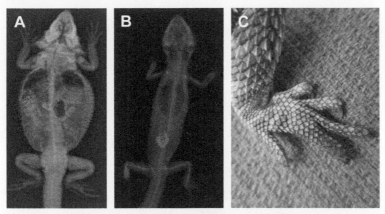

Fig. 9. Husbandry-related diseases of reptile neonates. (*A*) A 2-month-old male bearded dragon (*Pogona vitticeps*) that presented with signs of weakness has radiographic evidence of diffuse osteopenia suggestive of nutritional secondary hyperparathyroidism. There is also radiopaque material within the gastrointestinal tract, which likely represents pica behavior of substrate. (*B*) A 4-month-old female leopard gecko (*Eublepharis macularius*) presented with lack of defecation for several days and licking at the vent region. Radiographs show radiopaque material within the gastrointestinal tract indicating ingestion of substrate material (sand) used in enclosure. (*C*) The claw of digit IV of the right hind limb of this young bearded dragon has been traumatically amputated from a suspect bite wound. The markedly swollen digit indicates ascending infection. The claw of digit V is also missing. This bearded dragon lived in a 20-gallon tank with 10 other bearded dragons.

and incidence of malformations was 2.3% in pit vipers and 11.1% in rattlesnakes.[35] Diagnosis of a congenital lesion should prompt evaluation of the breeding stock and artificial incubation parameters.

Treatment Considerations

In general, a sick neonate should be afforded the same treatments as a similarly ill adult. These include administration of appropriate analgesic and antibiotic medications as well as nutritional, thermal, and fluid support. Due to the small size of neonates, medication administration can be challenging. Dosages for neonates that take into consideration differences that may exist in pharmacokinetics are lacking and judicial use of dosages used in adults are often used. Concentrations of medications may not be amenable to dosing and may require dilution. Consultation with a veterinary pharmacist may aid in developing medication-specific dilution recipes that are safe and efficacious to administer. For instance, at least 1 injectable form of ivermectin (Ivomec, 1% sterile solution, Merial, Duluth, GA, USA) is suspended in a lipid carrier. Because it is not aqueous, dilution with saline or sterile water may lead to nonhomogeneous distribution of the medication and potential patient overdose. Ivermectin is contraindicated in chelonian patients regardless of age.

Injectable, oral, or rectal administration of medications can be safely performed using the same guidelines as used in adults but with smaller instrumentation and care to prevent trauma to the fragile neonatal tissues. Injections can be given using insulin syringes that are available to measure to the nearest 0.01 mL, BD Ultra-Fine Short Needle, 0.3 mL or 0.5 mL (Becton, Dickinson and Company, Franklin Lakes, New Jersey), or to the nearest 0.005 mL, BD Ultra-Fine Short Needle with half-unit scale; the latter has the added benefit of a removable needle, allowing use of the

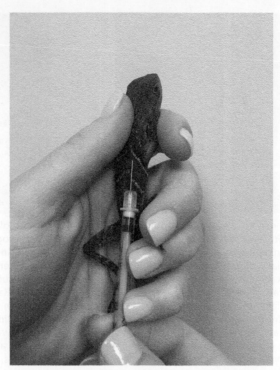

Fig. 10. Subcutaneous injection of a hatchling Chinese water dragon (*Physignathus cocincinus*) with a long-acting antibiotic to treat clinical signs of pneumonia. A commercially available insulin syringe and needle are used to prevent excessive tissue trauma.

syringe for oral administrations of medications. Both syringes have a small needle size (31 g) that reduces the incidence of tissue trauma (**Fig. 10**). A guitar pick can be an excellent tool to open small mouths.

REFERENCES

1. Pezaro N, Doody JS, Green B, et al. Hatching and residual yolk internalization in lizards: evolution, function and fate of the amnion. Evol Dev 2013;15(2):87–95.
2. Nechaeva MV, Makarenko IG, Tsitrin EB, et al. Physiological and morphological characteristics of the rhythmic contractions of the amnion in veiled chameleon (*Chamaeleo calyptratus*) embryogenesis. Comp Biochem Physiol A Mol Integr Physiol 2005;140(1):19–28.
3. Sartori MR, Taylor EW, Abe AS. Nitrogen excretion during embryonic development of the green iguana, *Iguana iguana* (Reptilia; Squamata). Comp Biochem Physiol A Mol Integr Physiol 2012;163(2):210–4.
4. Aubret F, Blanvillain G, Kok PJ. Myth busting? Effects of embryo positioning and egg turning on hatching success in the water snake *Natrix maura*. Sci Rep 2015; 5:13385.
5. Webb GJ, Manolis SC, Whitehead PJ, et al. The possible relationship between embryo orientation opaque banding and the dehydration of albumen in crocodile eggs. Copeia 1987;1:252–7.

6. Andrews RM. Effects of incubation temperature on growth and performance of the veiled chameleon (*Chamaeleo calyptratus*). J Exp Zool A Ecol Genet Physiol 2008;309(8):435–46.

7. Dang W, Zhang W, Du WG. Incubation temperature affects the immune function of hatchling soft-shelled turtles, *Pelodiscus sinensis*. Sci Rep 2015;5:10594.

8. Aïdam A, Michel CL, Bonnet X. Effect of ambient temperature in neonate aspic vipers: growth, locomotor performance and defensive behaviors. J Exp Zool A Ecol Genet Physiol 2013;319(6):310–8.

9. Fisher LR. Incubation temperature effects on hatchling performance in the loggerhead sea turtle (*Caretta caretta*). PLoS One 2014;9(12):e114880.

10. Van damme R, Bauwens D, Brana F, et al. Incubation temperature differentially affects hatching time, egg survival, and hatchling performation in the lizard *Podarcis muralis*. Herpetologica 1992;48(2):220–8.

11. Hulin V, Girondot M, Godfrey MH, et al. Mixed and uniform brood sex ratio strategy in turtles: the facts, the theory and their consequences. In: Wyneken J, Godfrey MH, Bels V, editors. Biology of turtles. Boca Raton (FL): CRC Press; 2008. p. 279–300.

12. Ewert MA, Etchberger CR, Nelson CE. Turtle sex-determining modes and TSD patterns, and some TSD pattern correlates. In: Valenzuela N, Lance VA, editors. Temperature-dependent sex determination in vertebrates. Washington: Smithsonian Books; 2004. p. 21–32.

13. Deeming DC. Prevalence of TSD in crocodilians. In: Valenzuela N, Lance VA, editors. Temperature-dependent sex determination in vertebrates. Washington: Smithsonian Books; 2004. p. 33–41.

14. Nelson NJ, Cree A, Thompson MB, et al. Temperature-dependent sex determinations in tuataras. In: Valenzuela N, Lance VA, editors. Temperature-dependent sex determination in vertebrates. Washington: Smithsonian Books; 2004. p. 42–52.

15. Harlow PS. Temperature-dependent sex determinations in lizards. In: Valenzuela N, Lance VA, editors. Temperature-dependent sex determination in vertebrates. Washington: Smithsonian Books; 2004. p. 42–52.

16. Miller JD, Dinkelacker SA. Reproductive structures and strategies of turtle. In: Wyneken J, Godfrey MH, Bels V, editors. Biology of turtles. Boca Raton (FL): CRC Press; 2008. p. 225–61.

17. Zhao B, Chen Y, Wang Y, et al. Does the hydric environment affect the incubation of small rigid-shelled turtle eggs? Comp Biochem Physiol A Mol Integr Physiol 2013;164(1):66–70.

18. Du WG, Ye H, Zhao B, et al. Patterns of interspecific variation in the heart rates of embryonic reptiles. PLoS One 2011;6(12):e29027.

19. Moreeira PL, Barata M. Egg mortality and early embryo hatching cased by fungal infection of Iberian rock lizard (*Lacerta monticola*) clutches. Herpetol J 2005;15: 265–72.

20. Vergne AL, Mathevon N. Crocodile egg sounds signal hatching time. Curr Biol 2008;18(12):R513–4.

21. Mack EW. Delayed neonatal feeding and growth in the Lake Erie Watersnake, Nerodia sipedon insularum. DeKalb (IL): Northern Illinois University; 2015. Available at: http://gradworks.umi.com/10/00/10008862.html.

22. Kelly TR, McNeil JB, Avens L, et al. Clinical pathology reference intervals for an in-water population of juvenile loggerhead sea turtles (*Caretta caretta*) in Core Sound, North Carolina, USA. PLoS One 2015;10(3):e0115739.

23. Casal AB, Camacho M, Lopez-Jurado LF, et al. Comparative study of hematologic and plasma biochemical variable s in Eastern Atlantic juvenile and adult nesting loggerhead sea turtles (*Caretta caretta*). Vet Clin Pathol 2009;38(2):213–8.
24. Divers SJ. Endoscopic sex identification in chelonians and birds (Psittacines, Passerines, and Raptors). Vet Clin North Am Exot Anim Pract 2015;18(3):541–54.
25. Hernandez-Divers SJ, Stahl SJ, Farrell R. An endoscopic method for identifying sex of hatchling Chinese box turtles and comparison of general versus local anesthesia for coelioscopy. J Am Vet Med Assoc 2009;234(6):800–4.
26. Martínez-Silvestre A, Bargalló F, Grífols J. Gender Identification by cloacoscopy and cystoscopy in juvenile chelonians. Vet Clin North Am Exot Anim Pract 2015; 18(3):527–39.
27. Bosch S, Tauxe RV, Behravesh CB. Turtle-associated salmonellosis, United States, 2006-2014. Emerg Infect Dis 2016;22(7):1149–55.
28. Lowther SA, Medus C, Scheftel J, et al. Foodborne outbreak of Salmonella subspecies IV infections associated with contamination from bearded dragons. Zoonoses Public Health 2011;58(8):560–6.
29. Pees M, Rabsch W, Plenz B, et al. Evidence for the transmission of Salmonella from reptiles to children in Germany, July 2010 to October 2011. Euro Surveill 2013;18(46):20634.
30. Izadjoo MJ, Pantoja CO, Siebeling RJ. Acquisition of Salmonella flora by turtle hatchlings on commercial turtle farms. Can J Microbiol 1987;33(8):718–24.
31. Goe A, Heard DJ, Fredholm DV, et al. Management of a patent urachus and yolk coelomitis in a prehensile-tailed skink (*Corucia zebrata*). J Zoo Wildl Med 2015; 46(4):909–12.
32. Rival F. Congenital ankyloblepharon in a leopard gecko (*Eublepharis macularius*). Vet Ophthalmol 2015;18(Suppl 1):71–3.
33. Charruau P, Nino-torres CA. A third case of amelia in Morelet's crocodile from the Yucatan peninsula. Dis Aquat Organ 2014;109(3):263–7.
34. Palmieri C, Selleri P, Di Girolamo N, et al. Multiple congenital malformations in dicephalic spur-thighed tortoise (*Testudo graeca ibera*). J Comp Pathol 2013; 149(2–3):368–71.
35. Sant-Anna SS, Grego KF, Lorigados CA, et al. Malformations in neotropical viperids: qualitative and quantitative analysis. J Comp Pathol 2013;149(4):503–8.

Veterinary Aspects of Bird of Prey Reproduction

Tom A. Bailey, BVSc, MRCVS, CertZooMed, MSc, PhD, DECZM,
RCVS Specialist in Zoo and Wildlife Medicine[a],*, Michael Lierz, DZooMed, DECZM(WPH), DECPVS[b]

KEYWORDS

- Raptor • Bird of prey • Falcon • Aviculture • Veterinary • Reproduction
- Assisted reproduction • Insemination

KEY POINTS

- Reproductive failure is a common occurrence in raptor breeding projects; if a veterinary investigation is needed by a breeding project the practitioner should assess the complete avicultural facility and review its management.
- The adult breeding stock should be examined annually; projects should have isolation and health screening protocols established to screen incoming breeding stock for infectious diseases.
- Avicultural record keeping is a core component of managing a breeding program; closed-circuit television camera systems with playback are widely used to observe and manage breeding pairs.
- Assisted reproduction techniques, such as artificial insemination (AI), play a key role in raptor breeding; semen assessment is an important tool to assess the fertility of males that are used in AI programs.
- Any birds that have had issues with lowered or absent fertility during the preceding season require an evaluation of their reproductive tract; endoscopy is the most useful tool to investigate infertility.

 Video content accompanies this article at http://www.vetexotic.theclinics.com.

BREEDING BIRDS OF PREY

Birds of prey are bred in captivity for many reasons including conservation of endangered species, commercial production of large falcon species, and hobby breeding

---

Disclosure Statement: T.A. Bailey worked at International Wildlife Consultants from 2011 to 2014 as head of the falcon breeding department exporting captive bred falcons to the Middle East. M. Lierz has nothing to disclose.
[a] Origin Vets, Goetre Farm, Trelessy Road, Amroth, Nr Narberth, Pembrokeshire SA67 8PT, UK;
[b] Clinic for Birds, Reptiles, Amphibians and Fish, Justus-Liebig-University Giessen, Frankfurter Street 91-93, Giessen 35392, Germany
* Corresponding author.
E-mail address: drtomabailey@gmail.com

of a wide variety of species that are kept and flown by falconers and bird of prey keepers.

Captive breeding has contributed to the successful restoration of many species of birds of prey threatened with extinction including the Californian condor (*Gymnogyps californianus*), Mauritius kestrel (*Falco punctatus*), and peregrine falcon (*Falco peregrinus*).[1-3] The restoration of peregrine falcon populations by the Peregrine Fund (Boise, ID) made conservationists aware that captive breeding could be used as a tool for conservation. Avicultural techniques that have been pioneered by raptor breeders include double clutching, direct fostering, cross-fostering, hatch and switch, hacking, imprinting male and female falcons for semen collection, and artificial insemination (AI) techniques (**Table 1** for explanations).[4-11]

Since the 1990s falcon breeding projects in the Middle East, Europe, and North America have used AI, egg-pulling from pairs, and artificial incubation to maximize number of offspring, breeding thousands of peregrines (*F peregrinus*), saker falcon (*Falco cherrug*), gyrfalcon (*Falco rusticolis*), and mixed species (so-called hybrid) falcons (usually gyr × peregrine or gyr × saker hybrids) for the lucrative Middle East falconry market (**Figs. 1** and **2**).

Falconry is popular as a field sport and for public displays in many countries and a wide range of species are bred by hobby breeders and falconry centers.

This article provides an overview of veterinary contributions that can maximize the reproductive success of raptor breeding projects.

EVALUATION OF BIRD OF PREY BREEDING FACILITIES

Veterinarians are often consulted when reproductive success is not as high as expected or for last ditch "fire brigade" medical intervention on sick falcons. It is interesting that despite the high value of large falcons most commercial projects have limited veterinary involvement. This along with commercial sensitivities and a culture of secrecy accounts for the paucity of veterinary information published from these projects.

Table 1	
Avicultural term explanations	
Term	**Explanation**
Double clutching	Removal (and artificial incubation) of the first clutch of eggs by a breeder so that the pair recycles and lays a second clutch of eggs.
Direct fostering	Placing an artificially hatched chick with a foster parent who is the biologic parent
Cross-fostering	Placing a chick with a foster parent who is not the biologic parent
Hatch and switch	Placing a chick that has hatched under its biologic mother with another parent
Hacking	A method used to release young captive bred raptors from trees or specially constructed towers. Birds are permitted to fly free for a period of time before being recaptured and before they begin hunting on their own and can live totally independently. Wildlife rehabilitators use this method to release injured raptors back into the wild. Falconers use this method to develop the flying skills of their birds.
Imprinting	The learning mechanism that occurs during a specific sensitive period, after hatching until about the 14th day in raptors, which establishes a long-lasting behavioral response to a specific individual or object. Falcon chicks used for breeding using semen collection or artificial insemination are imprinted on human handlers as future sexual partner.

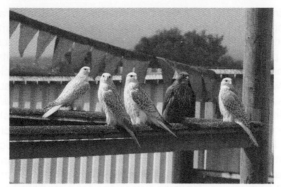

Fig. 1. Captive bred gyrfalcons in a hack pen. (*Courtesy of* Tom A. Bailey, Origin Vets, Pembrokeshire, United Kingdom.)

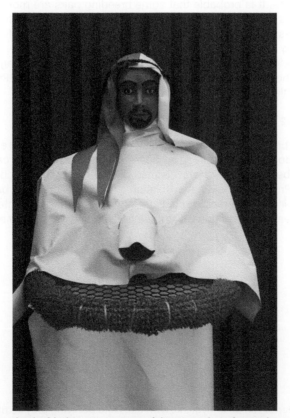

Fig. 2. A novel method of habituating young falcons to their future human environment. The "fake sheikh," a mannequin of an Arab falconer. This is a method of habituating young falcons to associate the presentation of food with a human-shaped mannequin. This is believed to contribute to the training of these birds for falconry in the Middle East. (*Courtesy of* Tom A. Bailey, Origin Vets, Pembrokeshire, United Kingdom.)

If a veterinary investigation is needed by a breeding project the practitioner should assess the complete avicultural facility and review its management. Protocols, including preventive medicine, food preparation, diet schedules (plus supplementation details), AI procedures, egg collection, incubation, biosecurity, pest control, photoperiod management and manipulation, pen cleaning, and chick rearing should be critically reviewed. Although aspects of avicultural management, such as maintaining clean aviaries, seem to be mundane, a hygienic environment in which a breeding bird spends its entire life is critically important. Chronic immune system response is considered to be a factor in the development of amyloidosis,[12] which in captive gyrfalcons could be linked to chronic exposure to environmental pathogen loads in aviaries. In their natural Arctic tundra habitat free-living gyrfalcons are unlikely to be exposed to the same pathogen loads. Although it seems simple to state that breeding chambers should be hygienic, feces and decaying food readily accumulate and the laboriousness of cleaning regimens can easily be overlooked (**Figs. 3** and **4**).

In addition attention should be paid to the providence of the breeding stock and the parentage of the stock. Captive lines of gyrfalcons had small founder populations taken from the wild and some breeders have performed line breeding, selectively breeding for a desired commercial features ("super" white) by mating them within a closely related line. It is probable that some breeding pairs are more closely related than the breeders imagine. Veterinarians assessing reproductive performance in large breeding projects should have a strong avicultural background and first-hand experience of breeding birds, ideally raptors.

Poor health and management are closely interrelated and management failures, even by experienced aviculturalists, are common reasons for reproductive failure.[13,14] The type of problems are listed in **Box 1**.

EVALUATING THE HEALTH OF BREEDING BIRDS

In any breeding project the adult breeding stock should be examined annually (**Fig. 5**). This is usually done after the breeding season when the birds are caught and their breeding chambers or aviaries are cleaned. Hematology and biochemistry should be performed. Projects should have isolation and health screening protocols established to screen incoming breeding stock for infectious diseases. Bacterial avian pathogens to be screened for include *Chlamydophila* spp and *Salmonella* spp. In addition,

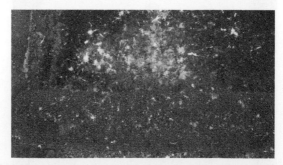

Fig. 3. Raptor aviaries can be unhygienic with feces and decaying prey accumulating during the breeding season. Annual aviary cleaning and maintenance are important avicultural tasks. Regular cleaning of drinking and bathing water along with surfaces that come into contact with food items are essential to reduce the pathogen load that birds are exposed to in their aviaries. (*Courtesy of* Tom A. Bailey, Origin Vets, Pembrokeshire, United Kingdom.)

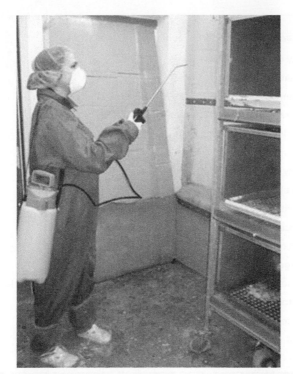

Fig. 4. Thorough cleaning of breeding facilities should include jet washing pens and spraying facilities with disinfectant. (*Courtesy of* Michael Lierz, Justus-Liebig-University Giessen, Giessen, Germany.)

birds that are imported from countries where there is a risk of avian influenza or paramyxovirus should be isolated and screened using diagnostic tests approved by national veterinary agencies. Feces and oral/crop swabs should be examined for parasitic pathogens, such as *Caryospora* spp, *Strigea* spp, *Capillaria* spp, *Serratospiculum* spp, *Ascaridia*, and trichomoniasis. It is recommended to screen for parasites at least two to three times annually. Endoparasite loads may increase over a relatively short time period caused by fecal contamination of the breeding chambers (**Fig. 6**). **Table 2** lists the minimum health screening samples for raptor breeding projects. Control measures for coccidia and helminth parasites should be included as part of an annual preventive medicine program.

BEHAVIORAL INFLUENCES ON RAPTOR FERTILITY

Aggression between incompatible pairs, asynchronous breeding activity, injuries, and behavioral disorders can result in failed breeding in natural pairs. Avicultural record keeping is a core component of managing a breeding program. The provision of observation holes into breeding chambers and good old-fashioned observation by staff with a knowledge of species-specific breeding behaviors is an essential avicultural skill. Observation records by staff in notebooks, on charts outside aviaries, and breeding log books is essential to enable productivity to be fine-tuned during and at the end of the season (**Fig. 7**). Closed-circuit television camera systems with playback are widely used in breeding chambers enabling the breeding behavior of pairs to be

---

Box 1
Management issues responsible for breeding failures in birds of prey.

Age and maturity of breeding stock

Artificial insemination protocols

Aviary cleaning and disinfection protocols

Aviary, nest substrate, and aviary furniture deficiencies

Biosecurity procedures for incoming birds

Breeding pair setup

Facility biosecurity failures

Facility security failures

Food supply, quality, and provision to breeding stock

Genetic providence of the breeding stock

Inbreeding issues of breeding stock

Incubation management

Management issues of staff handling imprinted birds for artificial insemination

Photoperiod protocols and manipulation

Power failure issues during breeding season affecting critical equipment

Rearing history of the breeding stock

Record keeping

---

reviewed (**Fig. 8**). **Fig. 9** shows an example of a closed-circuit television camera record sheet that is used to monitor breeding in a large falcon project. Systematic recording of aggression, food passing, calling, copulations, and egg laying times is important to maximize productivity from natural pairs and identify breeding problems that can be investigated. When establishing new pairs it is important to take account of the age and previous reproductive experience and history of the birds. Male raptors are about one-third smaller than females and pair aggression can be significant. For example,

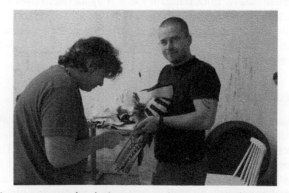

Fig. 5. When falcons are caught during pen maintenance and cleaning they should be examined. In this example morphometrics for a falcon pedigree are being collected before a health examination. (*Courtesy of* Tom A. Bailey, Origin Vets, Pembrokeshire, United Kingdom.)

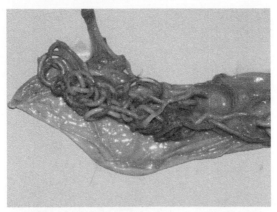

Fig. 6. *Ascaridia* infestation contributed to the death of this falcon in a breeding facility. (*Courtesy of* Michael Lierz, Justus-Liebig-University Giessen, Giessen, Germany).

placing a young inexperienced male with an aggressive female can stress the male so that he will not breed and may lead to injury or death. Therefore, experienced males should be paired with young females. The selection, training, and behavior of breeding stock is one of the major factors in successful breeding and is often overlooked by the breeders.[13] The rearing history of birds of prey is also highly relevant to breeding success. Likewise trying to ensure that the type of nest and breeding chamber a sexually mature falcon is placed in for breeding is similar to the environment the bird was reared in is considered to be important in ensuring future breeding success. Most fertility problems within a breeding project are not medical and require interventions by skilled aviculturalists.

ARTIFICIAL INSEMINATION AND SEMEN ASSESSMENT IN MALE RAPTORS

Assisted reproduction techniques, such as AI, plays a key role in raptor breeding, and it is a popular technique to propagate hybrid falcons, which are crosses of species that would not naturally breed if kept as natural pairs (eg, gyr × peregrine falcons). Inseminations is voluntary or forced. Voluntary insemination is when an imprinted female raptor stands for insemination and is inseminated intracloacally. Forced insemination occurs when an untrained or unwilling falcon is physically restrained and is inseminated directly into the oviduct. Video 1 shows a falcon being voluntarily inseminated. **Fig. 28** and Video 2 show a falcon being force inseminated. Semen assessment is an important tool to assess the fertility of males that are used in AI programs, and to

Table 2	
Minimum health screening samples for raptor breeding projects	
Sample	**Test**
Feces[a]	Parasitology and *Salmonella* spp
Oral swab	Parasitology
Blood	Hematology Biochemistry

[a] Microbiology and *Chlamydophila* may be appropriate if there has been a history of poor productivity, or respiratory or digestive tract disease.

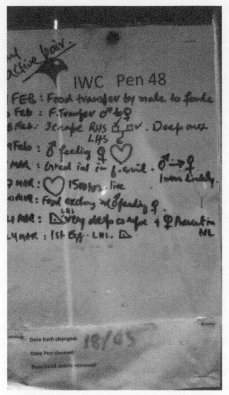

Fig. 7. Observation record sheet outside aviary to record key breeding behaviors. (*Courtesy of* Tom A. Bailey, Origin Vets, Pembrokeshire, United Kingdom.)

assess the fertility of males in natural pairs where infertile eggs have been produced.[11,15,16] Semen is collected either as voluntary samples from semen donors (**Fig. 10**) or as forced by massaging untrained males (**Fig. 11**).[17] Sperm concentration and motility are assessed according to standard methods[15,17,18] using hemocytometer chamber or fertility semen counting chambers (Hawksley, Lancing, Sussex, UK).

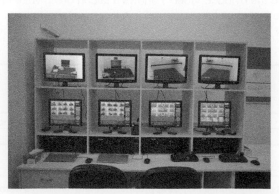

Fig. 8. Closed-circuit television camera bank. (*Courtesy of* Jaime Samour.)

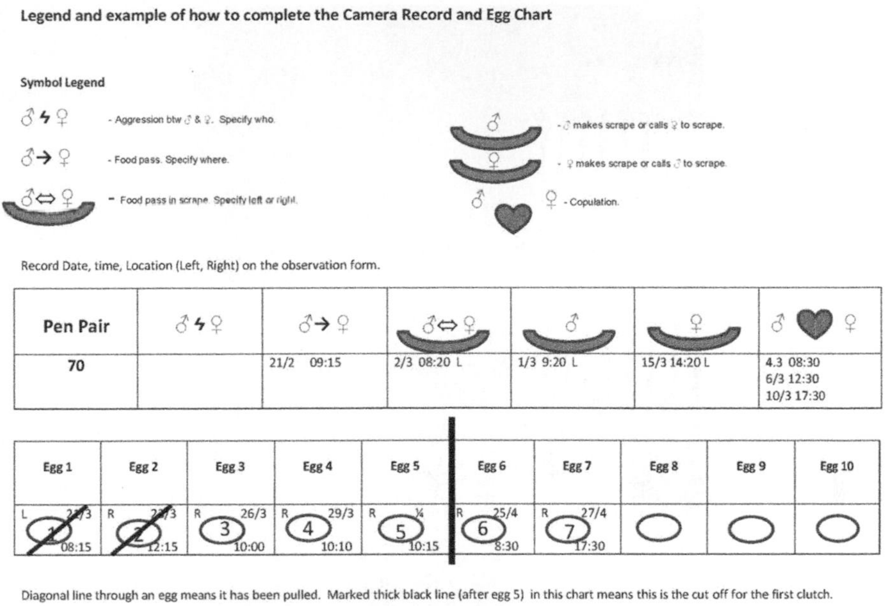

Legend and example of how to complete the Camera Record and Egg Chart

Symbol Legend

Record Date, time, Location (Left, Right) on the observation form.

Pen Pair	♂ ↯ ♀	♂ → ♀	♂ ⇔ ♀	♂	♀	♂ ♥ ♀
70		21/2 09:15	2/3 08:20 L	1/3 9:20 L	15/3 14:20 L	4.3 08:30 6/3 12:30 10/3 17:30

Egg 1	Egg 2	Egg 3	Egg 4	Egg 5	Egg 6	Egg 7	Egg 8	Egg 9	Egg 10
L 24/3 R 08:15	22/3 R 12:15	26/3 R (3) 10:00	29/3 R (4) 10:10	¼ R (5) 10:15	25/4 R (6) 8:30	27/4 R (7) 17:30	○	○	○

Diagonal line through an egg means it has been pulled. Marked thick black line (after egg 5) in this chart means this is the cut off for the first clutch.

Fig. 9. Closed-circuit television camera record and egg chart. (*Courtesy of* Tom A. Bailey, Origin Vets, Pembrokeshire, United Kingdom.)

Semen viability is assessed using Eosin B stains.[11] There are few published semen characteristic values in raptors (**Table 3**). There is variability in semen parameters between different males of the same species and between individual samples from the same male.[11,15] Falcon semen with 60% progressive motility and a concentration of 30,000 sperm/μL used for AI was able to fertilize eggs.[11]

Computer-assisted semen analysis is being more widely used in assisted reproduction in avian species[18] and along with advances in semen cryopreservation this technique will play an important role in more objective assessments of male fertility in the future. However, at present this technique has limitations in falcon semen, because the sperm size is similar to round bodies occurring in the semen fluid. This interferes with the automated counting and the software of the computer system must be adapted accordingly. Likewise recently developed electrostimulated semen collection techniques developed in parrots[20] may have a role to play with species of raptors where semen stripping is not possible because of size or safety issues. Apart from semen evaluation, functionality tests, such as the periviteline membrane penetration assay, may be helpful to see if the semen is able to fertilize an egg,[21] information that cannot gathered from semen motility or live/death rate.

AI protocols should be reviewed paying particular attention to hygiene and storage conditions. Semen is collected on latex hats (**Fig. 12**) or by massage techniques, transferred to capillary tubes, mixed with diluents, transferred to plastic AI tubes, and stored in a refrigerator at 5°C to 6°C before insemination. Refrigerated semen should be warmed to body temperature before insemination. Most breeders prefer to use semen on the same day of collection, but refrigerated diluted semen can be used for up to 2 days after collection. These steps offer opportunities for contamination if hygiene is suboptimal and bacteria (*Enterococcus faecalis* and *Staphylococcus* sp) were isolated from fresh semen samples collected at one breeding project.[15] Poor-quality semen samples and urine and bacterial contamination can contribute

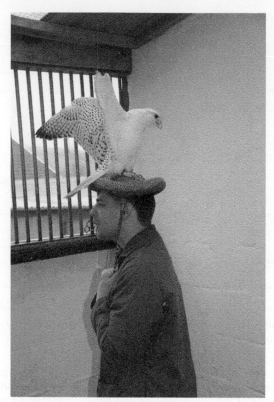

Fig. 10. Imprinted male gyrfalcon copulating on a latex hat designed to collect semen from indentations. (*Courtesy of* Tom A. Bailey, Origin Vets, Pembrokeshire, United Kingdom.)

to fertility failures or infections of the female reproductive tract. Cleaning protocols for semen collection and handling equipment along with storage protocols should be reviewed if there are concerns that hygiene deficiencies exist. Pathogens are transmitted via semen and the health status of semen donors and their negative status for some pathogens is vital. An example is the detection of mycoplasmas in falcon semen samples, even though their pathogenic potential is currently unclear.[22] Transmission to the female may potentially result in transmission into the egg and therefore interfere with embryonic development, which is well known for mycoplasmas in poultry.

ASSESSMENT OF THE DIET

Raptor projects need a reliable supply of healthy, nutritionally balanced prey items.[23] In countries where the supply of disease-free prey items cannot be ensured large breeding projects breed their own quail and rats to eliminate risks of introducing highly infectious avian diseases, such as Newcastle disease or avian influenza virus. Poultry adenoviruses has been linked with mortality episodes in some small falcons species that have ingested avian prey.[24] Externally sourced food should be purchased from reputable animal food wholesalers. Suppliers should have preventive medicine programs including vaccination and antiparasitic treatments and disease screening protocols in place for the breeding stock and offspring. The method of

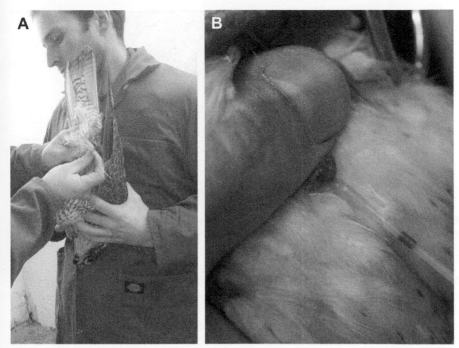

Fig. 11. (*A*) Semen being forcibly stripped from a male gyrfalcon. (*B*) Semen being collected in a capillary tube after being stripped from a male gyrfalcon. (*Courtesy of* [*A*] Tom A. Bailey, Origin Vets, Pembrokeshire, United Kingdom; and [*B*] Michael Lierz, Justus-Liebig-University Giessen, Giessen, Germany.)

killing the prey should also be known. This information prevents intoxications or foods that may be contaminated by medicines or euthanasia drugs. Nutritional analysis of the food and supplements fed to the food animals should be available for scrutiny. Some breeders feed vitamin E–enhanced quail to breeding birds 6 to 8 weeks before the breeding season starts. Vitamin E can be supplemented in the diet to quail flocks at a concentration of 200 IU/kg dry matter.[9] If feeding standard quail the vitamin E levels are boosted by injecting vitamin E into the quail pectoral muscle

Table 3
Selected spermatologic values of birds of prey

Species	Large Falcon[a]	Indian White Backed Vulture (*Gyps Bengalensis*)
Number of birds	115	4
Volume (μL)	72.4 ± 40.64	340 ± 260
Sperm concentration (n/μL)	73,500 ± 40,520	58,400 ± 33,200
Total sperm count (n/ejaculate)	5,260,000 ± 4,999,000	—
pH	6.4–8.0	7.1 ± 0.21
Total motility	—	46.8 ± 16.5
Reference	Fischer et al,[11] 2011	Umapathy et al,[19] 2005

[a] Large falcon species: *Falco rusticolis*, *Falco cherrug*, *Falco peregrinus*, and hybrids of these species.

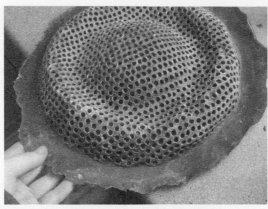

Fig. 12. Latex copulation hat showing indentations where the ejaculated semen is collected for artificial insemination. (*Courtesy of* Tom A. Bailey, Origin Vets, Pembrokeshire, United Kingdom.)

fed to the raptors at a concentration of 44 IU/100 g quail.[9] It is important that suppliers are aware that some preventive medicines (eg, the coccidiostat nicarbazin) have been linked with avian infertility,[25] so they should not be used in prey animals destined to be fed to breeding raptors. In addition cold storage facilities should have their temperatures monitored by sensors and alarms and provision of a backup generator can provide security against the risks of power failure that causes food spoilage. Attention should also be paid to food transport and storage. Thawing and freezing during transport and long-term storage, even freezing, reduces the vitamin content of the food.

Avicultural staff preparing food should follow strict hygiene protocols and quality control should be rigorous to ensure that substandard food items are rejected and returned to wholesalers (**Figs. 13** and **14**). Food should also be shock frozen and slowly thawed dry, to avoid food contact with thawing water, which leads to an increased bacterial load.

It is tempting for projects to reduce costs associated with feed. This might mean feeding of shot or otherwise sourced free-living animals, such as wild rabbits (*Oryctolagus cuniculus*) and pigeons (*Columba livia*) to raptors with the attendant risks of lead toxicity, agricultural toxins, and infectious diseases, such as trichomoniasis and herpesvirus.[26]

Attention to detail is paramount. Diets for all species of raptors should always include bone and the bone has to be available to the bird's digestive tract. Captive raptors should be offered crushed bone on a weekly basis.[9] Calcium deficiency can also occur when birds are overfed whole prey items (eg, pigeons) because they usually prefer meat and may not ingest the bones. The pure meat is also fed to the chicks, so calcium deficiency in adults, but particularly metabolic bone disease (nutritional secondary hyperparathyroidism) in chicks, can occur when pigeons are fed, especially in falcons.

Vitamin E deficiency in captive avian species, including raptors, has been associated with low fertility; low hatchability; immunosuppression; and specific clinical abnormalities, such as encephalomalacia and muscular myopathies.[27,28] In birds a diagnosis of vitamin deficiencies (eg, thiamine[29] or vitamin E[28]) was traditionally based on clinical signs and the clinical response to supplementation. Now that tests measuring vitamin levels in tissues and blood are more widespread, the ability of

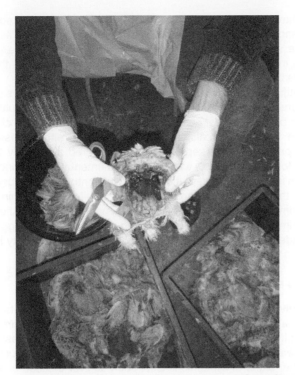

Fig. 13. It is important that avicultural staff are trained to identify quality control issues in the food fed to captive raptors. (*Courtesy of* Tom A. Bailey, Origin Vets, Pembrokeshire, United Kingdom.)

veterinarians to diagnose deficiencies and to provide more rational supplementation will improve. If there is concern about the nutritional status then assessment of blood vitamin levels may be beneficial. Inadequate vitamin E, selenium, and vitamins B_1 and B_{12} can cause decreased reproductive success.[14,28–30] Biotin (vitamin B_7) deficiency has been associated with a reduction in hatchability without adversely affecting egg production.[9]

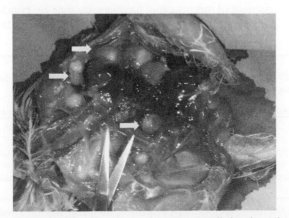

Fig. 14. Aspergillomas (*arrows*) in the carcass of a commercially bred quail supplied as falcon food. (*Courtesy of* Tom A. Bailey, Origin Vets, Pembrokeshire, United Kingdom.)

Carotenoids have been shown to contribute to beak coloration in some avian species and carotenoid signals have the potential to reveal important aspects of mate quality.[31,32] One successful project breeding New Zealand falcons, a small raptor that specializes in feeding on small birds in the wild, supplements the captive diet with carotenoids before the breeding season.[5]

Current scientific knowledge on the dietary requirements of raptors should then be translated into practical and economic diets for the birds. Menus should be developed and adapted for breeding birds, nonbreeding birds, and developing chicks. Likewise supplementation should be calculated rationally and either dosed individually (possible for imprinted falcons kept singly) or measured accurately to supplement batches of food for groups of birds where oversupplementation and undersupplementation may be an issue. Supplementation should take into account specific nutritional requirements of the sex, age, and breeding status of birds (eg, vitamin E supplementation of male semen donors providing multiple semen samples for AI or calcium supplementation of imprint female falcons laying sequences of up to 12 eggs). An example of a menu provided to large falcons at a commercial breeding facility is presented in **Table 4**.

INFERTILITY AND REPRODUCTIVE DISEASES IN BREEDING BIRDS

Any pairs or individual imprinted birds used for AI programs that have had issues with lowered or absent fertility during the proceeding season require an evaluation of their reproductive tract. Endoscopy is the most useful tool to investigate infertility. Endoscopy allows examination of the gonads, oviduct, or deferent duct, in addition to checking for other signs of systemic illness, such as liver disease or airsacculitis. In females in addition to inspecting the ovary, the oviduct and supporting ligament crossing the cranial division of kidney must be seen to ensure that eggs can be laid and females are not anatomically rendered sterile.[14] Likewise in males the deferent duct should be assessed along its complete length from the epididymis to the cloaca. Biopsies should be collected if abnormal findings are noted. **Tables 5** and **6** summarize endoscopic findings in 28 female and 12 male falcons investigated for infertility by the author (T.A.B.) at a large commercial breeding project. Medical issues were observed in 46% of female and 16% of male falcons examined for infertility investigations (**Figs. 15–19**).

If the bird is assessed and is considered systemically and anatomically healthy a more detailed assessment of reproductive functionality may be conducted. Females that have laid eggs in previous seasons have demonstrated the potential to

Table 4
Weekly menu including details on supplementation for a large commercial falcon breeding project during the breeding season

Monday	Tuesday	Wednesday	Thursday	Friday	Saturday	Sunday
Quail	Rat	Poussin	Rat	Quail	Poussin	Chicks
+	+	+	+	+	+	
Nekton E/S	Carophyll	Cod liver oil	Carophyll	Nekton E/S	Extra Ca/E	
	+	+	+		for imprint	
	Nutrobal	Extra Ca/E for	Nutrobal		females	
		imprint females				

Supplements used: Nekton-E (Nekton GmbH, Pforzheim, Germany), Nekton-S (Nekton GmbH), Carophyll (Carophyll Yellow, DSM Nutritional Products, Derbyshire, UK), Nutrobal (Vetark, Winchester, UK), Zolcal D (Vetark), cod liver oil (Equimins, Devon, UK).

Table 5
Endoscopic findings in 28 female falcons investigated for infertility issues at a falcon breeding project

	Imprint Females	Natural Pair Females	Total
Normal	2	13	15
Salpingitis	1	2[a]	2
Oviduct cyst	0	2	2
Ovarian cyst	0	1	1
Senescence	1	1	2
Immature	2	0	2
Other	0	5[b]	5
Total	6	22	28

[a] One bird also had a low-grade airsacculitis.
[b] Hepatic hemosiderosis (1), coelomitis/airsacculitis (4).
Data from Bailey, unpublished data.

successfully produce eggs and therefore, offspring. Females that have not previously laid eggs may not necessarily do so.

The timing of when the endoscopic examination is performed can also be critical to establishing possible reasons for infertility. If the birds are examined during the breeding season gonadal development can be scored. In **Table 6** some males examined for infertility had been paired with aggressive females and endoscopically it was observed that their testes were smaller and less developed compared with other male falcons examined at the same point in the season. It is hypothesized that the suppressed testicular development may have been related to the female aggression. Endoscopy combined with semen collection and examination is a useful tool in the fertility assessment of males.

Adenovirus has caused mortality in projects breeding small falcon species, such as New Zealand falcons (*Falco novaeseelandiae*), Mauritius kestrels, Aplomado falcons (*Falco femoralis septentrionalis*), orange-breasted falcons (*Falco deiroleucus*), teita falcons (*Falco fasciinucha*), merlin (*Falco columbarius*), Vanuatu peregrine falcon (*F peregrinus nesiotes*), and gyr × peregrine falcon hybrids.[33] In such species as aplomado falcons[34] and New Zealand falcons neonatal birds seem most susceptible to infection based on the author's (T.A.B.) experience (**Fig. 20**). In other species, such as Mauritius kestrel, adults are highly susceptible to infection.[24] Clinically affected birds exhibit hemorrhagic enteritis rapidly followed by death. Projects breeding smaller falcon species should modify their husbandry to

Table 6
Endoscopic findings in 12 male falcons investigated for infertility issues at a falcon breeding project

	Natural Pair Males
Normal	10[a]
Coelomitis/airsacculitis adjacent to testis	2
Total	12

[a] Four of the 10 testes examined were significantly smaller and less developed compared with other male falcons examined at the same point in the season.
Data from Bailey, unpublished data.

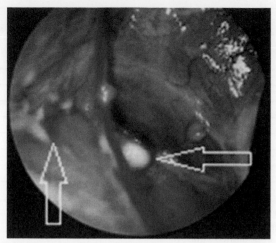

Fig. 15. Endoscopic image showing speckling (*arrows*) of the caudal thoracic airsacs of a female falcon that had produced infertile eggs the previous season. Adhesions were present from the pancreas to the adjacent abdominal organs. This bird had a previous coelomitis episode with a chronic air sacculitis. (*Courtesy of* Tom A. Bailey, Origin Vets, Pembrokeshire, United Kingdom.)

avoid all direct and indirect contact between different species and subspecies in the genus *Falco*.[33] Outbreaks in Mauritius kestrels were linked to feeding avian-derived food.[24]

INVESTIGATING INCUBATION PROBLEMS

Many breeders use artificial incubation to hatch raptor eggs. A full discussion of equipment used and incubation techniques is beyond the scope of this article and they are described elsewhere.[4,5,13,35,36] Commercial falcon breeding facilities can expect hatchabilities exceeding 85% of fertile eggs. When hatchability falls below expected percentages the incubation facility and its management should be investigated. Well-run breeding facilities have records, not only incubation data for each individual

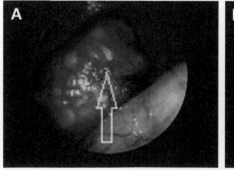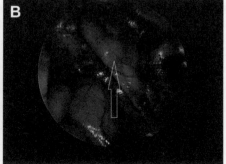

Fig. 16. Endoscopic images showing area of hemorrhage (*arrow*) on the ovary (A) and a distended oviduct (arrow) (B) of a female falcon that had produced fertile thin-shelled eggs that had not successfully hatched (early embryonic death). (*Courtesy of* Tom A. Bailey, Origin Vets, Pembrokeshire, United Kingdom.)

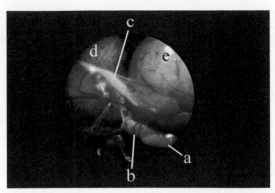

Fig. 17. Small immature ovary in a juvenile female falcon (*a*) ovary, (*b*) adrenal, (*c*) suspensory ligament of the ovary, (*d*) lung, and (*e*) kidney. (*Courtesy of* Michael Lierz, Justus-Liebig-University Giessen, Giessen, Germany.)

egg, but also records of incubators and the incubation room. An example of an incubation record sheet is presented in **Fig. 21**.

Suboptimal temperatures and humidity can directly cause incubation failure in avicultural facilities. Raptor eggs are incubated at a lower temperature (37.2°C–37.4°C) than poultry eggs.[13] Breeder's recommendations regarding incubator humidity vary considerably and the most important thing is that the incubated egg loses the appropriate amount of weight because of evaporation.[6] Dataloggers are readily available and represent an inexpensive and versatile tool that is used by veterinarians and aviculturists to monitor and investigate problems in the incubation unit.[37] Dataloggers are used to map temperature and humidity profiles in incubators, and in the room housing the incubation equipment (**Fig. 22**). Small variations of humidity and temperature during the incubation period can affect hatchability. Inadequate control of humidity in incubation rooms can result in knock-on problems within the incubator. In our experience optimal temperature and humidity in incubation rooms should be 18°C to 20°C and 25% to 35% relative humidity.

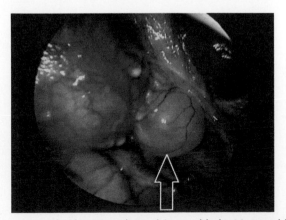

Fig. 18. Senescent ovary with a large cyst (*arrow*) in an elderly, 14-year-old imprinted peregrine falcon that had stopped laying. (*Courtesy of* Tom A. Bailey, Origin Vets, Pembrokeshire, United Kingdom.)

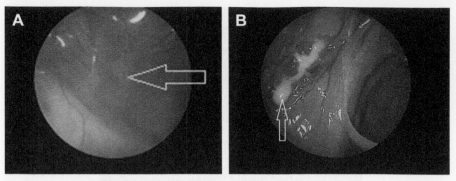

Fig. 19. (*A, B*) Male falcon in an infertile pair with airsacculitis (*arrows*) caused by aspergillosis in the airsacs adjacent to the gonad. (*Courtesy of* Tom A. Bailey, Origin Vets, Pembrokeshire, United Kingdom.)

EGG PATHOLOGY AND HATCHING PROBLEMS

Egg post mortem should be conducted on all unhatched eggs to assess fertility or the stage of death[13,35] (**Figs. 23–25**). Unhatched eggs are a common phenomenon in raptor breeding projects and are often referred to as being infertile, which can mean first that the ovum has not been fertilized or second that the embryo has died during development. These two broad categories of hatching failure are difficult to distinguish by gross egg post mortem, particularly in the early stages of embryo development. Techniques to distinguish between infertility (caused by insufficient sperm) and early embryo mortality in Zebra finch (*Taenlopygia guttata*) by assessing the germinal disk for cell nuclei and the perivitelline membrane for sperm or holes have been developed.[38] These methods have been used in raptor projects to determine accurate fertility levels and to identify early embryonic deaths. Raptor pediatrics are beyond the scope of this article and are reviewed elsewhere.[39]

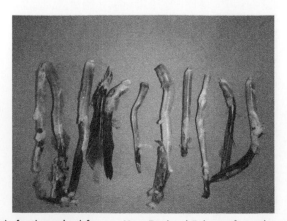

Fig. 20. Dystrophic feathers shed from a New Zealand Falcon after adenovirus infection in the second week of life. (*Courtesy of* Tom A. Bailey, Origin Vets, Pembrokeshire, United Kingdom.)

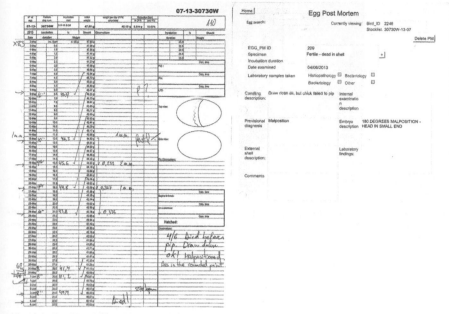

Fig. 21. Egg record chart and accompanying egg postmortem record for the same egg. (*Courtesy of* Tom A. Bailey, Origin Vets, Pembrokeshire, United Kingdom.)

GONADS

Infections of the ovary or the testes occur as part of systemic infections. In particular *Chlamydophila* and *Salmonella* occasionally cause disease of the gonads.[13] Although *Chlamydophila* is infrequently reported in raptors compared with psittacines, breeding projects need to be vigilant to this condition because it can easily be introduced following the feeding of infected prey, such as pigeons and waterfowl. Vertical transmission of *Chlamydophila* through the egg has been demonstrated in many avian species and following active infection the agent is shed via feces for more than a year.[40] Systemic viral infections, such as paramyxovirus or influenza A, can

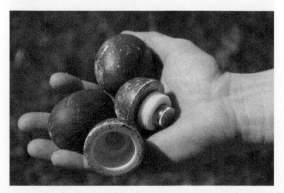

Fig. 22. Dataloggers can also be inserted in dummy eggs to monitor incubation parameters within an incubator or under female falcons used for natural incubation. (*Courtesy of* Tom A. Bailey, Origin Vets, Pembrokeshire, United Kingdom.)

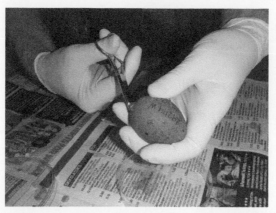

Fig. 23. Conducting egg postmortem examinations on unhatched eggs is a vital tool in understanding infertility issues in a project. (*Courtesy of* Tom A. Bailey, Origin Vets, Pembrokeshire, United Kingdom.)

cause gonad pathology (petechial bleeding) in other avian species, but usually the bird's general clinical signs are of greater importance. Such conditions as aspergillosis can cause fertility issues. Low-grade infection by *Aspergillus* spp of airsacs adjacent to gonads caused male infertility in gyrfalcons (see **Fig. 19, Table 6**). Gonadal neoplasia (**Fig. 26**), such as adenocarcinomas of the oviduct, have been occasionally reported.[12,41,42]

PRODUCTIVITY, SENESCENCE, AND MANAGEMENT OF BREEDING STOCK

Male falcons continue to be fertile until they are elderly. The authors are aware of one imprinted male gyrfalcon that produced semen when he was 22 years old.

In comparison the fertility of female falcons declines with age. Generally with the larger falcon species (sakers, gyrs, peregrines) the fertility starts to decline after 8 to 10 years and from 12 years of age onward they often cease laying. Females laying eggs until 18 years are reported, but clutches usually get smaller when aging. This

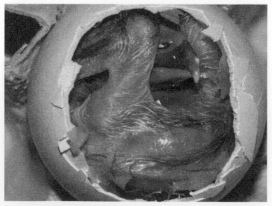

Fig. 24. The egg is opened at the blunt end. This demonstrates the correct position of the embryo in the egg immediately before pipping. (*Courtesy of* Michael Lierz, Justus-Liebig-University Giessen, Giessen, Germany.)

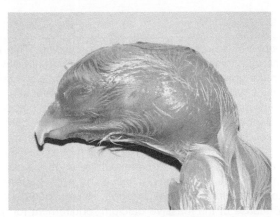

Fig. 25. Gyrfalcon embryo that died shortly before pipping demonstrating severe neck edema. A common cause of this is insufficient loss of water/weight during the incubation period. (*Courtesy of* Michael Lierz, Justus-Liebig-University Giessen, Giessen, Germany.)

highly depends on the amount of eggs the female has laid in her life because repeated clutching per year and especially egg pulling reduces age for reproduction. Endoscopy of such cases is diagnostic revealing senescent ovarian tissue that has a large pink ovary and the almost complete absence of follicles (see **Fig. 18**).

Annual reviews of breeding stock should include assessment of the age profile of the breeder flock to determine the numbers of replacements that are needed. Other information that should be included in any review are mortality rates (species, sex, and age class), productivity of pairs, and individual imprints (number of eggs and egg fertility and hatchability data). Managing a breeding project also means ensuring there is sufficient aviary space for replacement nonbreeding birds and a policy for dealing with nonproductive birds. Although some imprinted female falcons can still be used for rearing chicks or sold as falconry birds, surplus birds may need to be culled if they cannot be housed adequately. Euthanasia of healthy animals is against the law in many countries, so breeders must have spare aviaries for birds that do not reproduce but are otherwise healthy.

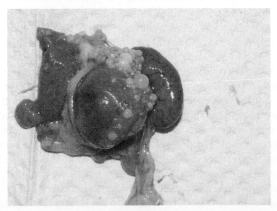

Fig. 26. Hemangiosarcoma adjacent to the ovary of a great horned owl (*Bubo virginianus*). (*Courtesy of* Michael Lierz, Justus-Liebig-University Giessen, Giessen, Germany.)

OVIDUCT
Egg Binding

The most common problem of the oviduct is egg binding. This means that the bird cannot lay the egg. In some cases the egg is only partially developed (without shell) and stays in the upper oviduct. This is caused by calcium deficiency; inflammation of the oviduct, which may be a result of systemic infection; or in imprint falcons by contaminated semen used in AI. In most cases the egg is fully developed and stays in the lower oviduct. Therefore egg binding is more common in late season or during the second clutch, in particular when calcium deficiency plays a role. Although oviduct inflammation might be a reason, hypocalcaemia or stress caused by disturbance are possible causes. In cases where eggs are being pulled before the clutch is complete, the female might leave the nest, causing egg binding if she does not accept an alternative nest scrape. Hypocalcaemia can occur if egg pulling is used. Because of the massive calcium requirement for shell production, some commonly used food items may be deficient. Reproductive neoplasms, skeletal deformities, and deformed and rarely overlarge eggs are rare causes of egg binding.

Clinical signs include reduced activity of the female. She may remain in the nest with closed eyes for several hours. It is hard to distinguish between egg-laying lethargy, which may occur before the first egg, and real egg binding. If the inactivity occurs after the first egg then egg binding is more likely. In egg binding, leg weakness also might occur. The egg can increase pressure on vessels and nerve and even intestine causing urinary or intestinal obstructions.

The history is important to distinguish between an unwell bird not laying the egg, from a case of egg binding. Information that is needed includes how many clutches the female laid during the last and current season, which egg number is expected, previous egg-laying problems, and diet and feeding of calcium and vitamin D supplements.

Radiographs (ventrodorsal and lateral) are essential to evaluate the eggshell, form and size and the pelvic bones, and the occurrence of medullary bones of the bird. In cases where the eggshell is developed but no medullary bone is present, calcium deficiency is possible. Ionized calcium is analyzed to confirm hypocalcemia. In these cases calcium gluconate (50–100 mg/kg intramuscular, intravenous slow bolus, intra osseus) and vitamin D (6600 U/kg intramuscular once) is administered by injection in addition to supplementing the diet and the bird is placed back in the breeding chamber. The use of oxytocin is questionable because it increases the blood pressure of the female and might lead to circulatory problems.[13] Some authors recommend the use of prostaglandin E_2 gel applied topically per cloacum to the uterine sphincter as an aid to dilating this sphincter and inducing uterine contractions.[13]

In cases where sufficient medullary bone is noted on radiographs calcium deficiency is unlikely and reasons why the egg cannot be laid naturally should be evaluated (eg, malformed pelvic bones, eggshell deformation, no eggshell present). In these cases and under anesthesia, manipulation of the egg within the abdomen can be performed using lateral pressure on each side of the bird's body; downward pressure can cause damage to the kidneys and also can reduce their blood supply. Gentle pressure can maneuver a shelled egg down the oviduct to present at the exit to the oviduct and with sustained pressure, lubrication, and by gently easing the oviduct over the egg it is possible to remove the impacted egg. These eggs often have no cuticle. Without a cuticle, the egg's surface is relatively rough and these eggs do not therefore pass out as easily as a normal egg.

If the eggshell is thin, the egg can be collapsed by aspiration of the egg contents after the shell has been punctured with a large 19G needle and then delivered through the cloaca. Once the egg is delivered, blood samples (chemistry and hematology) are useful. Administration of antibiotics (to prevent infections of the oviduct), fluids (subcutaneously and orally), calcium, and warmth are recommended.

If the egg cannot be delivered surgical intervention is necessary because torsion of the oviduct may be present. All manipulations are performed under general anesthesia. When the bird is weak the owners must be informed that anesthesia carries an increased risk. After any intervention, it is advisable to keep the bird away from the breeding pen and its partner to interrupt the laying cycle. Repeated egg binding in the female or oviduct tissue necrosis should be managed by surgical removal of the oviduct.

Failure to lay can also be caused by ectopic eggs (**Fig. 27**). Clinical management of ectopic eggs has been described in parrots.[43] Rarely birds can prolapse an egg into the urodeum. These eggs are difficult to remove and also the egg obstructs the ureters and the bird can develop renal failure. This should be considered after removal of the egg.

Infection and thickening or scarring of the vent may prevent the egg from being laid. An episiotomy may be needed. After such intervention some birds are not able to lay reliably and should be removed from the breeding program, as should birds with a recurrence of egg binding or irreversible physical abnormalities.

Salpingitis

Bacterial infection of the oviduct may occur after AI or egg binding. There are little data on the prevalence of oviduct infections after AI. If insemination, particularly forced AI (**Fig. 28**), is not carried out by skilled practitioners there is potential for trauma to the lining of the oviduct. Likewise semen contamination with feces, urine, or an

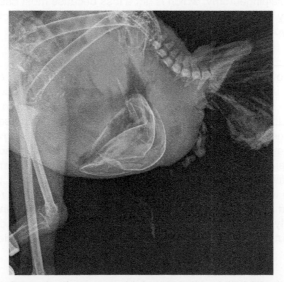

Fig. 27. Lateral radiograph of a 3-year-old female yellow billed kite (*Milvus aegyptius*) showing the outline of broken mineralized egg fragments in the ventral-caudal coelomic cavity. This was an ectopic egg. (*Courtesy of* Tom A. Bailey, Origin Vets, Pembrokeshire, United Kingdom.)

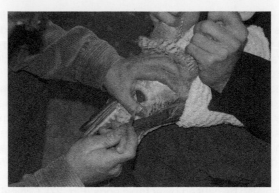

Fig. 28. This image shows a falcon being inseminated forcibly. It is easy to see that hygienic insemination techniques are essential to avoid infections of the oviduct. (*Courtesy of* Tom A. Bailey, Origin Vets, Pembrokeshire, United Kingdom.)

introduction of a contaminated tube into the oviduct has the potential to cause oviduct infections. Salpingitis may be more common if AI procedures are performed by untrained people and the equipment hygiene is poor. Inseminations have also been performed intracloacal, which carries a lower risk for oviduct infection by inseminations, especially if the semen is contaminated by feces, blood, or urine. However, if cloacal inseminations are used, resulting fertility is usually lower compared with intravaginal inseminations.[18] Cloacal infections can also lead to ascending infection of the oviduct, as do ruptured eggs or undetected egg binding. Such infections are often fatal because they are recognized too late for treatment. In some cases alterations of the eggshell (depigmentation, rough or irregular shell) might be detectable. If the bird is only used for breeding intensive antibiotic treatment might be tried. The treatment of choice is the salpingectomy, which is not a loss because most cases of salpingitis result in infertility of the female. An experienced breeding bird can often be used for crèche-rearing young birds even if she is unable to lay eggs herself.

Prolapse

Prolapse of the oviduct is sometimes difficult to differentiate from a cloacal prolapse (proctodeum or urodeum or both can prolapse) and often both occur. Outside the breeding season, oviduct prolapse is rare because the oviduct is too small. Prolapse of the oviduct can occur because of egg binding as the bird increases its abdominal pressure to lay the egg. It may also occur in older females after laying an egg because suspensory ligaments of the oviduct can be stretched or weakened and torn. Prolapses have been seen in imprint females that have laid large numbers of eggs in sequence. Oviduct neoplasms or infections are other causes. A prolapse of the oviduct requires immediate surgical intervention. Additionally, birds require intensive fluid therapy and antibiotic treatment. Because the reproductive, urinary, and intestinal tract all empty into the cloaca, pushing a prolapse back inside and retaining it with a purse-string suture, instead of proper diagnostics, frequently condemns the bird to death.

Egg Peritonitis

Egg peritonitis is rare in birds of prey compared with other birds laying more eggs, such as chickens. Yolk material in the abdominal cavity causes inflammatory reactions and may be absorbed without any further problems. A larger amount of yolk material or the bacterial colonization of the foreign material leads to a rapid and extensive inflammatory process resulting in severe illness. If untreated it is usually fatal. Yolk material enters the abdominal cavity by oviduct rupture or if the infundibulum fails to gather the yolk at the time of ovulation. Clinically the signs may be noticed during the egg-laying period, but sometimes signs are detected after the breeding season. In these cases the owner may observe that the female either laid no or less eggs than expected. Radiography shows the presence of an amorphous mass and fails to demonstrate an egg. An increased white blood cell count and elevated serum fibrinogen confirm an inflammatory process. Ultrasound is useful and a fine-needle aspirate of the abdominal contents is informative and is used for bacteriology (often *Escherichia coli*). If possible the bird should be stabilized before surgical removal of the egg yolks and possible salpingectomy. The prognosis for these cases is guarded.

CONGENITAL PROBLEMS

Congenital disorders are occasionally seen and unfortunately issues associated with inbreeding may become increasingly frequent in the future. Inbreeding has been shown to cause early embryonic death in passerine species.[44] It is becoming more difficult or impossible in Europe and North America because of import restrictions for breeders to legally acquire wild-caught unrelated breeding stock. Given that only a few raptor breeders have good record systems and unscrupulous breeders sell related birds as unrelated it is inevitable that the limited captive pool of birds used for breeding will become more inbred with each passing generation. Splayed legs, scoliosis, lordosis, opisthotonus, cerebellar defects, eye abnormalities (**Fig. 29**), joint deviations, and stunted birds are examples of congenital and growth problems seen in psittacines and raptors.[45] It is likely that genetic testing will become an important tool for diagnosing genetic and inbreeding issues in the future. Relatedness is tested through multiple gene loci comparison between birds and it may be helpful to identify the genetic variety within a breeding collection. Such tools are used to manage breeding in controlled stud books for species conservation breeding programs.

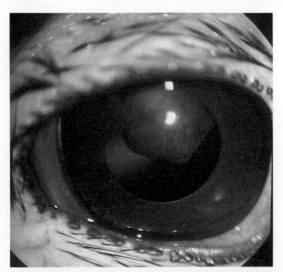

Fig. 29. Congenital malformed lens in a juvenile falcon. (*Courtesy of* Michael Lierz, Justus-Liebig-University Giessen, Giessen, Germany.)

HORMONAL THERAPY

Most companion birds are kept purely as pets and the owners have no interest in breeding. Indeed because many diseases of the female reproductive tract (egg binding, dystocia, yolk coelomitis, and cloacal prolapse) are life-threatening, hormonal therapy with gonadotropin-releasing hormone agonists is commonly used to suppress ovarian activity.[46] The use of gonadotropin-releasing hormone agonists may also be appropriate to suppress reproduction during the breeding season in female birds of prey that are not required for breeding and who have experienced reproductive disorders that could represent as life-threatening conditions (eg, egg binding, prolapses). Deslorelin acetate (Suprelorin, 4.7 mg, Virbac) implants have been used in chickens and psittacines to suppress ovarian activity for 3 to 4 months,[46] but no reports on the use of these agents in raptors are available.

Hormonal therapy has been anecdotally used in avian breeding projects to improve reproductive success, but there are few published reports on the efficacy of such treatment.[47,48] Buserelin, a gonadotropin-releasing hormone analogue (Receptal, MSD Animal Health) is a neurohormone that regulates reproduction and is used in mammals and fish, although its use has not been reported in birds of prey. It is used to stimulate ovulation in mammals and has been used in pigeons (Stacey Gellis, personal communication, 2016) and raptors anecdotally (Bailey, unpublished data; Samour, unpublished data). Clomifene citrate is another hormone that has been shown to increase follicular development in female sheep[49] and has been used in raptors anecdotally (Bailey, unpublished data; Marino Garcia-Montijano, personal communication, 2016). A summary of hormonal agents used in raptors is presented in **Table 7**.

Table 7 Examples of reproductive hormones used in raptors		
Pharmaceutical Agent	**Potential Uses in Raptors**	**Dose and Administration**
Buserelin (Receptal, MSD Animal Health)	1. Extending the breeding season of imprint males. 2. Stimulating reproductive activity in pairs in which there is little breeding interaction. Treatment of the females may stimulate egg laying.	0.25 mL/kg or 0.001 mg/kg given IM twice 10–14 d apart (extrapolated from pigeon dose). Samour (personal communication, 2016) used 0.6 mL for female gyrfalcons and 0.4 mL for males three times 1 wk apart.
Clomifene citrate (Clomid tablets, Sanofi)	Stimulate reproductive activity in unpaired females offering the potential for forced AI opportunities.	Marino Garcia-Montijano (personal communication, 2016) used in female raptors for 2–3 wk and noted it contributed to ovarian and oviduct development. Variable results: some birds laid, but not consistent. Seemed to promote sexual behavioral activity in female raptors. Treatment started at onset of reproductive season. 12.5 mg/kg once a day for 14–21 d

ACKNOWLEDGMENTS

Dr. T.A. Bailey thanks Martyn Paterson from Desert Falcons and Nick Fox, Oscar Oliva, Sandor Sebastian, and Diana Durman-Walters for the avicultural knowledge they shared during the 3 years he worked at International Consultants breeding falcons.

SUPPLEMENTARY DATA

Supplementary data related to this article can be found at http://dx.doi.org/10.1016/j.cvex.2016.11.008.

REFERENCES

1. Toone WD, Risser AC. Captive management of the California condor *Gymnogyps californianus*. Int Zoo Yearb 1988;50–8.
2. Cade TJ, Temple SJ. Management of threatened bird species: evaluation of the hands on approach. Ibis 1994;137:161–72.
3. Jones CG, Heck W, Lewis RE, et al. The restoration of the Mauritius Kestrel *Falco punctatus* population. Ibis 1995;137:S173–80.
4. Weaver JD, Cade T. Falcon propagation; manual of captive breeding. Boise (ID): The Peregrine Fund Inc; 1991. p. 1–99.
5. Fox NC. Understanding the bird of prey. Blaine (Washington): Hancock House Publishers; 1995. p. 58–111.
6. Heidenreich M. Birds of prey; medicine and management. 1st English edition. Oxford (United Kingdom): Blackwell Science Ltd; 1995. p. 35–59.
7. Knowles-Brown A, Wishart GJ. Progeny from cryopreserved golden eagle spermatozoa. Av Poult Biol Rev 2001;12:201–2.
8. Blanco JM, Gee GF, Wildt DE, et al. Producing progeny from endangered birds of prey: treatment of urine-contaminated semen and a novel intramagnal insemination approach. J Zoo Wildl Med 2002;33(1):1–7.
9. Holland G. Eagles, vultures, falcons and kestrels. In: Holland G, editor. Encyclopedia of aviculture. Surrey (Canada): Hancroft Books; 2007. p. 513–36.
10. Blanco JM, Wildt DE, Höfle U, et al. Implementing artificial insemination as an effective tool for ex situ conservation of endangered avian species. Theriogenology 2009;71:200–13.
11. Fischer D, Garcia de la Fuente J, Wehrend A, et al. Semen quality and semen characteristics of large falcons with special emphasis on fertility rate after artificial insemination. Repro Dom Anim 2011;46:14.
12. Jones R. Raptors: systemic and non-infectious diseases. In: Chitty J, Lierz M, editors. Manual of raptors, pigeons and passerine birds. Gloucester (United Kingdom): British Small Animal Veterinary Association; 2008. p. 284–98.
13. Lierz M. Raptors: reproductive disease, incubation and artificial insemination. In: Chitty J, Lierz M, editors. Manual of raptors, pigeons and passerine birds. Gloucester (United Kingdom): British Small Animal Veterinary Association; 2008. p. 235–49.
14. Lierz M. Advancements in methods for improving reproductive success. In: Speer BL, editor. Current therapy in avian medicine and surgery. St Louis (MO): Elsevier; 2016. p. 433–45.
15. Bailey TA. The role of demographic and genetic resource management in maintaining small populations of falcons in captivity: the example of the New Zealand falcon (*Falco novaeseelandiae*) captive breeding programme and a pilot study to

cryopreserve semen from *Falconidae* using field techniques [MSc thesis]. London: University of London; 2002. p. 89.

16. Bailey TA, Holt W, Bennett P, et al. The management of small populations of falcons in captivity and the results of a pilot study to cryopreserve semen from *Falconidae* using field techniques. 7th European Association of Avian Veterinarians Conference, SpainTenerife 2003;104–12.

17. Bird D, Lague PC. Semen production of the American kestrel. Can J Zool 1977; 55:1351–8.

18. Fischer D, Neumann D, Wehrend A, et al. Comparison of conventioinal and computer assisted semen analysis in cockatiels (*Nymphicus hollandicus*) and evaluation of different insemination dosages for artificial insemination. Theriogenology 2014;82(4):613–20.

19. Umapathy G, Sontakke S, Reddy A, et al. Semen characteristics of the captive Indian white-backed vulture (*Gyps bengalensis*). Biol Reprod 2005;73(5): 1039–45.

20. Lierz M, Reinschmidt M, Muller H, et al. A novel method for semen collection and artificial insemination in large parrors (Psittaciformes). Sci Rep 2013;3:2066.

21. Krohn J, Schneider H, Meinecke-Tillmann S, et al. Technical Note: In vitro examination of the penetration ability in avian spermatozoa of different species. Repro Dom Anim 2014;49(Suppl 1):29–30.

22. Lierz M, Hafez HM. Occurrence of mycoplasmas in semen samples of birds of prey. Avian Pathol 2008;37(5):495–7.

23. Clum NJ, Fitzpatrick MP, Dierenfeld ES. Nutrient content of five species of domestic animals commonly fed to captive raptors. J Raptor Res 1997;31:267–72.

24. Forbes N, Simpson GN, Higgins RJ, et al. Adenovirus infection in Mauritius kestrels (*Falco punctatus*). J Avian Med Surg 1997;11(1):31–3.

25. Bynum K, Yoder C, Eisemann J, et al. Development of nicarbazin as a reproductive inhibitor for resident Canada geese. Wildlife Damage Management Conferences – Proceedings. 2005. p. 101. Available at: http://digitalcommons.unl.edu/icwdm_wdmconfproc/101. Accessed December 28, 2016.

26. Chitty J. Raptors: nutrition. In: Chitty J, Lierz M, editors. Manual of raptors, pigeons and passerine birds. Gloucester (United Kingdom): British Small Animal Veterinary Association; 2008. p. 195.

27. Dierenfeld ES, Sandfort CE, Satterfield WC. Influence of diet on plasma vitamin E in captive peregrine falcons. J Wildl Man 1989;53:160–4.

28. Schink B, Hafez H, Lierz M. Alpha-Tocopherol in captive falcons: reference values and influence of diet. J Avian Med Surg 2008;22:99–102.

29. Carnarius M, Hafez HM, Henning A, et al. Clinical signs and diagnosis of thiamine deficiency in juvenile goshawks (*Accipiter gentilis*). Vet Rec 2008;163:215–7.

30. Calle PP, Dierenfeld ES, Robert ME. Serum α-tocopherol in raptors fed vitamin E-supplemented diets. J Zoo Wildl Med 1989;20:62–6.

31. Morales J, Velando A, Torres R. Fecundity compromises attractiveness when pigments are scarce. Behav Ecol 2009;20:117–23.

32. Ouventin PJ, McGraw KJ, Morel M, et al. Dietary carotenoid supplementation affects orange beak but not foot coloration in gentoo penguins *Pygoscelis papua*. Waterbirds 2007;30(4):573–8.

33. Schrenzel M, Lindsay Oaks J, Rotstein D, et al. Characterization of a new species of adenovirus in falcons. J Clin Microbiol 2005;43:3402–13.

34. Oaks LJ, Schrenzel M, Rideout B, et al. Isolation and epidemiology of falcon adenovirus. J Clin Microbiol 2005;43:3414–20.

35. Deeming C. Birds, nest and incubators. Somerset (United Kingdom): Brinsea Products Ltd; 2002. p. 209.
36. Crosta L, Melillo A, Schnitzer P. Incubation. In: Samour J, editor. Avian medicine. 3rd edition. St Louis (MO): Elsevier; 2015. p. 539–46.
37. Bailey T, Jepson L, O'Donovan D. The use of dataloggers in zoos, breeding projects, exotic animal practice and fieldwork. Chester (United Kingdom): Proceedings of the British Veterinary Zoological Society; 2016.
38. Birkhead TR, Hall J, Schute E, et al. Unhatched eggs: methods for discriminating between infertility and early embryo mortality. Ibis 2008;150:508–17.
39. Jones M. Raptors: paediatrics and behavioural development and disorders. In: Chitty J, Lierz M, editors. Manual of raptors, pigeons and passerine birds. Gloucester (United Kingdom): British Small Animal Veterinary Association; 2008. p. 250–9.
40. Crosta L, Melillo A, Schnitzer P. Chlamydiosis. In: Speer BL, editor. Current therapy in avian medicine and surgery. St Louis (MO): Elsevier; 2016. p. 82–93.
41. Forbes NA, Cooper JE, Higgins RJ. Neoplasms of birds of prey. In: Lumeij JT, et al, editors. Raptor biomedicine III. Lake Worth (FL): Zoological Education Network; 2000. p. 127–45.
42. Zehnder A, Graham J, Reavill DR, et al. Neoplastic diseases in avian species. In: Speer BL, editor. Current therapy in avian medicine and surgery. St Louis (MO): Elsevier; 2016. p. 107–41.
43. Mans CL, Sladky KK. Clinical management of an ectopic egg in a Timneh African grey parrot (*Psittacus erithacus timneh*). J Am Vet Med Assoc 2013;242(7):963–8.
44. Hemmings N, Slate J, Birkhead JR. Inbreeding causes early death in a passerine bird. Nat Commun 2012;3:863.
45. Bailey TA, Magno MN. Neonatology. In: Samour J, editor. Avian medicine. 3rd edition. St Louis (MO): Elsevier; 2015. p. 549–58.
46. Petritz O, Lierz M, Samour J. Advancements in methods for decreasing reproductive success. In: Speer BL, editor. Current therapy in avian medicine and surgery. St Louis (MO): Elsevier; 2016. p. 446–60.
47. Costantini V, Carraro C, Bucci FA, et al. Influence of a new slow-release GnRH analogue implant on reproduction in the Budgerigar (*Melopsittacus undulatus*, Shaw 1805). Anim Reprod Sci 2009;111:289–301.
48. Lovas EM, Johnston SD, Filippich LJ. Using a GnRH agonist to obtain an index of testosterone secretory capacity in the cockatiel (*Nymphicus hollandicus*) and sulphurcrested cockatoo *(Cacatua galerita)*. Aust Vet J 2010;88:52–6.
49. EL-Sherry TM, Derar R, Hussein HA, et al. Effect of clomiphene citrate (CC) on follicular recruitment, development, and superovulation during the first follicular wave in Rahmani ewes. Int J Endo Metab 2011;9(3):403–8.

Reproductive Disorders in Parrots

Alyssa M. Scagnelli, DVM*, Thomas N. Tully Jr, DVM, MS, DABVP (Avian), DECZM

KEYWORDS

- Avian • Psittacine • Coelomitis • Egg-binding • Avian reproductive disease
- Dystocia

KEY POINTS

- Medicine pertaining to the avian reproductive tract is commonly a multimodal approach consisting of both physiologic and environmental management.
- Egg binding represents a common reproductive disorder of Psittacine species, which can predispose to serious life-threatening complications, including dystocia and oviduct rupture.
- Use of synthetic, long-acting gonadotropin-releasing hormone (GnRH) agonists may help with certain reproductive diseases, including chronic egg laying.
- Inflammatory conditions of the reproductive tract are often linked to oviduct rupture or tear, resulting in coelomitis.
- Coelioscopy is often the best diagnostic tool to help diagnose most reproductive disorders and allow for assessment of tissues through biopsy and histopathology.

AVIAN REPRODUCTIVE ANATOMY: A RAPID REVIEW
Female

With the exception of certain avian species, most birds demonstrate development of the left reproductive tract exclusively, whereas the right gonadal tissue remains a vestigial organ system. Anatomically, the left ovary lies between the cranial division of the kidney, the adrenal gland, and the caudal aspect of the lung. It is attached to the coelomic wall by the mesovarian ligament. The main blood supply to the left ovary arises from the left cranial renal artery, which then branches into the ovario-oviductal artery, supplying the ovary and oviduct. Coming from the ovary are numerous vessels that allow return of blood to the vena cava. In a sexually active bird, these vessels may be difficult to distinguish due to follicular development.

The authors have nothing to disclose.
Veterinary Clinical Sciences, School of Veterinary Medicine, Louisiana State University, Skip Bertman Drive, Baton Rouge, LA 70810, USA
* Corresponding author.
E-mail address: ascagnelli@lsu.edu

Vet Clin Exot Anim 20 (2017) 485–507
http://dx.doi.org/10.1016/j.cvex.2016.11.012
1094-9194/17/© 2016 Elsevier Inc. All rights reserved.

vetexotic.theclinics.com

For avian species that are seasonal layers, follicular development occurs in separate stages. In birds classified as seasonal layers, as the numerous follicles begin to develop, they do so based on a "tier system," whereby the more developed follicles reach maturity first.[1] This system allows for the passing of a follicle along with its primary oocyte into the oviduct without immediate competition.[2,3] Changes in appearance to the ovary are observed during the different stages of development and are easily perceived via coelioscopy. A quiescent ovary (during the nonbreeding season) will be small, have a coarse surface, and is typically uniform in color, whereas an active ovary may look like a bunch of variably sized and colored spheres. As follicular development advances, yolk proteins are deposited, giving the maturing follicles a yellow appearance. Species variation is also appreciated with some parrots having more melanistic follicles than others.

The avian oviduct is composed of 5 separate regions that are mainly distinguished on the cellular level. The funnel-like infundibulum receives the ovum directly from the ovary and is the location of fertilization. During the approximately 1-hour transit time in the infundibulum, the outer yolk membranes and chalazae are added.[4,5] The ovum then reaches the magnum, where sodium, calcium, and magnesium are added. The magnum is easily distinguished from the rest of the oviduct due to its large size, coiled appearance, and large mucosal folds, all of which can be observed macroscopically. Microscopically, the magnum is associated with glandular tissue, consistent with its secretory role in egg development. After several hours in the magnum, the egg enters the isthmus, where the inner and outer shell membranes are added. The uterus (shell gland) is very short in avian species and is the site of shell deposition. The egg remains in the uterus for the longest period of time, whereby it accumulates salts, water, and shell pigment. The last segment of the oviduct, the vagina, is the shortest, but thickest-walled section and is solely responsible for oviposition. In a reproductively active bird, the left oviduct will grow markedly in size and may incorporate a large portion of the left coelom. Conversely, in young reproductively inactive birds, the oviduct may be small enough to be confused with the ureters coursing nearby. In most psittacine species, the interval between subsequent oviposition is 48 hours.[5]

Male

The oblong pair of testes is located in the dorsal coelomic body cavity between the cranial pole of the kidneys and the caudal aspect of the lungs. The avian testes are suspended from the body cavity by the mesorchium and are surrounded by an abdominal air sac. The male avian reproductive organs may appear light or dark in color depending on age, species, and reproductive activity. It is common for melanistic testes to be observed in some Psittaciformes (eg, conures, macaws, cockatoos).[5] The outer capsule of the testes is smooth due to lack of lobation (an observation in most mammalian species). Unlike their female counterparts, both testes are hormonally active and functional in birds.

The epididymis in birds is much smaller than the mammalian equivalent. Located at the dorsomedial aspect of the testes, the epididymis is often difficult to observe during coelioscopy, even when engorged due to reproductive activity. The epididymis functions as a conduit for spermatozoa from the rete testes to the ductus deferens. The ductus deferens will be tortuous, which will help distinguish it from the nearby tracking ureters. The distal-most aspect of the ductus deferens joins the urodeum, creating an ejaculatory papilla. Although some avian species have a phallus for copulatory function, Psittaciformes do not have a phallus. Instead, copulation is achieved through eversion of the cloacal wall and transfer of sperm from the ejaculatory papilla to the female cloaca.[2,5] Although the ejaculatory papilla can serve as a potential aid in sex determination in some avian species, this technique is difficult and is not consistent across Psittaciformes.

SEX DIFFERENTIATION

When trying to successfully reproduce parrots, it is extremely important to set up the breeding pair with a confirmed male and female of that particular species. Many parrot species are monomorphic, making sex determination difficult without gender-specific external characteristics. Differentiating between male and female parrots of monomorphic avian species has become increasingly accessible due to advances in DNA sexing. Submission of avian blood or feathers is sufficient for most tests, often heralded with accuracy rates greater than 99.9%. However, clinical experience of the authors places the accuracy rates of DNA sexing closer to 90%. Before DNA testing, sexing via celioscopy was the primary method used to determine male or female sex. Although "surgical sexing" through endoscopic viewing of the gonad is more involved than DNA sex determination and requires general anesthesia, it is still recommended for birds that are established as reproductive pairs. The internal examination of the coelom and gonad(s) is very important in determining the health of the animal and likelihood of it being reproductively active. If the owner of a bird is not interested in reproduction and only wants to determine the animal's sex, DNA testing is sufficient. Although some parrot owners may not want to know the sex of their companion bird, determination of sex is recommended to help elucidate medical and behavioral issues.

Although most parrots are monomorphic, some species are sexually dimorphic, displaying certain traits that are characteristic to either male or female sex. Most of these phenotypic traits are variances in color or pattern of the plumage; however, others include beak and cere color variances between sexes. The most widely known example for avian sexual dimorphism is the eclectus parrot (*Eclectus roratus*), whereby the male and female display green and red plumage, respectively (**Fig. 1A**). Changes in plumage in other psittacine species are relatively common, but can be subtle. Often, other traits can be used to determine sex. In the Derbyan parakeet (*Psittacula derbiana*), the male will have a yellow-orange–colored beak and the female will have an all-black beak (**Fig. 1B**). Characteristics, such as the previously mentioned examples, in a sexually dimorphic species, are enough to identify the sex of a bird and thus DNA sexing is not required.

REPRODUCTIVE BEHAVIOR

Environmental stimuli and behavior (between a pair of birds or the bird and the owner) are of prime importance when discussing psittacine reproductive medicine. Despite being maintained indoors, most parrots will still show seasonally dependent reproductive behavior due to changes in photoperiod.[6,7] This is even true of equatorial psittacine species. One can make the argument that although maintained indoors, parrots are still capable of responding to changes in temperature, rainfall, and other outdoor environmental cues. Often, the presence of another bird has a significant effect on reproductive behavior, regardless of species. Ultimately, these environmental variables will precipitate changes in endocrinology and result in subsequent reproductive activity. Although out of the scope of this text, understanding of the hypothalamic-pituitary axis and steroidogenesis are essential when considering treatment for certain reproductive diseases. Clinically, it is important to ask owners if the bird has been exhibiting signs of reproductive behavior because this information can help direct one toward differential disease diagnoses for the presenting problem(s). Behaviors such as nest-building (eg, paper shredding, accumulation of other items in an area),

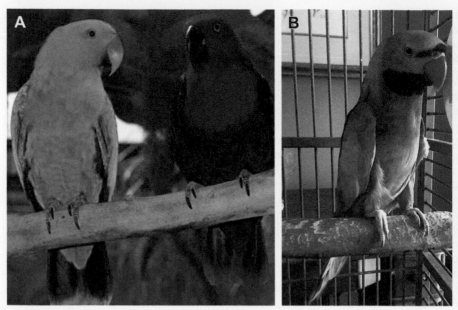

Fig. 1. (A) Image of the sexually dimorphic male (*left*) and female (*right*) Eclectus parrot. (B) Image of the male Derbyan parakeet. The beak is yellow-orange in the male bird (*pictured*) as opposed to the all-black beak in the female (*not shown*).

hiding, seeking out dark places, regurgitating for a mate, and copulation with objects should all be considered a valuable part of the patient history.

REPRODUCTIVE DISEASE IN COMPANION BIRDS

Disease affecting the reproductive tract in companion birds is not an uncommon presenting complaint for avian cases treated by veterinarians. As previously stated, reproductive diseases are frequently multifactorial; therefore, investigating a primary source or cause of the disease is often not rewarding. Although most pet birds are companion animals and not maintained for producing young, birds may still have undesirable reproductive behavior disease. The following section details some of the more common reproductive disorders in psittacine species, with a focus on reviewing methods of disease diagnosis as well as examining the current treatment recommendations for such disorders. Last, behavioral and environmental management is discussed as ancillary treatment for some reproductive disease conditions.

DISEASES AFFECTING THE FEMALE REPRODUCTIVE SYSTEM
Dystocia and Egg Binding

Dystocia involves a mechanical obstruction preventing normal oviposition from the caudal oviduct. In mammals, dystocia is often categorized into 2 separate headings: maternal and fetal causes. For birds, the egg is the equivalent of the fetus and abnormal presentation of the egg can certainly cause obstruction within the oviduct. Normal presentation of the egg within the caudal reproductive tract is with the blunted end of the egg exiting last.[4,5] Abnormal presentation of an egg may consist of rotation along the long axis resulting in the blunted end exiting first ("breach") or rotation along the short axis yielding neither blunted nor pointed end exiting first. Maternal causes of dystocia are often more medically challenging because of the multifactorial nature of the disease. Both primary reproductive tract disease (eg, oviduct torsion, oviduct neoplasia, salpingitis) and obstruction due to surrounding organ systems (eg, coelomic masses) must be considered. Anatomically, the most common regions associated with dystocia include the uterus, vagina, and vaginal-cloacal junction.[4,5,8,9]

Although the length of time between egg intervals can vary between species, in most companion psittacine species, subsequent eggs will be laid within a 48-hour period.[5] Egg binding is defined as the failure of an egg to pass through the oviduct within a normal time frame. It may be difficult to determine if egg binding is occurring unless obvious clinical signs have been directly observed in the patient, especially if the bird is considered a "first-time layer."

Although both dystocia and egg binding can be mutually exclusive, they are often discussed together because of the risk factors associated with both. Proper nutrition of the hen is of paramount importance, with calcium metabolism and vitamin E and selenium deficiency being of greatest concern.[4,5] Poor nutrition may not only result in inadequate smooth muscle contraction, but also improper egg formation resulting in soft or malformed eggs. Another common condition associated with egg binding is chronic egg laying, which may predispose to abnormalities and damage of the oviduct musculature. Other risk factors include systemic disease, obesity, lack of exercise, virgin hens, previous dystocia, and a persistent right oviduct. Although dystocia and egg binding can affect any species, smaller birds, such as canaries, lovebirds, finches, budgerigars, and cockatiels, seem to be overrepresented likely because of the size of the bird.[4,5,8,10]

Clinical signs

Common clinical signs associated with dystocia or egg binding are summarized in **Table 1**. Signs can vary depending on the size of the bird affected and the length of time associated with the problem. Because a bird can present obtunded or near death, the anamnesis and physical examination (including cloacal assessment) may be the only diagnostic information available to the practitioner. Attention to the diet of the bird is of particular importance and may help elucidate the potential cause of dystocia. Precaution should be observed for critical patients that may not survive prolonged handling and/or advanced diagnostic testing (eg, imaging).

Table 1
Clinical signs commonly associated with dystocia and egg binding

Clinical Sign	Comments
Acute depression/sudden death	Smaller birds may be at increased risk
Straining, tail-wagging, wide stance, drooped wings	May occur singly or together; mechanical or physiologic dystocia
Coelomic distension	May be present with coelomitis
Dyspnea	Space-occupying lesion, pain, metabolic disturbances, egg yolk coelomitis
Cloacal prolapse	May complicate dystocia or be the primary cause of dystocia
Limb paralysis, lameness, paresis, unwillingness to perch	Compression of the ischiatic nerves
Palpable egg in the coelom	May or may not be possible depending on species and location in the oviduct

Diagnostic testing

Depending on the severity of clinical signs exhibited by the patient on presentation, the physical and digital cloacal examinations may be the only diagnostic tests one can safely perform. Contingent on the presence of a calcified shell, the egg may or may not be able to be palpated in the coelom. Cloacal palpation may reveal the positioning of the egg, which may help determine the cause of dystocia. If time allows, and the patient is stable, diagnostic imaging (eg, radiography, ultrasonography) should be performed to help locate the egg and determine its position. It is recommended that radiographic images be interpreted with caution because soft-shelled or collapsed eggs may not be well defined. A cue that may help aid in diagnosis of egg binding is the recognition of medullary hyperostosis (new medullary bone formation due to the presence of circulating estrogen).[9,11,12] For cases of avian dystocia that are not straightforward, a complete blood count (CBC) and serum biochemistry may aid by revealing other secondary disease processes, such as metabolic disturbances, renal compromise, and/or concurrent inflammation. Typical CBC results from birds diagnosed with egg binding include leukocytosis with concurrent heterophilia, whereas the serum biochemistry panel may reveal elevated alkaline phosphatase, hyperglobulinemia, hypercholesterolemia, hypercalcemia or hypocalcemia, and elevated creatine phosphokinase.[4,5] Most laying birds will have a marked elevation in blood calcium (levels may reach 30–40 mg/dL; 7.5–10.0 mmol/L) due to the mobilization of calcium from the bones for shell deposition. However, if the bird is a chronic layer or has any nutritional deficiencies, it may present hypocalcemic.[5]

Therapy

Due to the multifactorial nature of dystocia and egg binding, recommended treatment is often specific to the inciting cause of disease. Regardless of the inciting cause of the egg-binding condition, each patient should be provided with standard supportive care: supplemental heat to a temperature of 85 to 90°F (29.4–32.2°C), fluid therapy, analgesics, and proper nutrition, including parenteral calcium. Additional therapy, including antibiotic medication, may be warranted if there is suspicion of a ruptured oviduct, otherwise it is not considered necessary. Supportive care may be the only treatment required; however, it is important that the patient is closely monitored as any decline in overall condition demands further intervention.

Should the bird not respond to basic supportive care measures, prostaglandin and hormonal therapy could be initiated, provided there is zero suspicion for oviduct obstruction, adhesion, or perforation. Much of the research that has assessed the role of prostaglandins and hormone therapy for birds with dystocia/egg binding has been performed in poultry; however, the clinical application has been greatly translated to other avian species, including psittacines.[1,4,5] Depending on availability of products, the 3 therapies that have been studied include oxytocin, prostaglandin E2 (PGE2), and prostaglandin F2α (PGF2α). A brief review of these compounds and the pros and cons of their use is described in **Table 2**.

Use of these compounds may be precluded by availability of products as well as the safety for both the patient and clinician. Before using of any of these agents, it is important to determine the patency of the uterovaginal sphincter, as any obstruction or adhesion present may result in uterine rupture. Additionally, as all of these agents elicit muscle contraction, parenteral administration of calcium is necessary before treatment. These treatments are all relatively fast-acting and should produce results within 30 minutes to 1 hour, but maybe longer.[1,4] Oxytocin can be repeated every 30 minutes as necessary, keeping in mind that repeated muscle contraction would rapidly use the calcium and glucose reserves of the patient.

Table 2
Use of prostaglandins and oxytocin for treatment of avian reproductive disease

Compound	Product	Function	Comments
Oxytocin	—	Contraction of uterine smooth muscle exclusively	• Few systemic side effects • Does not relax the uterovaginal sphincter; therefore, use only if the sphincter is relaxed • Contraindicated if uterine adhesions or masses are present • Must provide calcium before use
Prostaglandin F2α	Dinoprost tromethamine (Lutalyse; Upjohn, Kalamazoo, MI)	Generalized smooth muscle contraction	• Does not relax the uterovaginal sphincter; therefore, use only if the sphincter is relaxed • *Large* systemic side effects observed in mammals (nausea, hypertension, bronchoconstriction, cardiac arrhythmias, severe contractions/rupture) • Caution with handling; can absorb through skin and cause spontaneous abortions in humans
Prostaglandin E2	Dinoprostone gel (Prepidil gel; Pfizer, Division of Pharmacia and Upjohn, New York, NY)	Relaxes the uterovaginal sphincter and vagina Increases uterine contractions and the effects of oxytocin and PGF2α	• Applied topically to uterovaginal sphincter • Caution with handling; can absorb through skin and cause spontaneous abortions in humans • Caution with renal and hepatic insufficiency • Less potential for systemic side effects unless overdosed • Not commercially available at this time

Data from Hudelson KS, Hudelson P. A brief review of the female avian reproductive cycle with special emphasis on the role of prostaglandins and clinical applications. J Avian Med Surg 2016;10(2):67–74; and Bowles HL. Reproductive diseases of pet bird species. In: Speer BL, editor. The Veterinary Clinics of North America exotic animal practice: reproductive medicine. 5th edition. Philadelphia: W.B. Saunders; 2002. p. 489–504.

If treatment results are not achieved with prostaglandin or hormonal therapy, more aggressive measures must be considered. Gentle massage of the lower coelom and vaginal opening may cause vaginal relaxation and subsequent oviposition. Digital manipulation of the egg within the caudal oviduct may also stimulate caudal movement of the egg, but this may predispose an oviductal tear and/or the egg's collapse. For the aforementioned procedure, the bird must be placed under general anesthesia for maximum relaxation. The clinician then applies digital pressure to the vagina and uterovaginal sphincter to aid in dilation. Once dilated, the clinician should direct the fingers above and partially behind the egg so that the fingers are between the egg and the caudoventral aspect of the keel bone. Gentle, but firm pressure is then applied to the egg, moving caudally to aid in oviposition.

If all previous treatments have failed, ovocentesis is then performed to deflate the egg with contents either being expelled immediately through the aid of lavage, or to pass later through normal muscular contractions of the oviduct and cloaca. Ovocentesis, or aspiration of the egg, can performed either transcoelomically or transcloacally, with the latter being the safer of the 2 options.[4,5,8,9,11] The outcome of ovocentesis partially depends on the mineral content of the shell; hard-shelled eggs pose a risk for uterine tear or rupture, as pieces often break off and are left behind, acting as a potential nidus for infection. Uterine lavage using warm, sterile saline may help decrease the risk associated with remaining shell pieces and is typically common practice in mammalian dystocia therapy. For transcloacal ovocentesis, a vaginal speculum is used to visualize the egg. A large-bore needle is then used to penetrate the egg and the yolk and albumen are aspirated into a syringe. The egg is gently crushed via external manipulation. The pieces can be manually evacuated if they are caudal enough within the reproductive tract. If the egg is located more cranial and cannot be visualized, the transcoelomic approach is used. The egg is positioned against the body wall and other organs are pushed away. A needle is then inserted through the skin and into the egg. The following steps are similar to those for the transcloacal approach. Radiographic imaging should be used to confirm that the bird has expelled all the shell fragments within a 24- to 36-hour time frame.

The therapies discussed are for specific cases in which oviduct tear/rupture, oviduct torsion, ectopic eggs, or mechanical obstruction are not suspected. If one of these conditions is believed to have occurred, a surgical approach may be necessary with concurrent salpingohysterectomy to significantly reduce the possibility of future reproductive disease. All hens should be closely monitored for the first 72 hours following the resolution of the egg-bound condition for additional reproductive activity, as many are hormonally "programmed" to lay another egg.

Prevention of egg binding/dystocia in avian species is aimed at eliminating reproductive activity via moderating behavioral and environmental factors in the patient's home environment. Medical management also can be instituted for those birds that are chronic egg layers.

Chronic Egg Laying

Chronic egg laying is a common disorder among some companion bird species (eg, cockatiels, budgerigars, lovebirds, finches) whereby a hen will either lay more eggs than the typical clutch size or will have sustained reproductive activity without the presence of a mate or outside the normal breeding season.[4,5,8–11] In a survey to avian veterinarians, chronic egg laying represented the second most common behavior problem with avian patients that were presented to their clinic.[13] Inadvertent handling and behavior between the bird and the mate (humans, inanimate objects, other birds) may induce reproductive behavior yielding inappropriate egg laying. Therefore, obtaining an appropriate anamnesis, which includes dietary intake, social interactions, other animals in the environment, and other environmental stimuli, is essential when trying to investigate the cause of this behavior.

Although not directly problematic, chronic egg laying can predispose the hen to egg binding/dystocia disorders due to chronic changes of the oviduct, nutritional deficiencies, physical stress, and an increased risk for ectopic eggs. The bird is also at risk for developing nutritional secondary hyperparathyroidism due to hypocalcemia, increasing the potential of pathologic fractures.

Clinical signs

An owner may not present their companion bird with the complaint of "chronic egg laying"; therefore, clinical signs are more related to whatever the owner's interpretation of the problem is on presentation. Depending on chronicity of disease, the bird may show little to no clinical signs or show signs of severe malnutrition and weakness. If excessive egg production has been occurring for a prolonged period of time, the bird may be in poor body condition and dehydrated. Feather loss and dermatitis near the cloaca may also be observed, secondary to masturbation behavior.[4,5] The bird may be weak or have pathologic fractures attributable to hypocalcemia and osteoporosis. The owner may state that the bird has been laying "abnormal looking" and/or soft-shelled eggs, which also can signify calcium depletion.

Diagnostic testing

The diagnostic evaluation should be tailored to the severity of the disease process at the time of presentation. If the problem is acute and there are obvious environmental stimuli that can be attributed to excessive reproductive behavior, then minimal diagnostic testing may be required. For birds suffering from chronic disease, a CBC and serum biochemistry panel should be performed to evaluate the metabolic status of the bird and current calcium levels.

Treatment

Treatment of chronic egg laying involves understanding the multifactorial nature of the etiology behind this disease condition. Both genetic predisposition (eg, cockatiels, budgerigars, lovebirds) and environmental stimuli may contribute to the disease process, with treatment often aimed at altering the environment and considering medical management through use of therapeutic agents.[4,5,8,11] Excessive egg laying is often impacted by normal environmental cues that would signal for reproductive activity in the wild animal. Photoperiod and seasonality may play a large role, even in captive companion birds. Stimulation from a mate also will induce reproductive activity yielding nesting behavior and chronic regurgitation. Dietary intake is often overlooked, but may contribute substantially, because many companion animals are fed high-energy diets on a consistent basis, contributing to enhanced reproductive status.[5,8]

Recommendations for environmental changes include decreasing the photoperiod to 8 to 10 hours of light per day, consistent with seasonal changes discouraging reproductive behavior. Additionally, any inanimate objects that serve as a potential mate for the bird should be removed and placed out of sight. Nesting boxes should be discarded; however, if the bird were to lay eggs despite removing nesting material, one should be encouraged not to remove the eggs because this will cause "double clutching" or the process by which a bird will lay another egg to replace the old one. If an egg is laid, it should remain with the bird for the full incubation period so as to not induce double clutching. If a human is the supposed "mate," that person should be educated to not rub the bird along its dorsum or near the cloaca, as these may sexually stimulate the bird. The bird also should be encouraged to interact with other members in the household and new environments and toys. The high fat content associated with seed diets is believed to support reproductive behavior and a transition to primarily a formulated or pelleted food would be ideal. Although not entirely understood, this practice is used in poultry medicine to decrease production of eggs and to induce molting.[5]

Pharmacologic management of chronic egg laying is highly controversial, with most hormonal therapeutics not being without their own risks and restrictions over and above the unknown efficaciousness of these agents between avian species. Historically, medroxyprogesterone acetate (eg, Depo-Provera; Pfizer, Pharmacia & Upjohn Co, New York NY) injections or implants have been used to disrupt the ovulatory cycle, thereby stopping egg laying.[4,5] Side effects associated with medroxyprogesterone acetate include hepatic lipidosis, weight gain/obesity, lethargy, and polyuria and polydipsia. Due to serious and potentially fatal side effects, medroxyprogesterone acetate has largely fallen out of favor for therapeutic use in birds. Other treatments for chronic egg laying, including human chorionic gonadotropin and testosterone, have been used in clinical cases and described, but the results were variable or induced serious side effects.[4]

The gonadotropin-releasing hormone (GnRH) synthetic agonist, leuprolide acetate (eg, Lupron Depot; TAP Pharmaceuticals, Inc, Lake Forest, IL), has become a commonly used hormone to treat chronic egg laying in birds.[4,5,14,15] The different formulations of Lupron allow for either slow and sustained release or short-acting use. The slow-release depot product is the form of leuprolide acetate primarily used in avian medicine. Initial treatment will induce an escalation of clinical signs and behavior, whereas prolonged use will downregulate the pituitary gonadotropin receptors, resulting in decreased gonadotropin release (follicular-stimulating hormone and luteinizing hormone [LH]) and subsequent cessation of reproductive activity. Initial studies in cockatiels have shown that the long-acting Lupron can safely inhibit egg laying, but is reversible on cessation of injections.[7,16] For cockatiels injected every 18 days with 100 µg/kg (45.4 µg/lb) Lupron, all egg laying would cease. When tested in budgerigars, a shorter duration of action was found with repeated injections needed every 12 to 14 days when using the same dose.[17] Plasma sex hormone concentrations were reduced for 21 days when Hispaniolan Amazon parrots (*Amazona ventralis*) were intramuscularly administered 800 µg Lupron.[18] In a group of racing pigeons (*Columbia livia domestica*), Lupron administration did not have any effect on egg production or plasma sex hormone levels when administered at 500 or 1000 µg/kg (227 or 454.5 µg/lb).[19] Large species variability exists with regard to efficacy of treatment, and the dose needed to produce results. Although effective, the duration of effect for most species is short, considering that these conditions are often considered chronic problems. Multiple depot formulations are available, with the 1-month formulation being used most in avian medicine.

More recently, another long-acting GnRH agonist has been used in avian medicine with the goal of decreasing reproductive activity by downregulating the pituitary gonadotropin receptors. Deslorelin acetate (eg, Suprelorin; Peptech Animal Healthy Pty Ltd, Macquarie Park, NSW, Australia) is available and approved for use in veterinary medicine for several companion exotic species, including ferrets, for adrenal endocrinopathy (**Fig. 2**). Although controlled studies have been performed in poultry, quail, and pigeons, prospective studies in Psittaciformes are not available at this time.[20–24] Implantation of a 4.7 or 9.5 mg deslorelin implant in 2-year-old laying chickens (*Gallus gallus domesticus*) resulted in 100% cessation of egg laying by 14 days.[14,23] For those chickens that received a 4.7-mg implant, the average time associated with suppressed ovarian activity was 180 days.[23] The group of chickens

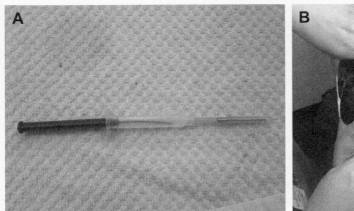
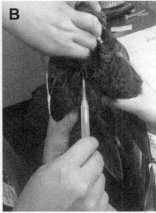

Fig. 2. (*A*) Applicator for deslorelin implant. (*B*) Subcutaneous injection of deslorelin implant into an avian patient.

that was administered the 9.5-mg implant did not produce any eggs for an average of 319 days.[23] This positive dose-dependent relationship conflicted with multiple studies performed in Japanese quail (*Coturnic japonica*), whereby the deslorelin implants did not eradicate ovarian activity in all test subjects. Reportedly, the 4.7-mg and 9.5-mg implants were approximately 60% to 70% efficacious depending on the study cited.[20,22] Duration of effect was also highly variable in Japanese quail, although long-term studies have not been performed. In male and female pigeons (*Columbia livia*) that were administered a long-acting 4.7-mg deslorelin implant, LH concentrations were significantly decreased compared with control subjects within 1 week of administration, and these effects lasted until the end of the study period at 84 days.[25] Additionally, the female birds that received the implant produced fewer eggs than the control animals for at least 49 days, with egg numbers reduced to zero within 2 weeks.[25]

Use of long-acting GnRH agonists, such as deslorelin, may offer treatment for chronic egg layers with little to no side effects. It is unclear, however, the duration of effect in other birds. Few clinical reports and retrospective studies in psittacine species exist. In one large study, 32 Psittaciformes were administered a 4.7-mg deslorelin implant that was 100% efficacious and suppressed egg laying for up to 3 months.[14,26] Other available reports are for male reproductive disease and are discussed later in this text.

Prolapse and Miscellaneous Disease of the Cloaca

Cloacal disease encompasses several processes, including prolapse, strictures, cloacal liths, and papillomas. Pathology to the cloaca often manifests in 1 of 2 ways: dystocia or inability to copulate.[5]

Prolapse of the cloaca may occur in birds during the normal egg-laying process, from straining as a part of more proximal dystocia, or due to hyperplasia of the oviduct. Extrareproductive causes of prolapse also may occur if a space-occupying mass within the caudal coelom pushes against the reproductive tract. Anatomically, the most common tissue associated with prolapse is the uterus, followed by the vagina and cloaca.[4,5] Predisposition to this condition may include malnutrition and concurrent weakness, causing increased abdominal contractions resulting in prolapsed tissue. Other risk factors include obesity, salpingitis or cloacitis, and malformed eggs.

Psittacine species more commonly afflicted by papillomas of the cloacal mucosa and to a lesser extent the choana, include Amazon parrots, macaws, and conures (**Fig. 3**).[5,27] Although discussion of viral disease is outside the scope of this text, it is important to note that presence of cloacal papillomas (presumed to be of viral etiology) is likely painful, generates a pathologic tissue presence inconsistent with successful reproductive activity, and creates an environment conducive for growth of infectious organisms.

Cloacal strictures often result from chronic cloacitis and birds will likely present for straining, possibly related to dystocia. This disease process is relatively uncommon, but justifies the importance of performing a cloacal examination using a speculum. Cloacal liths is another relatively rare condition in which uroliths form in the urodeum, coprodeum, or proctodeum of the cloaca. Birds with a large urolith may present for tenesmus and dystocialike signs. In a report of a blue-fronted Amazon parrot presenting with tenesmus, a uric acid urolith was deposited in the coprodeum.[28] The urolith was removed with forceps, assisted through cloacoscopy, and the bird recovered without complication.

Clinical signs

Prolapse of the cloaca and oviduct is clinically apparent at presentation (**Fig. 4**). Depending on the length of time since prolapse, the tissue may be completely viable or may show signs of devitalization with sloughing. In extreme cases in which the tissue has been exposed for prolonged periods of time, the bird may be clinically dehydrated, depressed, and/or obtunded. It is important to evaluate the patient's body condition when presented because this will help establish a treatment plan for concurrent disease. Strictures may develop from chronic cloacitis and are often easily diagnosed during the cloacal examination.[5]

Diagnostic testing

Diagnostic tests are not typically necessary for cases in which there is an acute history of prolapse; however, diagnostic evaluation may be required if concurrent disease processes are suspected. In the case of the bird with devitalized oviduct tissue, a CBC and serum biochemistry panel may be useful to establish metabolic status of the patient and determine if concurrent systemic inflammatory processes are present. If an infection or salpingitis is suspected, culture and sensitivity of the reproductive tract should be performed before replacement of tissues. In the case of dystocia

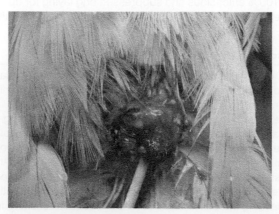

Fig. 3. Cloacal papilloma in an Amazon parrot.

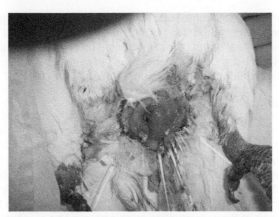

Fig. 4. Cloacal prolapse, as noted in this cockatoo, can be a consequence of reproductive tract disease that results in difficulty laying an egg.

causing prolapse, diagnostic imaging should be performed to assess for coelomic masses or the presence of eggs within the oviduct.

Therapy

Therapy is aimed at rapidly returning the prolapsed tissue back to correct anatomic positioning and manually breaking down any strictures, if present. If an egg is present in the caudal reproductive tract, it should be removed before replacement of tissues. The tissue should be lubricated and topical hyperosmotic agents may be applied to the tissue to help decrease edema or desiccation and aid in replacement. Broad-spectrum antibiotic therapy should be used while waiting on culture and sensitivity results if a bacterial infection is suspected. Because prolapses often recur, stay sutures may be necessary to retain the tissue within the reproductive tract until the uterine tissue regresses in size and returns to normal strength. Prognosis for animals with an acute history of cloacal prolapse due to egg laying is generally good if no other major complicating factors are diagnosed.[4,5] For animals in which the oviductal tissue is necrotic, a partial or complete salpingohysterectomy may need to be performed.

Coelomitis of Reproductive Origin

Coelomitis is a broad category of disease describing inflammation and possibly an infectious process present within the coelomic cavity. Reproductive disease is not always the cause of coelomitis; however, only reproductive etiologies are discussed in this text.

Coelomitis may be caused by a large list of avian reproductive disease. The following diseases are often implicated: salpingitis, metritis, oophoritis, ovarian cysts, cystic hyperplasia of the oviduct, oviduct rupture, ectopic eggs, septicemia, neoplasia, and granulomatous disease.[4,5,8] It is important to note that most of the listed reproductive conditions do not occur as a single disease process. Frequently, one disease will influence the initiation of another, resulting in a multifactorial patient presentation. This is especially true of coelomitis, which can be either the cause or result of other reproductive disease.

Clinical signs

Birds may present with nonspecific symptoms of illness, including lethargy, anorexia, and depression. A detailed set of questions, including reproductive history, may help establish a primary list of differential disease diagnoses. For birds that have laid eggs in the past, the owner may report that the bird has suddenly stopped laying eggs. For birds that are chronically affected, more specific signs of illness (eg, labored breathing [from free fluid within the coelom], coelomic distension, sudden death) may be observed and may be the primary complaint by the owner.

Diagnostic testing

Birds suffering from coelomitis should have a thorough workup, including hematology, diagnostic imaging, and coelomic fluid analysis, if applicable. Often, a CBC will reveal a leukocytosis with associated heterophilia in a patient presenting with coelomitis. Hypercalcemia (or hypocalcemia for chronic egg layers or malnourished birds), hyperglobulinemia, and hypercholesterolemia also may be observed and are typical findings in reproductively active birds.[4,5] Radiographic images may show a shelled egg within the coelom or loss of serosal detail, an observation consistent with free fluid. Soft tissue opacity in the region of the reproductive tract also may be evident, although this is not always indicative for oviductal disease because this finding is also considered normal during ovulation. Ultrasonography is a much more sensitive imaging modality for the reproductive tract and may help diagnose neoplasia, unshelled eggs, ectopic ova, cystic ova, free fluid, and collapsed eggs. Guided aspirates of any soft tissue pathology and coelomocentesis for any free fluid should be performed when indicated, followed by both cytology and bacterial culture and sensitivity of the aspirate. To achieve a definitive ante mortem diagnosis, coelioscopy is often required to aid in the visualization of affected tissues and assist in the harvest of biopsy samples.

Therapy

Treating coelomitis depends entirely on the secondary disease process. For birds that present with few clinical signs and without the suspicion of bacterial infection, supportive care may be all that is required. Standard care provided for these birds should include appropriate hydration, nutrition, and a heated/humid environment. For cases in which an infection is suspected, broad-spectrum antibiotic therapy should be initiated while culture and sensitivity results are pending. Birds presenting with dyspnea should be immediately assessed for free fluid in the coelom and a therapeutic coelomic aspiration performed (**Fig. 5**). Most reproductive disease will benefit by cessation of ovarian activity. Therefore, administration of a long-acting GnRH agonist should be considered, to try to stop ovulation.[4,5] For cases in which neoplasia, granulomatous disease, or cystic disease are diagnosed, treatment will involve obtaining a

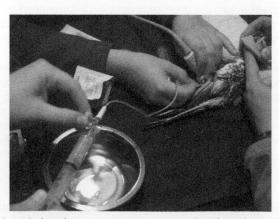

Fig. 5. Ultrasound-guided coelomocentesis in a cockatiel with coelomic fluid.

definitive diagnosis (often through coelioscopy and biopsy) followed by mass removal or salpingohysterectomy. Coelomitis should be treated similar to peritonitis, with the body cavity being thoroughly lavaged with sterile saline when performing an exploratory surgical procedure. It is important to remember that many avian cases in which coelomitis is diagnosed are not infectious in nature but aseptic.

Salpingitis, Metritis, and Oophoritis

Salpingitis, or inflammation of the avian oviduct, may arise from infectious or noninfectious causes. Noninfectious causes of salpingitis include trauma to the oviduct from egg binding, dystocia, foreign material, or neoplastic disease. Salpingitis can develop from an ascending bacterial infection or from a blood-borne pathogen affecting nearby structures and organs. Infectious organisms that may be identified through routine culture include *Escherichia coli, Salmonella* spp, *Pasteurella multocida, Streptococcus* spp, and *Mycoplasma gallisepticum*.[5] These pathogens may be introduced through copulation, environmental contamination, or even iatrogenic causes, such as lavage of the reproductive tract. Although not always the case, older and more reproductively mature birds appear to be more affected than younger animals.

When a local inflammatory process affects the uterine and ovarian tissues, the terms metritis and oophoritis are used, respectively. Metritis and oophoritis may arise from a multitude of causes associated with infectious or noninfectious disease processes and are similar to those listed for salpingitis. Inflammation of the uterine tissue commonly results in changes in shell formation and should be a differential disease diagnosis for birds presenting with malformed or soft shells.

Clinical signs

A bird may present with nonspecific symptoms of illness, but certain cues in the anamnesis may help one formulate a working list of differential disease diagnoses. Any abnormal changes to the eggs should increase suspicion for metritis, especially if dietary intake is deemed appropriate and the bird is considered to be in good body condition. Birds also may present in dystocia or exhibit egg binding, whereby the cause of these disease conditions may be due to inflammation or an infection associated with the reproductive tract. Some birds may present with coelomic distension or with cloacal discharge. Ultimately, the variation in presentation is due to other concurrent disease conditions or systemic processes.

Diagnostic testing

A complete diagnostic evaluation is often necessary to determine the underlying disease process affecting the ovary and/or uterus. More commonly, infectious etiologies predominate over noninfectious origins. Performing a CBC and serum biochemistry panel may reveal a leukocytosis and heterophilia with or without toxic changes, increasing the suspicion for an underlying infectious etiology. Radiographic and ultrasonographic imaging also may be useful when evaluating for secondary disease processes (eg, egg binding, dystocia). The left oviduct will enlarge when reproductively active. Therefore, observing a large soft tissue opacity in the region of the reproductive tract is not definitive of disease in this area of the coelom. One must consider that this observation may simply increase suspicion of disease associated with the reproductive tract. In certain instances, loss of serosal detail on radiographs may indicate free fluid within the coelom; therefore, performing a coelomocentesis may provide more information toward a diagnosis. Although the diagnostic testing described previously often aids in the development of a treatment plan, a definitive diagnosis is primarily determined through cytology, bacteriology, or biopsy of the affected tissues. This can be performed via coelioscopy-guided biopsies, cytology, or culture and sensitivity of the oviductal lumen or free fluid.

Therapy
If an infectious etiology is diagnosed, therapy is aimed at using appropriate pharmaceuticals based on culture and sensitivity results. It is important to follow up treatment with repeat cultures of the oviductal tissue because pathogens are often hard to completely eradicate and may change their sensitivity patterns. In addition to antibiotic therapy, administration of long-acting GnRH agonists may be useful to help mitigate ovarian activity, thus minimizing inflammation to the reproductive tract mucosa associated with egg development. This is especially true of oophoritis, whereby ovulation itself can exacerbate an inflammatory condition within the ovary.[12] If a noninfectious etiology is suspected, recommendations are provided based on the underlying cause of the disease condition(s), with emphasis to simultaneously address any required husbandry changes. For refractory cases, salpingohysterectomy may be necessary depending on the tissues affected and severity of the disease.

Oviduct Impaction

Impaction of the oviduct is often a sequela from inflammatory conditions of the reproductive tract (salpingitis or metritis) or from egg binding/dystocia.[5] Disease associated with the oviduct can cause the abnormal accumulation of mucous, albumen, and/or content from ruptured eggs, including calcified portions of the shell. Obtaining an appropriate anamnesis is key to disease diagnosis because clinical signs are often nonspecific and diagnostic testing is often unrewarding. If the bird has recently laid an egg or has been displaying broody behavior, but no egg has passed, oviduct impaction should be ruled out.

Clinical signs
Because oviduct impaction may be more chronic in nature if related to salpingitis or metritis, birds may present nonspecific clinical signs (eg, lethargy, anorexia, weight loss, weakness). Occasionally tenesmus and coelomic distension can be appreciated with impaction of the oviduct. If the bird is showing broody behavior, but no egg has passed, and no egg is palpated in the coelom, this may be indicative of oviduct impaction. Radiograph imaging should be performed to confirm that an egg is not involved, because eggs located in a cranial oviductal location may not always be palpated.

Diagnostic testing
A complete diagnostic evaluation, including CBC, serum biochemistry panel, and radiographic imaging, should be performed to rule out dystocia or egg binding. A CBC may reveal the patient with an oviduct impaction having a leukocytosis with or without heterophilia, depending on if local, systemic, or other disease processes are present. Elevated total serum calcium and alkaline phosphatase may provide evidence of a reproductively active bird.[4,5] If available, ultrasonography should be performed because this is often a useful modality for diagnosing radiolucent obstructions within a lumen. Performing celioscopy or an exploratory celiotomy may provide the only means by which to definitively diagnose oviduct impaction. If present, celioscopy may reveal a focally enlarged oviduct, which often is an indication for surgical intervention.

Therapy
When performing a celiotomy for an oviduct impaction, the oviduct may need to be resected if the tissue is not viable or adhesions are present. In extreme cases, a

salpingohysterectomy may be necessary. Microbial cultures of the affected tissue and/or coelomic/oviduct fluid should be taken at the time of the procedure. Broad-spectrum antibiotic therapy should be initiated while culture and sensitivity results are pending. Supportive care of the patient, including isotonic fluids, supplemental heat, and nutritional supplementation, should be included in the treatment regimen. Long-term management of oviduct impaction involves reinforcing the required husbandry changes, similar to those discussed for birds with chronic egg-laying disorders.

Cystic Hyperplasia of the Oviduct and Ovary

Hyperplastic change to the left oviduct and the vestigial remnant of the right oviduct may occur in some birds afflicted by endocrinopathy or by congenital anomalies. For birds with cystic ovarian disease, certain species appear to be overrepresented. Budgerigars, cockatiels, and canaries have been reported as being predisposed to cystic changes of the ovary, whereas endocrinopathy, neoplasia, or congenital anomalies are disease conditions attributed to the development of this condition.[4,5,8,10] Although cystic hyperplasia of the oviduct and/or ovary are often benign on their own, these pathologic changes to the reproductive tract often result in egg binding or salpingitis.

Clinical signs

When birds become clinical for illness, it is often the secondary disease process that is the cause of the clinical signs, and cystic hyperplasia of the oviduct and/or ovary is no different. Therefore, most signs will be similar to those listed for other reproductive diseases; however, ovarian cysts may produce somewhat different clinical signs, including expression of broody behavior without egg production.[4] Another common historical finding is that the bird may have suddenly ceased producing eggs, despite always being a good layer. Additionally, coelomitis is a more common sequela with cystic ovarian disease. Therefore, coelomic distension and dyspnea may be evident if the bird has free fluid within the coelom.

Diagnostic testing

Similar to other conditions of the reproductive tract, diagnostic imaging is often useful not only to rule out other diseases, but also to gain insight toward cystic hyperplasia of the oviduct and/or ovary. Ultrasonography may be the preferred diagnostic imaging modality because it is probable that one will observe the cystic tissue associated with the reproductive tract. Fluid-filled structures may be noted within the walls of the oviduct or with ovarian tissue, keeping in mind that normal ovarian follicles may be present.[5] In some circumstances, the cysts may be very large, making interpretation difficult. However, it is important to note that if cysts are not diagnosed through ultrasonography, this does not rule out cystic hyperplasia of the oviduct and/or ovary. Radiographic images may reveal an increase in soft tissue opacity in the region of the reproductive tract, with or without concurrent loss of serosal detail, implicating free fluid. Coelomocentesis should be performed to obtain any free fluid in the coelom, which should then be submitted for bacterial culture and sensitivity. If fluid from the cyst is directly obtained, the aspirate also should be submitted for bacterial culture and cytologic evaluation. Typical fluid from these cysts will be clear to straw-colored and should have a low cellularity.[5] Performing a CBC and serum biochemistry panel may reveal changes consistent with inflammation and an active reproductive status. A leukocytosis and heterophilia along with hypercalcemia, hyperglobulinemia, and hypercholesterolemia may be evident. Even if cystic tissue is observed though diagnostic imaging, a definitive diagnosis is made only with biopsy and histopathology of the affected tissue. Either celioscopy or celiotomy must be performed to achieve this diagnosis. Tissues collected through the invasive procedures should be submitted for bacterial culture and sensitivity along with the histopathological evaluation.

Therapy

In birds that are not used as breeding animals, a salpingohysterectomy may be the best treatment option because the removal of the oviduct will significantly reduce the chance for a reoccurrence of cystic hyperplasia of the oviduct and/or ovary. Regardless of breeding status, cystic ovarian tissue is prone to tears and rupture; therefore, administration of a long-acting GnRH agonist will help by diminishing ovulation, thus decreasing the risk of damage within the oviduct.[4,5] During this time, the bird should be treated with appropriate antibiotic medication if an infection is present. For birds that are used as breeding animals, the GnRH agonist always can be discontinued after necessary rechecks to ensure that the disease condition has resolved.

Treatment for cystic ovarian disease is aimed at aspiration of the cysts and concurrent management of secondary disease syndromes. If the bird presents in respiratory distress, performing abdominocentesis is not only diagnostic, but also therapeutic. Pharmacologic therapy (aimed at decreasing ovarian activity) along with dietary, behavioral, and environmental husbandry changes is recommended. For reoccurring cases of cystic ovarian disease, a salpingohysterectomy should be performed on these patients.

Oviduct Rupture

Rupture of the reproductive tract may be a result of a primary disease process or by iatrogenic means. Dystocia is the most common cause of rupture, whereby the mechanical obstruction itself or the therapies used to treat dystocia can result in trauma to the wall of the oviduct.[5] One should be cautious with administration of prostaglandins and oxytocin in an animal that may be obstructed, because strong contractions of the smooth muscle against a physical barrier can promote a tear in the tissue. Clinical signs associated with oviduct rupture can fall within a relatively large spectrum; lethargy, decreased appetite, and weakness can be observed in some patients with oviduct rupture, whereas birds presenting with respiratory difficulty and in stages of shock can be seen in more severe cases. Radiographic imaging may reveal a shelled egg in the coelom, although occasionally it can be difficult to determine if the egg is actually in the oviduct or not (**Fig. 6**). For a case in which a shelled egg is not identified via radiography, but clinical suspicion of reproductive disease still exists, ultrasonography is required. There may be evidence of free fluid within the coelom, at which point coelomocentesis should be performed. If coelomitis is evident, an exploratory celiotomy is then indicated, and surgical repair of the oviductal tissue may be performed; however, in other cases, a complete salpingohysterectomy may be necessary.

Ectopic Ovulation

Ectopic ovulation is defined as egg laying or ovulation occurring outside the oviduct and occurs when the infundibulum fails to catch the ova. This process can occur rather often in some avian species (eg, chickens) and when it occurs, the ova and its yolk proteins are resorbed within the coelom and do not pose any threat for disease.[5,6,9] When occurring pathologically, the ectopic egg or ova may result in a coelomitis and subsequent systemic disease. The abnormal deposition of ova outside of the reproductive tract may be triggered by several conditions that will result in weakening of the oviduct, including dystocia, oviduct rupture, cystic pathology, trauma, neoplasia, or

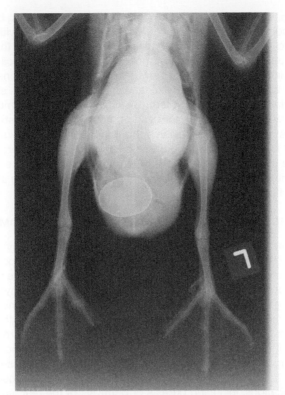

Fig. 6. Egg in coelom due to oviduct rupture. The position and location of the egg aid in determining if the egg is in the oviduct.

malnutrition. Clinical signs of ectopic ovulation can be nonspecific, but for cases in which coelomitis is present, birds can present with coelomic distension and may be depressed, weak, and dyspneic (**Fig. 7**). Depending on the maturity of the egg, radiography may show a shelled egg within the coelom, although it is often hard to discern

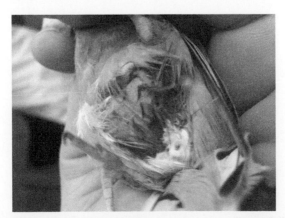

Fig. 7. Distended coelom in a budgerigar due to internal ovulation following the initial removal of fluid though coelomocentesis.

if it is truly ectopic. A coelomic ultrasound scan may reveal that an egg is outside of the oviduct and is recommended for radiolucent ova that have ovulated within the coelom. Therefore, the bird should be monitored over the next 12 to 48 hours for oviposition or any progression/development of clinical signs. If the bird begins to clinically decline, an exploratory celiotomy is indicated. If salvageable, damaged portions of the oviduct should be surgically repaired, otherwise a salpingohysterectomy should be performed. Even if the oviduct does not look diseased grossly, it is important to take appropriate biopsy samples to look for cystic pathology or neoplastic disease. It is important to remember that certain avian species will continue to ovulate (eg, ducks) when the oviduct has been surgically removed. Therefore, it is imperative that therapeutic means are used to stop ovulation. With patients that continue to ovulate, it is imperative that therapy to prevent ovulation is administered as long as the animal is reproductively active.

NEOPLASIA OF THE REPRODUCTIVE TRACT IN FEMALE AND MALE COMPANION BIRDS

Neoplastic disease affecting the reproductive tract may affect any bird; however, prevalence seems to be much higher in budgerigars, cockatiels, and poultry.[29] Various types of tumors have been associated with the female reproductive tract, including adenomas, adenocarcinomas, lymphosarcoma, leiomyomas, leiomyosarcoma, and hormone-secreting tumors (eg, granulosa cell neoplasms).[29] One report of an orange-winged Amazon parrot described a hemangiosarcoma of the reproductive tract with metastasis to the pericardium and epicardium.[30] Male reproductive tumors include Sertoli cell tumors, seminomas, Leydig (interstitial) cell tumors, adenocarcinoma, leiomyosarcoma, and lymphosarcoma.[29] Clinical signs of disease can range from nonspecific signs, such as lethargy, decreased appetite, and behavior change, to serious complications, including paresis or paralysis of the rear leg(s) (**Fig. 8**). For cases in which the tumor grows large and impacts the ischiatic nerves, it is important to note that the tumor also may compress the local blood supply to the limbs, resulting in necrosis of the distal tissues. Some clinical signs may be pathognomonic for certain diseases, including color change to the cere in budgerigars, which typically occurs with hormone-secreting testicular neoplasms (**Fig. 9**).[4,5,8] A bird also may present with signs similar to those described in other reproductive conditions, alluding to the fact that a thorough workup is often needed to accurately diagnose neoplastic

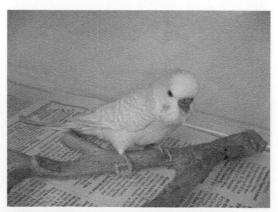

Fig. 8. Budgerigar with unilateral leg lameness. A common presentation with this species diagnosed with a gonadal tumor that is impinging on the ischiatic nerve.

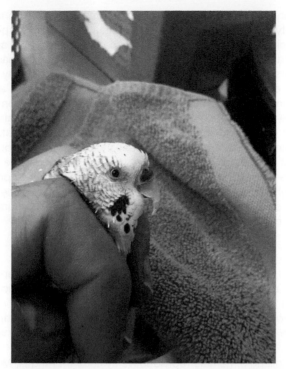

Fig. 9. Cere coloration change due to gonadal tumor. The cere was originally blue and the bird had significant coelomic distension.

disease. It is not entirely uncommon for 2 disease processes to occur simultaneously. For instance, a growing tumor may cause weakening of the oviduct, resulting in oviduct rupture and subsequent coelomitis.

Treatment for most neoplastic diseases affecting avian reproductive organs has typically been unrewarding, especially because it is common for birds to present when the tumor is large or when other secondary clinical conditions (including metastasis) are present. Removal of diseased tissue through complete ovariohysterectomy or orchiectomy is ideal because little information is available on chemotherapeutics; however, these surgeries on small avian patients are not practical. There have been several published reports and clinical anecdotal descriptions regarding the use of synthetic long-acting GnRH agonists as ancillary management for ovarian neoplasia; however, there is little evidence to support its use at this time.[12]

DISEASES AFFECTING THE MALE REPRODUCTIVE SYSTEM

Orchitis, or inflammation associated with the testicular tissue, may arise from local disease afflicting the testicle or nearby structures, hematogenous spread of an infectious organism, or as an ascending infection from the cloaca.[4,5,8] Clinical signs associated with orchitis may be vague in the early stages of disease unless the bird is used as a breeding animal. An owner might state that the bird has decreased or declining fertility, similar to mammals suffering from this disease. Other signs might include lethargy or decreased appetite, consistent with chronic pain or a chronic infectious process. Although the infection may stay localized to the testicular tissue, it can also spread to adjacent organs, air sacs, and coelom, with ability to cause coelomitis and related clinical signs. A typical diagnostic approach for an avian patient suspected of having orchitis would include a CBC that commonly indicates a leukocytosis and heterophilia. Radiographic images of the patient with orchitis may reveal an increase in soft tissue opacity in the dorsal coelom, cranial and ventral to the proximal kidney lobe, indicating the possibility of enlarged testes. Ultrasonography is more sensitive and can provide more accurate information regarding the shape, contour, and consistency of the testes, which may help discern between neoplastic disease and certain infectious processes. Because of the location of the avian testes and size of the patient, an ultrasonographic examination often requires an experienced examiner to obtain diagnostic quality images of the gonads. Celioscopy is often required and is the diagnostic procedure of choice that allows one to visualize the testes as well as provide definitive diagnosis through biopsy techniques. Broad-spectrum antibiotic therapy should be initiated on all birds suspected of having orchitis while bacterial culture and sensitivity results from any collected fluid or tissues are pending.

REFERENCES

1. Hudelson KS, Hudelson P. A brief review of the female avian reproductive cycle with special emphasis on the role of prostaglandins and clinical applications. J Avian Med Surg 2016;10(2):67–74.
2. Witschi E. Biology and comparative physiology. In: Marshall A, editor. Biology and Comparative Physiology of Birds. vol. II. New York: Academic Press; 1961. p. 10–36.
3. King A, McLelland J. Female reproductive system. In: King A, McLelland J, editors. Birds: their structure and function. 2nd edition. Philadelphia: Bailliere Tindal; 1984. p. 145–65.
4. Bowles HL. Reproductive diseases of pet bird species. In: Speer BL, editor. The Veterinary Clinics of North America exotic animal practice: reproductive medicine. 5th edtion. Philadelphia: W.B. Saunders; 2002. p. 489–504.
5. Joyner KL. Theriogenology. In: Ritchie BW, Harrison GJ, Harrison LR, editors. Avian medicine: principles and application. Lake Worth (FL): Wingers Publishing; 1994. p. 748–75.
6. Rosskopf WJ, Woerpel RW. Avian reproductive endocrinology. Vet Clin N Am Small Anim Pract 1991;21:1346–59.
7. Millam JR. Reproductive management of captive parrots. Vet Clin N Am Exotic Anim Pract 1999;4:93–110.
8. Powers L. Avian reproductive tract disorders. DVM-360. http://webcache. googleusercontent.com/search?q=cache:NQnMQJuyVP8J:www.dvm360storage. com/cvc/proceedings/dc/Avian%2520Medicine/Powers/Powers,%2520Lauren_ Avian_reproductive_tract_disorders_STYLED.pdf+&cd=2&hl=en&ct=clnk&gl=us &client=safari. Accessed August 14, 2016.
9. Romagnano A. Avian obstetrics. Semin Avian Exot Pet Med 1996;5(4):180–8.
10. Rich GA. Syndromes and conditions of parrotlets, pionus parrots, poicephalus, and mynah birds. Semin Avian Exot Pet Med 2003;12(3):144–8.
11. Rosen LB. Avian reproductive disorders. J Exot Pet Med 2012;21(2):124–31.
12. Keller KA, Beaufrère H, Brandão J, et al. Long-term management of ovarian neoplasia in two cockatiels (*Nymphicus hollandicus*). J Avian Med Surg 2012; 27(1):44–52.
13. Gaskins L, Bergman L. Surveys of avian practitioners and pet owners regarding common behavior problems in psittacine birds. J Avian Med Surg 2010;25(2):111–8.

14. Mans C, Pilny A. Use of GnRH agonists for medical management of reproductive disorders in birds. Vet Clin North Am Exot Anim Pract 2014;17:23–33.

15. Mitchell MA. Leuprolide acetate. Semin Avian Exot Pet Med 2005;14(2):153–5.

16. Millam J, Finney H. Leuprolide acetate can reversibly prevent egg laying in cockatiels. Zoo Biol 1994;13:149–55.

17. Straub J, Zenker I. First experience in hormonal treatment of Sertoli cell tumors in budgerigars (*M. undulates*) with absorbable extended release GnRH chips (Suprelorin). In: 1st International Conference on Avian, Herpetological and Exotic Mammal Medicine. Wiesbaden, April 20-26, 2013. p. 299–301.

18. Klaphake E, Fecteau K, DeWit M, et al. Effects of leuprolide acetate on selected blood and fecal sex hormones in Hispaniolan Amazon parrots (*Amazona ventralis*). J Avian Med Surg 2016;23(4):253–62.

19. De Wit M, Westerhof I, Pefold L. Effect of leuprolide acetate on avian reproduction. In: Proceedings of the Association of Avian Veterinarians. New Orleans, August 16, 2004. p. 73–4.

20. Petritz OA, Guzman DS, Paul-murphy J, et al. Evaluation of the efficacy and safety of single administration of 4.7-mg deslorelin acetate implants on egg production and plasma sex hormones in Japanese quail (*Coturnix coturnic japonica*). Am J Vet Res 2013;74(2):316–23.

21. Petritz OA, Lierz M, Samour J. Advances in methods to decrease reproductive success. In: Speer BL, editor. Current therapy in avian medicine and surgery. St Louis (MO): Elsevier; 2016. p. 446–53.

22. Petritz O, Guzman D, Hawkin M, et al. Evaluation of deslorelin acetate implant dosage on egg production and plasma progesterone in Japanese quail (Coturnix coturnix japonica). Proceedings of the 25th Annual Conference of the Association of Avian Veterinarians 2013;17.

23. Nooan B, Johnson P, Matos D. Evaluation of egg-laying suppression effects of the GnRH agonist deslorelin in domestic chicken. Proceedings of the 24th Annual Conference of the Association of Avian Veterinarians 2012;4.

24. Molter CM, Fontenot DK, Terrell SP, et al. Use of deslorelin acetate implants to mitigate aggression in two adult male domestic turkeys (*Meleagris gallopavo*) and correlating plasma testosterone concentrations. J Avian Med Surg 2015; 29(3):224–30.

25. Cowan M, Martin GB, Johnston SD, et al. Inhibition of the reproductive system by deslorelin in male and female pigeons (*Columba livia*). J Avian Med Surg 2014; 28(2):102–8.

26. Van Sant F, Sundaram A. Retrospective study of deslorelin acetate implants in clinical practice. Proceedings of the 25th Annual Conference of the Association of Avian Veterinarians 2013;211–20.

27. Hoppes SM. Viral diseases of pet birds. Merck Man. 2015. Available at: http://www.merckvetmanual.com/mvm/exotic_and_laboratory_animals/pet_birds/viral_diseases_of_pet_birds.html. Accessed August 14, 2016.

28. Beaufrère H, Nevarez J, Tully T. Cloacolith in a blue-fronted Amazon parrot (*Amazona aestiva*). J Avian Med Surg 2016;24(2):142–5.

29. Reavill D, Schmidt R. Tumors of the psittacine ovary and oviduct: 37 cases. Pittsburgh (PA): Proceedings of Association of Avian Veterinarians 2003;67–9.

30. Mickley K, Buote M, Kiupel M, et al. Ovarian hemangiosarcoma in an orange-winged Amazon parrot (*Amazona amazonica*). J Avian Med Surg 2008;23(1): 29–35.

Reproductive Disorders in Commonly Kept Fowl

Daniel Calvo Carrasco, LV CertAVP(ZooMed), MRCVS[a],*,
Mikel Sabater González, LV CertZooMed, DECZM(Avian)[b]

KEYWORDS

- Reproductive disease • Egg coelomitis • Egg bound • Fowl • Chicken
- Backyard poultry

KEY POINTS

- Backyard poultry and other commonly kept fowl species are often kept for their ability to lay eggs.
- Reproductive disease is common in fowl species.
- Despite being classified as food-producing species, they can be considered valuable pets and the demand for adequate veterinary care is constantly increasing.
- The clinician should be familiar with the different abnormalities and the potential treatment options.
- Fowl species have been traditionally an anatomic, physiologic and experimental model for avian medicine; however, information about treatment options is often limited and extrapolated from other species.

INTRODUCTION

The term fowl include birds of 2 different biological orders closely related[1]: the Galliformes, commonly called game birds or land fowl, and the Anseriformes, or waterfowl. Commonly kept fowl species include quails (eg, *Coturnix japonica*, **Fig. 1**, and *Colinus virginianus*), pheasants (eg, *Phasianus colchicus*), partridges (eg, *Alectorix chukar*, *Perdix perdix*, and *Alectoris rufa*), turkeys (eg, *Meleagris gallopavo*, **Fig. 2**), Guinea fowls (*Numida meleagris*, **Fig. 3**), peafowls (eg, *Pavo cristatus*, **Fig. 4**), ducks (eg, *Anas platyrhynchos*, **Fig. 5**), geese (eg, *Anser anser*, **Fig. 6**, and *Anser cygnoides*), and swans (eg, *Cygnus olor*, **Fig. 7**, *Cygnus buccinator*, and *Cygnus cygnus*). Many of those species have been domesticated for centuries, not exclusively for their abilities as layers, but also for other socioeconomic reasons (meat source, game, feather,

Disclosure Statement: The authors have nothing to disclose.
[a] Great Western Exotics, Vets-Now Referrals, Unit 10 Berkshire House, County Business Park, Shrivenham Road, Swindon SN1 2NR, UK; [b] Avian, Reptile and Exotic Pet Hospital, University of Sydney, 415 Werombi Road, Brownlow Hil, New South Wales 2570, Australia
* Corresponding author.
E-mail address: danicalvocarrasco@gmail.com

Vet Clin Exot Anim 20 (2017) 509–538
http://dx.doi.org/10.1016/j.cvex.2016.11.009
1094-9194/17/© 2016 Elsevier Inc. All rights reserved.

vetexotic.theclinics.com

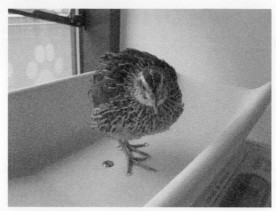

Fig. 1. Japanese quail (*C japonica*). (*Courtesy of* Minh Huynh, DVM, DipECZM (avian), MRCVS, Paris, France.)

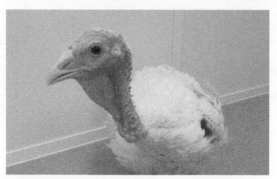

Fig. 2. Domestic turkey (*M gallopavo*). (*Courtesy of* Minh Huynh, DVM, DipECZM (avian), MRCVS, Paris, France.)

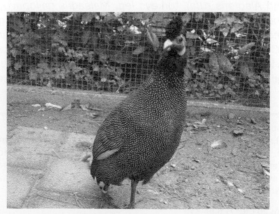

Fig. 3. Guineafowl (*N meleagris*). (*Courtesy of* Minh Huynh, DVM, DipECZM (avian), MRCVS, Paris, France.)

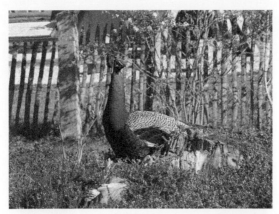

Fig. 4. Peacock (*P cristatus*). (*Courtesy of* Minh Huynh, DVM, DipECZM (avian), MRCVS, Paris, France.)

or display).[2] Centuries of selection have achieved excellent layer breeds, which inevitably translates to certain complications given the physically and energetically demanding nature of the process, all together with shortened rest periods.[3] For these reasons, fowl are legally considered egg- and meat-producing animals in most countries, which significantly influences the clinical approach, and particularly, the treatment options (even when considered as valued pets and not as food sources).

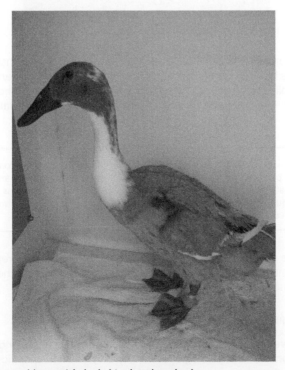

Fig. 5. Indian runner (domestic) duck (*A platyrhynchos*).

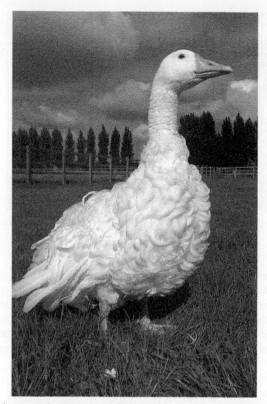

Fig. 6. Sebastopol (common) goose (*A anser*).

Moreover, the increasing popularity of backyard fowl, very often considered not only as a food source but also as companion pets, means that there is an increased demand of the public for advanced veterinary care,[3] and clinicians should be familiar with their anatomic and physiologic particularities, common abnormalities and therapeutic options.

Reproductive disease is one of the most common abnormalities in commonly kept fowl (Petritz-Samour, 2016),[118] partially influenced by the fact that most backyard poultry are initially maintained for their ability to lay eggs (Greenacre 2015),[3] particularly chickens (*Gallus gallus*). Despite their frequency and relative ease to be diagnosed, some of these disorders and their treatment remain challenging (Mans & Pilny 2014).[12]

The aim of this article is to review the most frequently observed reproductive diseases in commonly kept fowl in noncommercial settings, including their cause, diagnosis, and treatment options.

ANATOMY AND PHYSIOLOGY

Fowl species have been thoroughly studied among avian groups, and they are often used as an anatomic and physiologic reference. Only relevant specific characteristics within the different fowl species are included in this section.

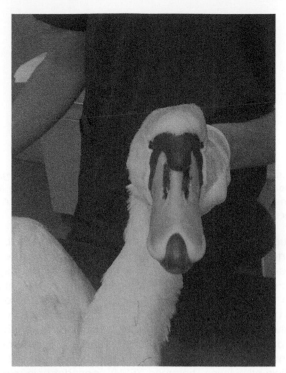

Fig. 7. Mute swan (*C olor*).

It is important to remember that, in birds, the female is the heterogametic (ZW) gender, whereas the male is the homogametic (ZZ) gender.[4]

Anatomy and Physiology of the Female Fowl Reproductive Tract

Whereas the other living representatives of the archosaurs, the crocodilians, have 2 symmetric ovaries and oviducts, in most avian species, the embryonic left ovary and oviduct soon exceed the right ones in their development, provoking a nonfunctional right ovary.[4,5] However, a right ovary in the absence of a right oviduct has been reported in at least 16 different orders assumed to have only one functional ovary. Right oviducts are not very often encountered, although in backyard poultry, it is not uncommon to find a cystic right oviduct.[6]

The general anatomy of the left ovary seems fairly constant across the avian species.[4] It is located in the coelomic cavity cranio-dorsally to the left kidney, and it is suspended by a short mesovarium (**Fig. 8**).[7]

The ovarian cortex is ill defined and contains immature follicles, whereas the medulla contains blood vessels, nerves, smooth muscle, and interstitial cells.[4] The vascular supply is via a branch of the left arteria renalis cranialis and drains via 2 ovarian veins ending in the caudal vena cava. These blood vessels and nerves enter the ovary at its hilum located on the roof of the coelom.[4] Some investigators consider ovariectomy difficult because of the short stalk of the cranial renal artery and the proximity to the aorta, whereas others suggest that the intimate and lengthy attachment to the overlying common iliac vein is what makes this procedure risky.[3]

The left oviduct has 5 parts[7]: infundibulum, magnum, isthmus, uterus (shell gland), and vagina. It is suspended from the roof of the coelomic cavity by the dorsal and ventral ligament. The blood supply for the oviduct is brought by the arteria oviductalis

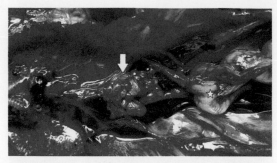

Fig. 8. Post-mortem examination a white-faced whistling duck (*Dendrocygna viduata*) after removal of the heart, liver, and gastrointestinal tract. The ovary (*white arrow*) is located caudoventral to the lungs and cranioventral to the kidneys (*black arrow*). Also note the relatively large oviduct (*star*) of a reproductively active female.

cranialis, a. oviductalis media, and the a. oviductalis caudalis.[8] In fowl, a cranial accessory oviductal artery, the a. oviductalis cranialis accessoria, may be found, and it is consistently present in ducks. The oviduct is innervated by both sympathetic and parasympathetic nerves, the most innervated parts being the uterus and its junction to the vagina. In fowl, the membrane that separates the cloaca from the vagina in juveniles breaks down during sexual maturity under hormonal control.

The reproductive physiology in avian species is, as in other vertebrates, under the control of the hypothalamic-pituitary-gonadal (HPG) axis,[9,10] which responds to environmental triggers and internal factors.[7] Ovarian function is regulated by luteinizing hormone (LH), follicle-stimulating hormone (FSH), gonadotropin-releasing hormone (GnRH), neuropeptide cytokines, and growth factors. GnRH seems to play a key role in the control of not only ovulation, incubation, and semen production but also sexual maturity, sexual maturity, and reproduction aging.[11] GnRH acts as the main link between the central nervous system, which receives environmental stimulus (eg, photoperiod, nutritional resources availability, and courtship display) and the HPG axis.[12] In birds, 3 types of GnRH have been described: avian GnRH-1 (aGnRH-1),[13] avian GnRHH-2 (aGnRH-2),[14] and avian GnRH-3 (aGnRH-3),[15] and they are thought to play different roles in reproduction: aGnRH-1 is the main regulator of LH/FSH expression and release in birds, whereas aGnRH-2 has been shown to control sexual behaviors.[9] Not only the type and levels of GnRH but also the pattern of excretion can differentiate their function: constantly elevated levels will lead to decreased gonadotropin production, whereas pulsatile GnRH stimulation increases gonadotropin production.[16]

The bird ovary secretes estrogens and androgens from its interstitial cells and progestogens from its granulosa cells. Follicular steroids stimulate sexual activity and have important roles in the induction of ovulation. The role of testosterone (T) has been controversial. However, there is now enough evidence to demonstrate the essential action of T in the ovulatory process.[17]

Sexual maturity can be reached as soon as several weeks after hatching (eg, Japanese quails) or after some months of life, depending on the species. In hens, this can be significantly advanced by increasing the photostimulation period, and it usually occurs at around 3 to 5 months of age.[4]

Seasonal reproduction is regulated by increasing photoperiods detected by photoreceptors within the brain, which will translate into a reduction to the melatonin and gonadotropin-inhibitory hormone (GnIH)[17] as the hours of light decrease. GnIH is a neuropeptide secreted by the paraventricular nucleus, with a negative effect on GnRH functions.[18] The decline of GnIH allows GnRH secretion to increase initiating the follicle growth.

The number of ovulations during a reproductive cycle depends on the species (eg, Galliformes have clutches containing 8–12 eggs, whereas Japanese quail can lay 365 eggs per year). Between 4 and 6 hours before ovulation, an increase of LH and progesterone plasma concentration occurs. Although progesterone naturally increases during ovulation, an injection of progesterone can induce a preovulatory surge of LH and premature ovulation.[7] Ovulation in fowl usually happens half an hour after the egg is laid. However, not all the ovulated oocytes are caught by the infundibulum, and internal (ectopic) laying happens relatively frequently.[5] The egg takes approximately 25 hours to traverse the oviduct, spending approximately 20 hours in the uterus where the shell is formed.[5,19] In fowl, the egg usually remains in the uterus with its sharp end pointing caudally. In ducks, the egg turns into the uterus just before oviposition in order to have the blunt end coming out first.

Oviposition, at least in the domestic hen and the quail, is controlled by neurohypophyseal hormones, prostaglandins, acetylcholine, galanin, and hormones of the preovulatory and postovulatory follicles.[4] Oxytocin and arginine vasotocin can both induce premature oviposition in laying hens. Release of arginine vasotocin from the neurohypophysis is stimulated by prostaglandins (PGF2α, PGE1, and PGE2), estradiol-17β, progesterone, angiotensin-II, and acetylcholine. Prostaglandins induce uterine contractions mediated by entry of extracellular calcium and myosin light chain kinase phosphorylation.[4]

Anatomy and Physiology of the Male Fowl Reproductive Tract

In birds, 2 testes are found caudal to the lungs and cranioventral to the kidney. Although traditionally it has been said that the left testis tends to be larger than the right one during the first months of life, recent data suggest that broiler chickens have 2 similar in size testes from 2 to 50 weeks of age.[20] It has also been described that the right testis can eventually become heavier than the left after 6 months of age.[21] Nevertheless, male avian birds have 2 functional testes. Some species or even some specific breeds (as the Leghorn breed) can have dark resting testes[22,23] that turn lighter when becoming sexually active.[24] The presence of melanoblast in the interstitium tissue gives them their dark color. The testes are suspended from the dorsal aspect of the coelomic cavity by the mesorchium, encapsulated by 2 fibrous tissue layers,[24] which also conduct the nerves and blood vessels of the testicle.[25] The tunica albuginea in birds is a thin layer immediately over the testicle and lacks the mediastinum testis (an incomplete vertical septum formed by a portion of the tunica albuginea, which reflects into the interior of the testis in mammals).[23]

Arterial blood is supplied by a testicular artery arising from the cranial renal artery, and it is drained by several testicular veins into the caudal vena cava. The pampiniform plexus, which helps with thermoregulation of the testes in mammals, is absent in birds.[23] Histologically, testes are similar to those of mammals except that the anastomoses of the seminiferous tubules are more numerous in birds. The epididymis is located dorsomedially to the testis and is composed of several ducts, including the rete testis, efferent ducts, connecting ducts, and epididymal ducts. The volumetric proportion of epididymal structures can vary among species.[26] In chickens, the epididymal appendix extends cranially to the epididymis and is firmly attached to the adrenal gland by connective tissue. This appendix contains aberrant ductules that can invade the adrenal gland. The epididymal appendix could be of clinical relevance after surgical castration because those aberrant ductules can secrete androgens.[23]

In fowl, the deferent ducts are anatomically similar to those of mammals. Birds do not possess accessory gland, such as prostate, seminal vesicles, or bulbourethral glands, but have specific accessory reproductive organs, including the paracloacal vascular bodies, the dorsal proctodeal gland, and lymphatic folds.[22,23] The accessory reproductive organs are located in the cloaca or in its proximity.[25]

Two types of phalli exist in fowl. The intromittent (or true phallus) is found in Anseriformes ventrally in the proctodeum of the cloaca and varies in length depending on the species (**Fig. 9**).[7]

In other species, a functional lymphatic intumescence called a nonintromittent (or nonprotruding) phallus passes the sperm to the female through the "cloacal kiss."[27] Whereas in mammals, erection is blood-vascular and semen is transported via the urethra, birds have a lymphatic erection, and semen is transported via the sulcus spermaticus.[28]

The sperm of birds is elongated compared with the sperm of mammals and can be stored in host glands in the vagina. Sperm can remain viable for 72 days in turkeys and 14 days in hens and pheasants.[29]

Avian gonadotropins (LH and FSH) are glycoproteins produced in the adenohypophysis of significant importance for the control of testicular function in the male bird.[7,30] As in other vertebrate species, FSH stimulates spermatogenesis, whereas LH increases the production of sexual hormones (T and androstenedione) by stimulation of the Leydig cells,[31] although the effects of FSH are potentiated by T.[25]

The preoptic area, located in the avian brain, plays an important role in male sexual behavior. It contains androgens and estrogens receptors, and its size decreases after surgical castration.[32] Androgens, especially T, secreted by interstitial cells, play a role in deferent duct growth and development of secondary sexual dimorphic characteristics (such as plumage and courtship behavior).[23]

The size of the testicle varies significantly depending on the levels of reproductive or nonreproductive activity. In some species, the testicle can be 300% bigger while active (**Fig. 10**).[7]

In response to elevated LH and FSH, there is an increased length and diameter of the seminiferous tubules and a higher number of interstitial cells. Many avian species, especially long-distance migrants, have seasonal gonadal recrudescence and regression (also called the seasonal reconstruction of the testis). Time and rate of gonadal maturation differ between species. In the Japanese quail, it has been demonstrated that a photoperiod longer than 12 hours significantly increases maturation.[33] In some tropical species, rainfall may also play a role in gonadal regression.[34]

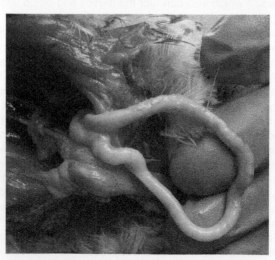

Fig. 9. Phallus of a black-bellied whistling duck (*Dendrocygna autumnalis*).

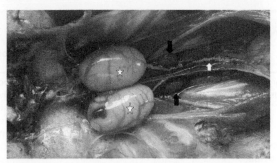

Fig. 10. Active testes (*stars*) of a black-bellied whistling duck (*D autumnalis*), cranial to the kidneys (*black arrows*). Also note the ductus spermaticus (*white arrow*).

ABNORMALITY/CONDITIONS
Reproductive Disorders in Females

Egg bound, egg binding, and dystocia
Difficulties with the oviposition (expulsion of the egg) are a common problem encountered in avian practice.[35] However, those are not as common in poultry and waterfowl when compared with other avian groups, with the exception of the small fowl species,[3] because most of the domesticated species have been selected for the purpose of laying. Young pullets laying an unusually large egg are most prone to develop these problems.[6] Some discrepancies are found when attempting to define the concepts of egg binding, egg bound, egg retention, and dystocia. Sometimes these terms are used as synonyms, whereas in other occasions they may be used to define slightly different pathologic processes or stages of the same abnormality. Echols[3] defines egg binding as prolonged oviposition, with an egg remaining in the oviduct longer than normal, whereas dystocia is used to define a more advanced process, in which the egg is located in the distal oviduct and causes a mechanical obstruction of the cloaca with or without an associated oviductal prolapse. The authors consider egg retention as a synonym of egg binding and egg bound as a synonym of dystocia. The most common anatomic areas for this to occur are the distal uterus, the vagina, and the vaginal-cloacal junction.[21,36,37]

> The most common anatomic areas for dystocia to occur are the distal uterus, the vagina, and the vaginal-cloacal junction. This condition is often linked to calcium imbalances, caused by a combination of dietary deficiencies, stress, and other husbandry-related problems.

Egg retention and dystocia can occur because of single or multiple causes (inflammatory processes, complete or partial paralysis of the muscles of the oviduct, or production of an egg so large that it is physically impossible to be laid), which have been included in **Table 1**. As in other avian species, this condition is often linked to calcium imbalances, caused by a combination of dietary deficiencies, stress, and other husbandry-related problems.[38]

A recent postmortem survey in backyard poultry[39] revealed Marek diseases (caused by Marek disease virus or Gallid herpesvirus 2) as the most common pathologic agent. Marek disease causes tumors in a variety of visceral organs, including the ovaries. Malignant reproductive neoplasia (also referred to as carcinomatosis) characterized by multifocal masses throughout the abdominal organs, including the gastrointestinal tract and reproductive tract, with or without the presence of ascites was also reported to be common (**Fig. 11**).[30]

Table 1 Causes of egg binding		
Physical Factors	**Environmental Factors**	**Metabolic and Other Factors**
• Double yolk, large and malformed eggs • Neoplasia • Cloacolith • Cloacitis • Mechanical tears or damage to the oviduct • Obesity • Oviductal torsion • Coelomic organomegaly • Early oviposition (before pelvic maturation) • Persistent right oviduct	• Temperature changes • Lack of exercise • Stressful events • Pecking • Breeding out of natural season	• Hypocalcemia • Hypovitaminosis E • Selenium deficiency • Malnutrition • Systemic disease • Genetic predisposition

Nonviral reproductive neoplasia reports are limited given the short lifespan of production animals.[40] The prevalence of spontaneous reproductive neoplasia in chickens increases with age (13% at 4 years and 40% at 6 years).[41]

Clinical signs commonly observed include straining, coelomic distension, weakness, ataxia, recumbency, cloacal or oviduct partial or complete prolapse, with or without a palpable, and/or visible egg.[42,43] Changes in egg production are frequently reported as suddenly occurring before showing other clinical signs. An egg lodged in the pelvic canal may compress the pelvic blood vessels, kidneys, and ischiatic nerves, causing circulatory disorders, lameness, paresis, or paralysis.[35]

A presumptive diagnosis can be achieved if an egg is visualized or palpated in the distal aspect of the oviduct or the coelomic cavity. Radiographs are indicated in order to obtain a more accurate diagnosis and understanding of any other ongoing processes. Hematology and biochemistry (including electrolytes) will also contribute to understand any underlying contributing findings and their adequate treatment.

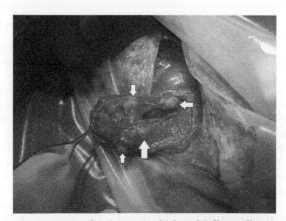

Fig. 11. Exploratory laparotomy of a domestic chicken (*Gallus gallus domesticus*) revealed the presence of multiple masses (*arrows*) in the coelomic organs, including the gastrointestinal tract. (*Courtesy of* Neil A. Forbes, BVetMed, Dip ECZM (avian), CBiol, MIBiol, FRCVS, Swindon, United Kingdom.)

Medical management is indicated for those cases with no obvious physical problems, based on fluid therapy (Hartmann solution at 50–100 mL/kg/d, with an initial bolus of 10 mL/kg), calcium, oxytocin (**Table 2** supplies further information), warmth (incubator at 30°C), and privacy. The efficacy of using oxytocin in birds is controversial because some investigators still do not consider it as an avian hormone.[44] Arginine vasotocin is not commercially available. In the authors' experience, oxytocin seems have some effect, although there is probably a dispair results depending on the species. Intracloacal PGE2 gel will usually produce uterovaginal sphincter dilation and straining within 5 to 10 minutes[44] and might facilitate manual manipulation of the egg. PGF2α will cause oviductal contractions without relaxing the uterovaginal sphincter and is therefore contraindicated. Prostaglandins should be handled carefully and always with gloves, in particular, with women, as it can cause undesired response. However, prostaglandin and hormonal therapy do require adequate calcium to be effective. Nutritional support and adequate analgesia are recommended. Broad-spectrum antibiotics are indicated if it is suspected that the integrity of the oviduct has been compromised.[35]

If initial medical management is unsuccessful and the egg can be reached, ovocentesis (either directly into the eggshell or via the coelomic wall) should be considered. It is best to avoid manual crash of the egg, as well as pulling pieces from the eggshell, as iatrogenic damage of the oviduct may occur. If the shell of the egg is not eliminated within 24 to 72 hours, salpingohysterectomy might be indicated because the remnants of the shell might adhere to the oviduct, inevitably causing further complications in future ovipositions.[36] Surgical intervention (primarily exploratory celiotomy) is rarely required in poultry and waterfowl[3] otherwise.

Oophoritis

Inflammation of the ovary results from neoplastic, mechanical, or infectious causes. Infectious oophoritis often occurs as a result of spread from adjacent organs or septicemia.[35] Bacteria cultured from cases of oophoritis with or without associated salpingitis and/or coelomitis in hens include *Escherichia coli* (colibacilosis), *Salmonella gallinarum* (fowl typhoid), and *Salmonella pullorum* (pullorum disease), *Gallibacterium anatis*, *Klebsiella* sp, *Proteus* sp, and *Pseudomonas* sp.[45–51] Clinical signs may include anorexia, weight loss, depression, cessation of egg production, egg binding, and sudden death. The case of an adult hen that laid eggs but subsequently developed tubercular oophoritis without associated neoplasia, underwent sex reversal, and was able to successfully fertilize eggs, was reported.[52] Diagnosis is made through history, physical examination, hematology (may demonstrate leukocytosis with heterophilia), radiography, ultrasonography, coelomocentesis with fluid analysis, coelioscopy (enlarged and hypervascularized ovary), coeliotomy, and biopsy of the ovary with bacterial culture and sensitivity and histopathologic analysis. Persistent or chronic oophoritis may progress to granulomatous disease. Treatment of oophoritis includes broad-spectrum antibiotics (co-amoxiclav, quinolones), pending sensitivity results in combination or not with pharmacologic therapy to stop ovulation temporarily or partial or complete ovariectomy.[35]

Cystic ovarian disease

Ovarian cysts have been known to occur in pheasants and domestic ducks.[35,53] Cyst development may be caused by endocrine disorders, anatomic abnormalities on the ovary itself, and pathologic conditions of the ovary. Clinical signs include chronic reproductive behavior without egg production or impaired reproductive performance in breeding hens, depression, inappetence and weight loss, and abdominal distension (often due to secondary coelomitis) (**Fig. 12**).[35,37]

Table 2
Common therapeutic agents used in reproductive disease

Drug	Therapeutic Group	Dosage	Route	Frequency	Species	Comments	References
Meloxicam	Analgesic (NSAIDs)	1 mg/kg	PO	Every 12 h	Chicken	Wait 12 d to ingest any egg	86
		0.5 mg/kg	IV	Single dose	Chicken, duck, turkey		87,88
		2 mg/kg	IM	Every 12 h × 14 d	Japanese quail		89,90
Butorphanol	Analgesic (opioid)	1 mg/kg	Intra-articular	Single dose	Chicken		91
		2 mg/kg	IV	Every 2 h	Chicken		92
		2 mg/kg	IM	Every 2 h	Chicken		93
		100 mg implant (141 µg/kg/h)	SC osmotic pump	Single SC implant	Peafowl	Maintained therapeutic levels for at least 7 d	94
		2–4 mg/kg	IV	Every 30 min	Helmeted Guinea fowl		95
		0.5 mg/kg	IM	Single dose	Turkey		96
Tramadol	Analgesic (opioid)	7.5 mg/kg	PO	Every 12–24 h	Peafowl		97
Co-amoxyclav	Antibiotic	125 mg/kg	IM, PO	Every 12 h	Chicken, turkey, pigeon	Oral and IM dose similar bioavailability and pharmacokinetic profile at 12 mg/kg	98–100
		500 mg/L	PO (drinking water)		Chicken		101

Drug	Class	Dose	Route	Interval	Species	Notes	References
Enrofloxacine	Antibiotic	10 mg/kg	PO, IM	Every 24 h	Chicken	Residues in egg up to day 10 after treatment	102–104
		50 ppm drinking water	PO	Every 24 h	Muscovy and Pekin (common) ducks		105
		10 mg/kg	PO, IV	Every 24 h × 5 d	Turkeys		106,107
		10 mg/kg	PO	Every 12 h	Japanese quail		108,109
		10 mg/kg	PO	Every 24 h	Common pheasant		108
Marbofloxacine	Antibiotic	2 mg/kg	PO	Every 24 h	Broiler chicken		110,111
		3–12 mg/kg	PO/IV		Turkey quail	2 mg/kg PO/IV effective against *E coli* O78/K80	108,109
Oxytocin	Hormone	3–5 IU/kg			Waterfowl	No real data, controversial	112
Prostaglandin E$_2$	Hormone	0.02–0.1 mg/kg	Topically to uterovaginal sphincter	Once	Waterfowl	No real data, controversial	112
Calcium gluconate		50–100 mg/kg	IM	Single administration, can be repeated		Anecdotic reports	112
Deslorelin acetate implants		4.7 mg	SC	6 mo	Chicken		113
		9.4 mg		10.5 mo			
		4.7 mg			Male domestic turkeys		114
		9.4 mg					
		4.7 mg			Female Japanese quail		115
Leuprolide Acetate	Hormone	60 µg/d for 14 d			Chicken	Ovarian regression and molt induction	116,117

Abbreviations: IM, intramuscularly; IV, intravenously; NSAIDs, nonsteroidal anti-inflammatory drugs; PO, orally; SC, subcutaneously.

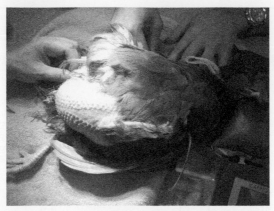

Fig. 12. Coelomic distension in a domestic chicken (*G gallus domesticus*) with coelomitis. (*Courtesy of* Neil A. Forbes, BVetMed, Dip ECZM (avian), CBiol, MIBiol, FRCVS, Swindon, United Kingdom.)

Diagnostic findings include leukocytosis with a relative heterophilia, peripheral hypercalcemia, hyperglobulinemia and hypercholesterolemia, polyostotic hyperostosis, a soft tissue density in the area of the ovary and/or oviduct, coelomic fluid, and displacement of coelomic viscera. Ultrasound may reveal a fluid-filled cyst or cysts in the area of the ovary or coelomic fluid of an undetermined origin. Abdominocentesis with cytology and bacterial culture and sensitivity should be performed if coelomitis is suspected. Definitive diagnosis may be achieved by coelioscopy/coeliotomy, ovarian biopsy, and microbiological cultures and sensitivity. Cytology of fluid aspirated from the cysts is clear to straw-colored and of low cellularity. Pharmacologic, behavioral, environmental, and dietary intervention to reduce ovarian activity are indicated because production of reproductive hormones may perpetuate ovarian cysts. Aspiration of cysts, salpingohysterectomy, and partial ovariectomy may be beneficial for complete resolution. Cryosurgical destruction may be beneficial. Long-term resolution may be difficult, and patients suffering from cystic ovarian disease should be regularly monitored for recurrence.[35]

Ovarian torsion
Ovarian torsion is an uncommon but a relevant cause of abdominal pain in women. This condition has only been reported once in birds, in a 14-month-old female ostrich (*Struthio camelus*) presented for postmortem examination.[54] A domestic duck (*A platyrhynchos domesticus*) was presented to one of the author's practice with a history of lethargy and abdominal distension. Exploratory laparotomy revealed the presence of an ovarian torsion that was treated successfully with salpingohysterectomy (**Fig. 13**).

Ovarian and oviductal neoplasia
A US Department of Agriculture Inspection Service study reported that 38% of mature fowl condemnated was due to neoplastic disease and that genital tract neoplasia was the commonest neoplasia reported.[55] Another study reported an incidence of 4% to 20% of ovarian cancer in 2.5- to 3.5-year-old hens,[56] and as mentioned, Namazi and Mosleh[41] reported an increase to 40% with 6 years of age. Clinical signs of ovarian and oviductal neoplasia may include abdominal distension, coelomic fluid, lameness, dyspnea, depression, inappetence, and chronic reproductive-associated behavior with or without egg production. Egg binding, oviductal impaction, ovarian cysts,

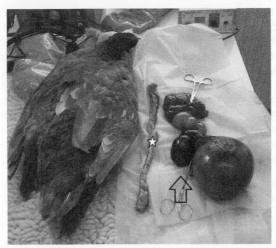

Fig. 13. Macroscopic appearance of the twisted ovary (*arrow*) and oviduct (*star*) following salpingohysterectomy. (*Courtesy of* Neil A. Forbes, BVetMed, Dip ECZM (avian), CBiol, MI-Biol, FRCVS, Swindon, United Kingdom.)

abdominal hernia, and coelomic fluid may be seen in conjunction with reproductive tract neoplasia.[35] Diagnosis is supported by history and physical examination, demonstration of enlargement in the area of the ovary or oviduct on radiographs, ultrasound, computed tomography, or MRI, and biopsy with histopathologic examination of abnormal tissues. Therapeutic options include chemotherapy, radiation therapy, and partial or complete ovariectomy. All the different neoplasia of the reproductive tract carries a guarded to poor prognosis unless the neoplastic tissue is completely removed.

Adenocarcinoma Adenocarcinomas may be originated in the ovary or in the upper portion of the magnum of the oviduct, with occasional cases occurring in the infundibulum or uterus (shell-gland). Adenocarcinomas show similar characteristics in chickens and mature turkey hens. Early lesions are found in hens with active ovaries, whereas abdominal metastases are associated with ascites and loss of body condition. Adenocarcinomas of the magnum are extremely malignant. Metastasis to the lungs and other viscera occurs via hematogenous emboli. Early stages of ovarian adenocarcinomas are small, round, white, and firm nodules on the ovarian surface, which may be mistaken for atretic follicles, whereas oviductal adenocarcinomas are individual or clustered sessile gray and firm masses. In advanced cases, these coalesce into a gray-white, firm cauliflower-like mass (ovarian ones) or irregular as protruding into the oviductal lumen (oviductal ones), and numerous transcoelomic implants on serosal surfaces of the pancreas, oviduct, mesentery, and/or intestines are commonly observed. Ascites usually develops when such tumorous growth is extensive. The walls of affected intestines are thickened and adhered together, and the intestinal lumina become constricted. Failure to detect tumor growth in the mucosal lining of the oviduct indicates that the tumor was not of oviductal origin and, therefore, probably arose from the ovary. Immunohistochemical studies showed that ovarian adenocarcinomas contained ovalbumin and retained their receptors for estrogen and progesterone. Adenocarcinomas of the magnum were estrogen responsive; their growth was maintained by potent estrogens and suppressed by antiestrogens. Ovarian myxomas have also been reported.[57]

Granulosa-theca cell tumor This tumor is yellow, round, and lobulated with an extremely friable consistency. This type of tumor may become very large. Metastasis to adjacent viscera occurs occasionally. The identification of a unique ultrastructural component known as the transosome allows the confirmation of their follicular granular cells origin. Hens with larger tumors present marked elevations of the concentration of estrogen in plasma. The high concentrations of circulating estrogen result in the oviducts being similar in size to those of laying hens. Comb development is as for hens in lay, but eggs are not produced. Granulosa cells from mature follicles normally produce progesterone, whereas theca cells produce estrogen. The presence of highly vacuolated thecalike cells may lead to the tumor being designated as luteinized, and if this is excessive, the tumor may be referred to as a luteoma.[57]

Arrhenoma and arrhenoblastoma Arrhenomas and arrhenoblastomas encompass a diverse group of virilizing ovarian tumors, but very few of the cases of virilism reported are due to ovarian tumors. In avian species, the male is the neutral sex, and the ovarian sexual hormones in the female chick demasculinize the individual. In the hen, only the left ovary normally develops, but rudimentary male medullary tissue and primordial cells are present in the normal ovary. Surgical removal of the functional ovary leads to hypertrophy of the vestigial right gonad into an organ resembling an ovo-testis or testis, depending on the age at treatment. The ovo-testis so formed has some areas of immature seminiferous tubules, but spermatogenesis is not normally a feature. Destruction of the left ovary by a nonsteroid-producing tumor or other pathologic processes may result in the formation of a right ovo-testis. It is not known if sex reversal is due to a lack of estrogens or the production of androgens. Arrhenomas are characterized by growth of seminiferous tubules within the ovarian stroma and appear as white, solid, lobulated masses within atrophic ovaries. In large tumors, there may be cystic cavitation and hemorrhage. Experimental induction of masculinizing arrhenoblastomas by injection of radioactive isotopes into the left ovary has been described.[57]

Ovarian sertoli cell tumors Sex reversal was not apparent, and circulating hormone concentrations were comparable to those of nonlaying hens. Some ovarian Sertoli cell tumors appeared to develop within granulose/theca cell tumors.[57]

Dysgerminomas Dysgerminomas are considered to originate from seminiferous elements within the left ovary or vestigial right gonad. Dysgerminomas have been reported in pseudo-hermaphrodites showing loss of external morphologic features of hens and acquisition of some male characteristics, such as enlarged combs and male-type saddle feathers. Sex reversal has not been yet reported for dysgerminomas.[57]

Leiomyoma Leiomyoma of the mesosalpinx, usually located centrally in the ventral ligament of the oviduct, is a common tumor in hens. Occasionally, leiomyomas may be found on the peritoneal surface of the oviduct or growing in the mesentery. They vary from small white nodules with a characteristic white, glistering appearance on the cut surface to large gray, heavily vascularized masses of several centimeters in diameter. These tumors may be referred to as leiomyofibromas or fibroleiomyomas, depending on which tissue predominates. Mitotic figures are rare. Leiomyomas are benign and appear to have little effect on the oviduct or its function, although they may predispose to ova escaping into the abdominal cavity. Affected hens had elevated concentrations of circulating 17-ß-estradiol.[57]

Cystic hyperplasia of the oviduct
Cystic hyperplasia of the left oviduct may occur from improper formation of the oviduct or secondary to an endocrine abnormality. It often contributes to salpingitis

and egg binding. Clinical signs may include depression, anorexia, abdominal distension, ascites, and dyspnea. A tentative diagnosis is made through history, physical examination, and supporting laboratory tests, similarly to that of salpingitis and metritis. Coelioscopy may show a dilated oviduct filled with a white or brown mucoid fluid. Definitive diagnosis requires laparotomy with biopsy, cytology, histopathology, and bacterial culture and sensitivity. Therapy to stop ovulation should be initiated due to increased risk of oviductal rupture during ovulation, oviposition, and possible hormonal contribution to the cystic state of the oviduct. If bacterial infection is suspected or documented by cytology and bacterial culture and sensitivity, appropriate antibiotic treatment is indicated. Salpingohysterectomy may be required to resolve the current problem or prevent future recurrence.[35]

Retained cystic right oviduct

In the female chicken embryo, 2 Müllerian ducts start to develop into oviducts. The left duct develops into a functional oviduct, whereas the right duct regresses. Incomplete regression may result in a cystic right oviduct. Cystic right oviducts are common incidental findings. Small cysts are of little consequence, but large cysts may compress the abdominal viscera.[6]

Salpingitis and metritis

Salpingitis, the inflammation of the oviduct, may be a consequence of infectious or noninfectious diseases, and despite being more common in adult hens, it may also occur in young birds. Inflammation of the oviduct caused by E coli results in decreased egg production and sporadic mortality, and it is one of the most common causes of mortality in commercial layer and breeder chickens but also affects other female birds, especially ducks and geese.[58] Streptococcus sp, Mycoplasma gallisepticum, Acinetobacter sp, Corynebacterium sp, Salmonella sp, and Pasteurella multocida have all been implicated in salpingitis in various species.[3] Venereal colibacillosis is an acute and frequently fatal vaginitis that affects turkey breeder hens shortly after they are first inseminated.[58] In Anseriformes, salpingitis due to non-lactose-fermenting, gram-negative bacteria (eg, Pseudomonas aeruginosa, Proteus mirabilis, Proteus vulgaris) has been reported.[37] A 10-year retrospective survey of salpingitis in 7-week-old domestic ducks revealed that Riemerella anatipestifer, E coli, and P multocida were the bacteria more commonly isolated, whereas E coli and P multocida dominated in geese of different ages. The same study reported a lower prevalence of salpingitis due to Actinobacillus spp, Aeromonas hydrophila, Bordetella avium, Citrobacter freundii, Enterococcus faecalis, Flavobacterium spp, Mycoplasma spp, Proteus spp, Salmonella spp, Staphylococcus aureus, Streptococcus spp, and Yersinia enterocolitica.[59] Newcastle disease also has been associated with salpingitis in several species.[21] Prosthogonimus ovatus and other related trematodes (flukes) can inhabit the oviduct of poultry and waterfowl and result in salpingitis with heavy infestations.[21,60–62] Specifically in poultry, vent cannibalism has been implicated as a precursor to salpingitis.[63]

Noninfectious salpingitis can also be seen, especially with chronic sterile oviductal impactions. Noninfectious causes of salpingitis include trauma and inflammation secondary to oviposition disorders, malnutrition, and foreign bodies.[37] Excessive abdominal fat has been associated with salpingitis in domestic fowl.[35]

Metritis is the inflammation within the shell gland portion of the oviduct and may result from or cause egg binding, chronic oviductal impaction and rupture, coelomitis, and septicemia. Birds with nonseptic salpingitis or metritis often show vague signs of illness, whereas septic birds are usually clinically ill. Eggshell deformities and embryonic and neonatal infections are often secondary to metritis.

Although leukocytosis with heterophilia may be observed in cases of oviductal disease, most forms of it have not been seen to correlate with significant hematologic or biochemical abnormalities.[64] Radiographs and ultrasonography may reveal an enlarged oviduct. Definitive diagnosis is made at celiotomy or endoscopy with aspiration of oviductal fluid for cytologic and microbiologic analysis or, if the oviduct has no liquid contents, biopsy with culture.

Use antibiotics based on culture and sensitivity results. If trying to spare the oviduct, repeated endoscopic evaluation, direct and indirect oviductal flushing, and long-term antimicrobials are recommended. Salpingohysterectomy is indicated for most cases.

Oviductal impaction
Occasionally, an oviduct is occluded by masses of yolk, coagulated albumen, shell membranes, and in some instances, fully formed eggs.[6] Oviductal impaction may occur following salpingitis, metritis, neoplasia, or dystocia.[21,65,66] Clinical signs may be vague and can include cessation of egg production, broody behavior without egg production, weight loss, anorexia, depression, constipation, diarrhea, abdominal distension, and reluctance to walk or fly.[35] Large masses of yolklike material may also be found in the oviduct, and upon transection, these masses have the appearance of concentric rings.[6]

Oviductal prolapse
Oviductal prolapse may occur secondary to any condition that causes chronic, excessive abdominal straining, such as normal physiologic hyperplasia, egg laying, dystocia, or large intracoelomic space-occupying masses. Predisposing factors may include abnormal or soft-shelled eggs, malnutrition, obesity, salpingitis, and cloacitis (**Fig. 14**).[35]

Lines of turkeys selected for rapid growth and high meat yield have an increased incidence of prolapse of the oviduct compared with unselected or traditional strains of turkeys, but in sire lines, it was not associated with any anatomic abnormalities or high plasma estradiol during reproductive development.[67] The uterus with or without partial prolapse of the vagina and cloaca protrudes through the cloaca and/or the vent. Rapid management is necessary to prevent necrosis of the prolapsed tissues. Any egg that may be present should be removed, and all exposed tissues cleaned, irrigated, and kept well moistened to prevent desiccation. Temporary stay sutures may be indicated to aid in preventing recurrence, because prolapse of the oviduct may recur, and repeated replacement is often required. Complete blood count, serum chemistries, microbiological culture and sensitivity, radiographs, ultrasonography, and coelioscopy are strongly recommended. Treatment should be

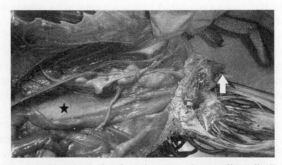

Fig. 14. Post-mortem examination of a female smew (*Mergellus albellus*) presented with cloacal prolapse (*arrow*), which revealed an egg-related coelomitis (*star*).

directed at clearing any bacterial infection and preventing further prolapse, decrease reproductive hormone levels to prevent further egg formation, decrease the size of oviductal tissue, and allow the reproductive tract to rest. Salpingohysterectomy may be considered to prevent recurrence. Predisposing factors should be corrected to prevent recurrence and secondary diseases addressed.[35]

Oviductal volvulus

Oviductal volvulus associated with a moderate amount of sero-hemorrhagic intracoelomic fluid has been reported as a postmortem finding in a chicken.[68]

Oviductal rupture

Oviductal rupture may occur secondary to dystocia or oviductal disease. Infection by the oviduct fluke *P ovatus* resulted in inflammation and rupture of the oviduct and peritonitis in chickens.[60] Prostaglandins, oxytocin, arginine vasotocin, and ovocentesis may cause traumatic rupture of the oviduct. Clinical signs may include depression, anorexia, and abdominal distension secondary to coelomitis or the deposition of egg or oviductal contents. Radiographs and ultrasonography may reveal osteomyelosclerosis, polyostotic hyperostosis (see **Fig. 8**), a soft tissue density in the region of the ovary, ovarian follicles, an enlarged or cystic oviduct, a shelled or non-shelled egg, and coelomic fluid if a concurrent coelomitis is present. Diagnosis is confirmed at coelioscopy or coeliotomy. The laceration may be repaired, depending on the integrity of the tissue, or salpingohysterectomy may be performed as a therapeutic and preventive technique (**Fig. 15**).[35]

Egg-related coelomitis

Egg-related coelomitis includes all of those involving egg yolk, albumin, and/or eggshell. This condition is not a primary reproductive disorder, but has been included as it is, in the authors' opinion, one of the most common clinical presentations in practice. This condition is often presented as a chronic generalized coelomitis, with or without bacterial infection. Fowl, and particularly chickens, might not always develop coelomitis after ectopic ovulation, and it is not uncommon to encounter follicles in the coelomic cavity in different stages of reabsorption at postmortem examination. In most cases, there is an underlying reproductive condition that has led to the ectopic ovulation or retrograde movement from the oviduct back into the coelomic cavity. This condition can be caused by an underlying disorder or can occur after a stressful event while the egg was forming within the oviduct. In both situations, the egg reaches the

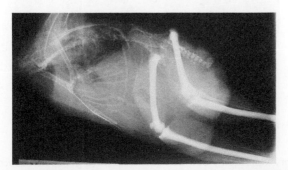

Fig. 15. Right lateral radiograph of a burrowing owl (*Athene cunicularia*) with significant hyperostosis in both femurs, with an egg-releated coelomitis. (*Courtesy of* Neil A. Forbes, BVetMed, Dip ECZM (avian), CBiol, MIBiol, FRCVS, Swindon, United Kingdom.)

coelomic cavity causing a coelomitis. Secondary bacterial colonization can occur; *E coli* is the most commonly found bacteria. Often this occurs because of pathologic changes in the oviduct, with either infectious or neoplastic causes, or because of oviductal damage in battery hens. Clinical signs are often unspecific and include lethargy, anorexia, and cessation of egg production. Ceolomic distension is a common clinical finding, which may cause dyspnea, lameness, or recumbency. The diagnosis is often based on imaging techniques (eg, radiographs or ultrasound) and cytology of samples obtained by coelomic centesis. Coelomic centesis not only guides toward a diagnosis but also can be therapeutic when dyspnea is observed. Fluid therapy, antibiotics, analgesia (see **Table 2** for further information), and assisted feeding are required at initial stabilization. Salpingohysterectomy is likely to be required for long-term treatment because this condition is likely to reoccur (**Figs. 16** and **17**).

Reproductive Disorders in Males

Orchitis and epididymitis

Orchitis may be infectious (ascending infections, hematogenous spread, or infected adjacent organs) or noninfectious. *S gallinarum* (fowl typhoid) and *S pullorum* (pullorum disease) may provoke orchitis in mature roosters and turkeys.[47] Orchitis, epididymitis, and epididymo-orchitis caused by *S aureus* and *E coli* have been reported in broilers.[69] *Chlamydia psittaci* causes orchitis and epididymitis in turkeys, which may provoke the death of the bird due to internal hemorrhage secondary to rupture of the testicular blood vessels.[70] Avian infectious bronchitis virus (IBV) and potentially avian metapneumovirus (aMPV) may have a role in the development of epididymal stones and low fertility in broilers.[71] Clinical signs may include infertility, depression, hyporexia, lethargy, and/or coelomic distension if a secondary coelomitis develops. Leukocytosis with a relative heterophilia may be noted.[35] Testicular enlargement may be identified by using imaging diagnosis techniques. Coelioscopy may reveal inflammation and hypervascularization of the enlarged testicle. Definitive diagnosis is made by cytology, bacterial culture and sensitivity, and histopathologic examination of samples from affected testis. IBV may be diagnosed by reverse transcriptase-polymerase chain reaction (RT-PCR), whereas aMPV may be detected by viral

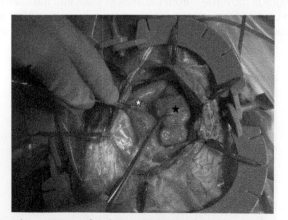

Fig. 16. Exploratory laparotomy of a domestic chicken (*G gallus domesticus*) with an egg-related coelomitis; please note the distended oviduct (*black star*) with an abnormal yellow coloration. Intracoelomic fat (*white star*). (*Courtesy of* Neil A. Forbes, BVetMed, Dip ECZM (avian), CBiol, MIBiol, FRCVS, Swindon, United Kingdom.)

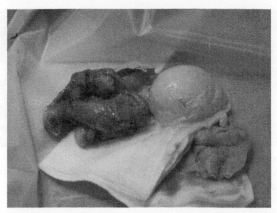

Fig. 17. Removed egg material and oviduct of a domestic chicken (*G gallus domesticus*) with egg-related coelomitis. (*Courtesy of* Neil A. Forbes, BVetMed, Dip ECZM (avian), CBiol, MI-Biol, FRCVS, Swindon, United Kingdom.)

isolation and/or RT-PCR.[71] Serology may be useful in the diagnosis of S gallinarum and S pullorum.[47] Therapy includes broad-spectrum antibiotics until results from bacterial culture and sensitivity are available. Vaccination may be used to control the S gallinarum and S pullorum.[47]

Testicular neoplasia
Testicular neoplasias are more often unilateral than bilateral. Sertoli cell tumor has been reported in Japanese quail, as a cause of feminization in an incompletely castrated brown leghorn wherein the tumor arose from the gonadal remnants tissue, and showing peritoneal and mesenteric metastases in a goose in which the other testicle was atrophied.[71–73] Seminomas have been reported solitary or associated with multiple metastases (visceral organs) in a monorchid Guinea fowl and (with hepatic, pancreatic, peritoneal, and pulmonary metastasis) Mallard duck.[74–77] Mixed germ cell–sex cord–stromal tumor (Sertoli, seminoma, and intersticial cell components) has been reported in a Pekin duck.[78] Arrhenoblastomas have been described in an Indian Desi hen and chukar partridge.[79,80] A testicular teratoma has been reported in domestic fowl.[81]

Clinical signs include chronic weight loss, coelomic distension, and/or unilateral paresis, cyanosis, and/or hypothermia of the pelvic limb due to compression of the ischiatic nerve and blood vessels.

Diagnostic imaging techniques may reveal testicular enlargement, air sac compression, and sometimes secondary polyostotic hyperostosis (**Fig. 18**). Definitive diagnosis is made by testicular biopsy and histopathologic examination. Orchiectomy is the recommended treatment and is associated with a good prognosis as long as metastasis is not present. In the case of cystic testicular tumors, aspiration of the cyst during surgery may reduce the mass size and facilitate its removal.[3]

Cystic dilation of the seminiferous tubules and testes
Nonneoplastic cystic testicular disease is very infrequently reported, and its significance is unknown. Cystic dilatation of the seminiferous tubules and/or testes has been observed in fowl fed a diet high in ionic sodium, in fowl fed with egg albumen as a source of protein, or in roosters affected with epididymal cysts and stones.[82–84] Cystic testes should be drained, biopsied, and potentially removed.

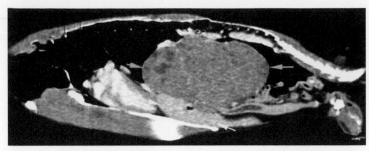

Fig. 18. Sagittal image of a common duck demonstrating the testicular enlargement (*green arrows*) and the dorsoventrally compressed liver (*yellow arrows*) in a khaki Campbell (domestic) duck (*A platyrhynchos domesticus*).

Phallus inflammation and prolapse

Phallus inflammation and prolapse may occur secondary to local bacterial infection, trauma, or excessive sexual stimulation. In geese, phallus inflammation has been associated with local *Mycoplasma* spp infection, whereas phallus erosions and prolapse have been associated with *Neisseria* spp infection (suspected to be sexually transmitted).[58,85] Frostbite and bacterial infection may occur as a sequela of phallus prolapse. Treatment may range from medical therapy (eg, local or systemic antibiotics or anti-inflammatories), debridement, or amputation in severe cases with or without partial closure of the cloaca (**Table 3**).

PHARMACOLOGIC TREATMENT OPTIONS

Avian and exotic clinicians deal with a higher number of species on a daily basis compared with the small animal clinician and are often familiar with prescribing medications "off license" (also called "off label"). However, it is important to highlight that some fowl species, and particularly chickens, might have commercially available drugs available. Therefore, the use of "off-label" medications must be justified and follow local legislation. Animals presented to the avian clinician are unlikely to be consumed, although their eggs frequently are. Therefore, the clinician should also be familiar with the maximum residue levels (MRL) and the withdrawal periods (including the ones for eggs) of the different medications before its use.

For US clinicians, the Web site, www.farad.org, is a valuable resource regarding extralabel drug use and might provide acceptable withdrawal time for off-label drug use.[42] Fluoroquinolone (eg, enrofloxacin), cephalosporin, chloramphenicol, and metronidazole are prohibited for use in any food animal in the United States, to prevent the formation of antibiotic-resistant *Campylobacter* spp.[42]

In the United Kingdom, the veterinary surgeon should always follow the "medication cascade" when prescribing any medication (https://www.gov.uk/guidance/the-cascade-prescribing-unauthorised-medicines), wherein it is stated that *"Any pharmacologically active substances included in a medicinal product administered to a food-producing animal under the cascade must be listed in Table 1 in the Annex to Commission Regulation (EU) NO. 37/2010."* Therefore, if a veterinary surgeon decides to prescribe a substance under the cascade for a food-producing animal, that active substance must be listed in Table 1 of EC 37/2010. This provision does not specifically require an MRL to be set for the species for which the veterinary surgeon intends to use it. Therefore, even if the MRL entry for that substance does not include eggs, a veterinary surgeon could consider it for use in chickens intended to produce eggs

Table 3
Commonly reported egg abnormalities

Egg Abnormality	Cause
Shell-less egg: Fully formed egg laid without the shell	Infectious (eg, infectious bronchitis, *M gallisepticum*, or adenovirus [egg drop syndrome, EDS]) Nutritional (eg, calcium, phosphorus, or vitamin D3 deficiency or overdose of phosphorus or vitamin D3) Age
Double yolk: Large eggs with 2 yolks; young flocks just starting into production	Light overstimulation (excessive increase in day length or an excessive increase in light intensity) Methionine overdose.
Discolored yolks (DY)/blood spots (BS)/meat spots (MS): Normally not indicative of flock problems	DY (eg, ingestion of high amounts of copper or Gossypol) BS (eg, stress or inadequate vitamin K levels) MS (ovarian or oviductal tissue incorporated into the egg during ovulation)
Abnormal shape: Misshapen or "wrinkled" eggshells seen; other clinical signs are usually not seen unless infectious bronchitis or EDS is involved, in which case respiratory signs and lesions along with egg production loss are seen	Change in lighting schedule that disrupts the ovulation pattern, resulting in double ovulation with 2 eggs developing at one time Infectious bronchitis EDS virus
Shell color loss: Only noticeable in brown egg layer flocks; the protoporphyrin-IX pigment that is secreted from the epithelial cells lining the uterus during the 90 min just before oviposition is responsible for the brown eggshell color	Strain of bird, age of bird, and stress levels can affect the shade of brown of the eggshell Nicarbazine (coccidiostat) EDS Infectious bronchitis. The pigment loss recovers in the case of infectious bronchitis infection but may take up to 6 wk
Poor eggshell quality: Thin shell (TS) Rough shells (RS) (flocks early or in the middle stages of production) Soft ends of the eggshell (SE) (early in production)	TS: Factors that interfere with calcium utilization (eg, inadequate mineral supplementation, inappropriate phosphorus levels in feed, inadequate vitamin A or D levels in feed) RS: May be associated with inadequate vitamin supplementation, especially vitamins A and D, or cracks occurring in the eggshell while it is still developing in the shell maker gland, which is covered by secretion of additional shell material in the shell maker gland and appears as ridged areas over the original breakage sites (this damage may occur after excessive vigorous activity in the flock) SE: May be associated with strain of chicken or nutritional factors
Parasites in the egg	Ascending migration of intestinal parasites from the cloaca to the oviduct in the hen (usually apparently healthy unless obstructing the oviduct): Roundworms (eg, *Ascaridia galli*) Tapeworms Flukes (eg, *Prosthogonimus* sp)

Data from Arundel JH, Kingston JL, Kerr PJ. Prosthogonimus pellucidus in domestic poultry. Aust Vet J 1980;56:460–1; and Stipkovits L, Szathmary S. Mycoplasma infection of ducks and geese. Poult Sci 2012;91:2812–9.

for human consumption. In this case, the veterinary surgeon should consider the risks of using this substance and is obligated to consider the time of use in relation to the stage of development of the eggs and the length of time between administration of the last dose and the first egg being laid and to the set an appropriate withdrawal period to ensure that residues of any substances administered will not enter the food chain. Doxycycline and enrofloxacin appear in Table 1 to 37/2010; neither have an MRL in eggs, but do have an MRL in other tissues. It is important to emphasize that if the active substance administered does not have an MRL in eggs, the presence of any residues of that substance in eggs (irrespective of the levels) will be illegal. The cascade requires that a minimum withdrawal period of 7 days is applied. However, it is the responsibility of the veterinarian to ensure the withdrawal period they specify for such products will ensure no residues will be present in the eggs collected for human consumption. The veterinarian may therefore wish to take a precautionary approach when specifying the withdrawal period in relation to the use of an active substance, which has no egg MRL. Where an egg MRL exists, the veterinarian should specify a withdrawal period that will ensure that any residues of the substance in eggs are below the MRL.

SUMMARY

Backyard poultry and other commonly kept fowl species are often kept for their ability to lay eggs. Reproductive disease is common in fowl species. Despite being classified as food-producing species, they can be considered valuable pets, and the demand for adequate veterinary care is constantly increasing. The clinician should be familiar with the different abnormalities and the potential treatment options. Fowl species have been traditionally an anatomic, physiologic, and experimental model for avian medicine; however, information about treatment options is often limited and extrapolated from other species. Egg-related coelomitis is commonly seen in fowl, often linked to abnormality of the oviduct, such as neoplasia.

Secondary bacterial infection is often caused by E coli. The clinician must be familiar with the local legislation before prescribing medications for fowl.

REFERENCES

1. Sibley CG, Ahlquist JE, Monroe BL. A classification of the living birds of the world base on DNA-DDNA hybridization studies. Auk 1988;105:409–23.
2. Eo SH, Bininda-Emonds ORP, Carroll JP. A phylogenetic supertree of the fowls (Galloansera, Aves). Zool Scr 2009;38:465–81.
3. Echols S. Soft tissue surgery. In: Greenacre CB, Morishita TY, editors. Backyard poultry medicine and surgery. A guide for veterinary practitioners. Ames (IA): Wiley-Blackwell; 2015. p. 220–59.
4. Johnson AL. Reproduction in the female. In: Scanes CG, editor. Sturkie's avian physiology. 6th edition. London: Elsevier; 2015. p. 635–65.
5. King AS, McLelland J. Female reproductive tract. In: King AS, McLelland J, editors. Birds: their structure and function, vol. 1. Eastbourne (United Kingdom): Bailliere Tindall; 1984. p. 145–65.
6. Crespo R, Shivaprasad HL. Developmental, metabolic, and other noninfectious disorders. In: Saif YM, editor. Diseases of poultry. 12th edition. Ames (IA): Blackwell Publishing; 2008. p. 1150–6. Available at: http://eu.wiley.com/WileyCDA/WileyTitle/productCd-0470958995.html.
7. Crosta L, Gerlack H, Bürkle M, et al. Physiology, diagnosis, and diseases of the avian reproductive tract. Vet Clin North Am Exot Anim Pract 2003;6(1):57–83.

8. Waibl H, Sinowatz F. Harn- und Geschlechtsapparat. In: Nickel R, Schummer A, Seiferle H, editors. Lehrbuch der Anatomie der Haustiere, Band V: anatomie der Vögel. Hamburg (Germany): Parey; 1992. p. 224–61.

9. Ubuka T, Bentley GE. Neuroendocrine control of reproduction in birds. In: David O, Norris DO, Lopez KH, editors. Hormones and reproduction of vertebrates, vol. 4. London: Elsevier; 2011. p. 1–25. Birds.

10. Mans C, Taylor WM. Update on neuroendocrine regulation and medical intervention of reproduction in birds. Vet Clin North Am Exot Anim Pract 2008; 11(1):83–105.

11. Dunn IC, Millam JR. Gonadotropin releasing hormone: forms and functions in birds. Avian Poultry Biol Rev 1998;9:61–85.

12. Mans C, Pilny A. Use of GnRH-agonists for medical management of reproductive disorders in birds. Vet Clin North Am Exot Anim Pract 2014;17(1):23–33.

13. King JA, Millar RP. Structure of chicken hypothalamic luteinizing hormone-releasing hormone. II. Isolation and characterization. J Biol Chem 1982; 257(18):10729–32.

14. Miyamoto K, Hasegawa Y, Nomura M, et al. Identification of the second gonadotropin-releasing hormone in chicken hypothalamus: evidence that gonadotropin secretion is probably controlled by two distinct gonadotropin-releasing hormones in avian species. Proc Natl Acad Sci U S A 1984;81(12): 3874–8.

15. Bentley GE, Moore IT, Sower SA, et al. Evidence for a novel gonadotropin-releasing hormone in hypothalamic and forebrain areas in songbirds. Brain Behav Evol 2004;63(1):34–46.

16. Millan JR. Reproductive physiology. In: Altman RB, Dorrestein GM, Clubb S, et al, editors. Avian medicine and surgery. Philadelphia: W.B. Saunders; 1997. p. 12–26.

17. Rangel PL, Gutierrez CG. Reproduction in hens: is testosterone necessary for the ovulatory process? Gen Comp Endocrinol 2014;203:150–261.

18. Calisi RM, Diaz-Munoz SL, Wingfield JC, et al. Social and breeding status are associated with the expression of GnIH. Genes Brain Behav 2011;10:557–64.

19. König HE, Walter I, Bragulla H, et al. Weibliche Geschlechtsorgane (Organa genitalia feminina). In: König HE, Liebich HG, editors. Anatomie und Propädeutik des Geflügels. Stuttgart (Germany): Schattauer; 2001. p. 133–42.

20. Vizcarra J, Alan R, Kirby J. Reproduction in males. In: Scanes CG, editor. Sturkie's avian physiology. 6th edition. London: Elsevier; 2015. p. 667–93.

21. Joyner KL. Theriogenology. In: Ritchie BR, Harrison GJ, Harrison LR, editors. Avian medicine: principles and application. Lake Worth (FL): Wingers Publishing; 1994. p. 748–804.

22. Smith RE. Reproductive disorders in birds. In: Rosskopf WJ Jr, Woerpel R, editors. Diseases of cage and aviary birds. 3rd edition. Baltimore (MD): Williams and Wilkins; 1996. p. 449–57.

23. King AS, McLelland J. Male reproductive tract. In: King AS, McLelland J, editors. Birds: their structure and function, vol. 1. Eastbourne (United Kingdom): Bailliere Tindall; 1984. p. 166–74.

24. Orosz S. Anatomy of the urogenital system. In: Altman RB, Dorrestein GM, Clubb S, et al, editors. Avian medicine and surgery. Philadelphia: W.B. Saunders; 1997. p. 614–22.

25. Kirby JD, Froman DP. Reproduction in male birds. In: Witthow GC, editor. Sturkie's avian physiology. 5th edition. San Diego (CA): Academic Press; 2000. p. 597–615.

26. Aire TA. The epididymal region of the Japanese quail (Coturnix coturnix japonica). Acta Anat 1979;103:305–12.
27. Briskie JV, Montgomerie R. Efficient copulation and the evolutionary loss of the avian intromittent organ. J Avian Biol 2001;32:184–7.
28. Brennan PL, Clark CJ, Prum RO. Explosive eversion and functional morphology of the duck penis supports sexual conflict in waterfowl genitalia. Proc Biol Sci 2010;277:1309–14.
29. Roberts V. Galliform birds: health and husbandry. In: Roberts V, Scott-Park F, editors. BSAVA manual of farm pets. Gloucester (United Kingdom): British Small Animal Veterinary Association; 2008. p. 190–214.
30. Orosz S. Anatomy of the endocrine system. In: Altman RB, Dorrestein GM, Clubb S, et al, editors. Avian medicine and surgery. Philadelphia: W.B. Saunders; 1997. p. 475–88.
31. Scanes CG. Introduction to endocrinology: pituitary gland. In: Witthow GC, editor. Sturkie's avian physiology. 5th edition. San Diego (CA): Academic Press; 2000. p. 437–60.
32. Seredynski AL, Ball GF, Balthazart J, et al. Specific activation of estrogen receptor alpha and beta enhances male sexual behaviour and neuroplasticity in male Japanese quail. PLoS One 2011;6:e1862.
33. Follett BK, Maung SL. Rate of testicular maturation, in relation to gonadotrophin and testosterone levels, in quail exposed to various artificial photoperiods and to natural daylengths. J Endocrinol 1978;78:267–80.
34. Deviche P. Reproduction behavior. In: Scanes CG, editor. Sturkie's avian physiology. 6th edition. London: Elsevier; 2015. p. 695–715.
35. Bowles HL. Evaluating and treating the reproductive system. In: Harrison GJ, Lightfoot LT, editors. Clinical avian medicine volume II. Palm Beach (FL): Spix Publishing; 2006. p. 519–40.
36. Romagnano A. Avian obstetrics. Journal of Exotic Pet Medicine 1996;5:180–8.
37. Speer B. Diseases of the urogenital system. In: Altman RB, Clubb SL, Dorrestein GM, et al, editors. Avian medicine and surgery. Philadelphia: WB Saunders Co; 1997. p. 625–44.
38. Calvo Carrasco D, Sabater González M. Emergencies and critical care of commonly kept fowl. Vet Clin North Am Exot Anim Pract 2016;19(1):543–65.
39. Crespo R, Senties-Cue G. Postmortem survey of disease conditions in backyard poultry. Journal of Exotic Pet Medicine 2015;24:156–63.
40. Johnson PA, Giles JR. The hen as a model of ovarian cancer. Nat Rev Cancer 2013;13:432–6.
41. Namazi F, Mosleh N. Intestinal metastasis of ovarian adenocarcinoma in a native chicken (Gallus domesticus). Journal of World's poultry research 2013;3:80–2.
42. Gingerich G, Shaw D. Reproductive diseases. In: Greenacre CB, Morishita TY, editors. Backyard poultry medicine and surgery. A guide for veterinary practitioners. 1st edition. Ames (IA): Wiley-Blackwell; 2015. p. 169–80.
43. Smith S, Rodriguez Barbon A. Waterfowl: medicine and surgery. In: Roberts V, Scott-Park F, editors. BSAVA manual of farm pets. Gloucester (United Kingdom): British Small Animal Veterinary Association; 2008. p. 250–73.
44. Doneley B. Disorders of the Reproductive tract. In: Doneley B, editor. Avian medicine and surgery in practice, companion and aviary birds. 2nd edition. Boca Raton (FL): CRC Press; 2016. p. 317–32.
45. Harry EG. Some observations on the bacterial content of the ovary and oviduct of the fowl. Br Poult Sci 1963;4:63–70.

46. Montgomery RD, Boyle CR, Lenarduzzi TA, et al. Consequences to chicks hatched from Escherichia coli inoculated embryos. Avian Dis 1999;43:553–63.
47. Shivaprasad HL. Fowl typhoid and pullorum disease. Rev Sci Tech 2000;19(2): 405–24.
48. Bojesen AM, Nielsen OL, Christensen JP, et al. In vivo studies of Gallibacterium anatis infection in chickens. Avian Pathol 2004;33:145–52.
49. Batra GL, Balwant S, Grewal GS, et al. Aetiopathology of oophoritis and salpingitis in domestic fowl. Indian Journal of Poultry Science 1982;52:172–6.
50. Bisgaard M, Dam A. Salpingitis in poultry. II. Prevalence, bacteriology, and possible pathogenesis in egg-laying chickens. Nord Vet Med 1982;33:81–9.
51. Sharma JK, Joshi DV, Baxi KK. Studies on the bacteriological etiology of reproductive disorders of poultry. Indian J Poult Sci 1980;15:78–82.
52. Fell HB. Histologic studies on the gonads of the fowl. I. The histological basis of sex reversal. Br J Exp Biol 1923;1:97–129.
53. Keymer IF. Disorders of the avian female reproductive system. Avian Pathol 1980;9(3):405–19.
54. Suárez-Bonnet A, Herráez P, Batista-Arteaga M, et al. Follicular ovarian torsion in an ostrich (Struthio camelus). Vet Q 2012;32(2):103–5.
55. United States Department of Agriculture. Food Safety and Inspection Service. Statistical summary of Federal Meat and Poultry Inspection. Washington, DC: Washington DC State (USA); 1984.
56. Ansenberger K, Richards C, Zhuge Y, et al. Decreased severity of ovarian cancer and increased survival in hens fed a flax-seed-enriched diet for 1 year. Gynecol Oncol 2010;117:341–7.
57. Fadly AM. Neoplastic Diseases. In: Saif YM, editor. Diseases of poultry. 12th edition. Ames (IA): Blackwell Publishing; 2008. p. 449–616.
58. Barnes HJ, Nolan LK, Vaillancourt JP. Colibacillosis. In: Saif YM, editor. Diseases of poultry. 12th edition. Ames (IA): Blackwell Publishing; 2008. p. 691–738.
59. Bisgaard M. Salpingitis in web-footed birds: prevalence, aetiology and significance. Avian Pathol 1995;24(3):443–52.
60. Arundel JH, Kingston JL, Kerr PJ. Prosthogonimus pellucidus in domestic poultry. Aust Vet J 1980;56:460–1.
61. Kingston N. Trematodes. In: Hofstad MS, Barnes HJ, Calnek BW, et al, editors. Diseases of poultry. 8th edition. Ames (IA): Iowa State University Press; 1984. p. 668–90.
62. Soulsby EJL. Helminths, arthropods and protozoa of domesticated animals. 7th edition. London: Bailliere Tindall; 1982. p. 32–4.
63. Reid GG, Grimes TM, Eaves FW. A survey of disease in five commercial flocks of meat breeder chickens. Aust Vet J 1984;61(1):13–6.
64. Speer B. Pet waterfowl medicine and surgery. Proceedings of the North American Veterinary Conference. Orlando (FL); 2006. p. 1585–8.
65. Davis MF, Ebako GM, Morishita TY. A golden comet hen (Gallus gallus forma domestica) with an impacted oviduct and associated colibacillosis. J Avian Med Surg 2003;17(2):91–5.
66. Srinivasan P, Balasubramaniam GA, Murthy TRGK, et al. Prevalence and pathology of oviduct impaction in commercial white leghorn layer chicken in Namakkal region of India. Vet World 2014;7(8):553–8.
67. Buchanan S, Robertson GW, Hocking PM. Development of the reproductive system in turkeys with a high or low susceptibility to prolapse of the oviduct. Poult Sci 2000;79(10):1491–8.

68. Ajayi OL, Antia RE, Omotainse SO. Oviductal volvulus in a Nera black chicken (Gallus gallus domesticus) in Nigeria. Avian Pathol 2008;37(2):139–40.

69. Monleon R, Martin MP, John Barnes H. Bacterial orchitis and epididymo-orchitis in broiler breeders. Avian Pathol 2008;37(6):613–7.

70. Beasley JN, Moore RW, Watkins JR. The histopathologic characteristics of disease producing inflammation of the air sacs in turkeys: a comparative study of pleuropneumonia-like organisms and ornithosis in pure and mixed infections. Am J Vet Res 1961;22:85–92.

71. Villarreal LY, Brandão PE, Chacón JL, et al. Orchitis in roosters with reduced fertility associated with avian infectious bronchitis virus and avian metapneumovirus infections. Avian Dis 2007;51(4):900–4.

72. Siller WG. A Sertoli cell tumour causing feminization in a brown leghorn capon. J Endocrinol 1956;14(2):197–203.

73. Gorham SL, Ottinger MA. Sertoli cell tumors in Japanese quail. Avian Dis 1986; 30(2):337–9.

74. Uetsuka K, Suzuki T, Doi K, et al. Malignant sertoli cell tumor in a goose (Anser cygnoides domesticus). Avian Dis 2012;56(4):781–5.

75. Kurkure NV, Pande VV, Thomas F, et al. A seminoma in a monorchid guinea fowl (Numida meleagris). J Vet Med A Physiol Pathol Clin Med 2006;53(1):22–3.

76. Golbar HM, Izawa T, Kuwamura M, et al. Malignant seminoma with multiple visceral metastases in a guinea fowl (Numida meleagris) kept in a zoo. Avian Dis 2009;53(1):143–5.

77. Mutinelli F, Vascellari M, Bozzato E. Unilateral seminoma with multiple visceral metastases in a duck (Anas platyrhynchos). Avian Pathol 2006;35(4):327–9.

78. Ganorkar AG, Kurkure NV. Bilateral seminoma in a duck (Anas platyrhynchos). Avian Pathol 1998;27(6):644–5.

79. Leach S, Heatley JJ, Pool RR, et al. Bilateral testicular germ cell-sex cord-stromal tumor in a Pekin duck (Anas platyrhynchos domesticus). J Avian Med Surg 2008;22(4):315–9.

80. Gupta BN, Langham RF. Arrhenoblastoma in an Indian Desi hen. Avian Dis 1968;12(3):441–4.

81. West JL. Arrhenoblastoma in a chukar partridge. Avian Dis 1974;18(2):258–61.

82. Helmboldt CF, Migaki G, Langheinrich KA, et al. Teratoma in domestic fowl (Gallus gallus). Avian Dis 1974;18(1):142–8.

83. Fulton RM. Other toxins and poisons. In: Saif YM, editor. Diseases of poultry. 12th edition. Ames (IO): Blackwell Publishing; 2008. p. 1231–12360.

84. Janssen SJ, Kirby JD, Hess RA. Identification of epididymal stones in diverse rooster populations. Poult Sci 2000;79:568–74.

85. Siller WG, Dewar WA, Whitehead C. Cystic dilatation of the seminiferous tubules in the fowl: a sequel of sodium intoxication. J Pathol 1972;107:191–7.

86. Souza MJ, White MS, Gordon KI, et al. Pharmacokinetics and egg residues after oral Meloxicam in poultry. Proceedings of the ExoticsCon. Portland (OR); 2016. p. 43.

87. Baert K, De Backer P. Comparative pharmacokinetics of three non-steroidal anti-inflammatory drugs in five bird species. Comp Biochem Physiol C Toxicol Pharmacol 2003;134:25–33.

88. Baert K, De Backer P. Disposition of sodium salicylate, flunixin and meloxicam after intravenous administration in broiler chickens. J Vet Pharmacol Ther 2000;25:449–53.

89. Sinclair KM, Paul-Murphy J, Church M, et al. Histopathologic renal changes induced by Meloxicam in quail. Proceedings of the Association of Avian Veterinarians. San Diego (CA); 2010: p. 287–8.

90. Sinclair KM, Church ME, Farver TB, et al. Effects of meloxicam on hematologic and plasma biochemical analysis variables and results of histologic examination of tissue specimens of Japanese quail (Coturnix japonica). Am J Vet Res 2012; 73(11):1720–7.

91. Gentle MJ, Hocking PM, Bernard R, et al. Evaluation of intraarticular opioid analgesia for the relief of articular pain in the domestic fowl. Pharmacol Biochem Behav 1999;63:339–43.

92. Singh PM, Johnson C, Gartrell B, et al. Pharmacokinetics of butorphanol in broiler chickens. Vet Rec 2011;168(22):588–92.

93. O'Kane PM, Connerton IF, White KL. Pilot study of long-term anaesthesia in broiler chickens. Vet Anaesth Analg 2016;43:72–5.

94. Clancy MM, KuKanich B, Sykes JM. Pharmacokinetics of butorphanol delivered with an osmotic pump during a seven-day period in common peafowl (Pavo cristatus). Am J Vet Res 2015;76(12):1070–6.

95. Escobar A, Valadão CAA, Brosnan RJ, et al. Effects of butorphanol on the minimum anesthetic concentration for sevoflurane in guineafowl (Numida meleagris). Am J Vet Res 2012;73(2):183–8.

96. Buchwalder T, Huber-Eicher B. Effect of the analgesic butorphanol on activity behaviour in turkeys (Meleagris gallopavo). Res Vet Sci 2005;79:239–44.

97. Black PA, Cox SK, Macek M, et al. Pharmacokinetics of tramadol hydrochloride and its metabolite O-desmethyltramadol in peafowl (Pavo cristatus). J Zoo Wildl Med 2010;41(4):671–6.

98. Escudero E, Vicente MS, Carceles CM. Pharmacokinetics of amoxicillin/clavulanic acid combination after intravenous and intramuscular administration to pigeons. Res Vet Sci 1998;65(1):77–81.

99. Jerzsele A, Nagy G, Semjen G. Oral bioavailability and pharmacokinetic profile of the amoxicillin–clavulanic acid combination after intravenous and oral administration in Turkeys. J Vet Pharmacol Ther 2010;34:202–5.

100. Jerzsele A, Nagy G, Lehel J, et al. Oral bioavailability and pharmacokinetic profile of the amoxicillin–clavulanic acid combination after intravenous and oral gavage administration in broiler chickens. J Vet Pharmacol Ther 2009;32:506–9.

101. Ziv G, Shem-Tov M, Glickman A, et al. Concentrations of amoxycillin and clavulanic acid in the serum of broilers during continuous and pulse-dosing of the drinking water. Journal of Veterinary Pharmacology and Therapeutics 1997; 20(Suppl 1):190–1.

102. Cornejo J, Lapierre L, Iragüen D, et al. Study of enrofloxacin and flumequine residues depletion in eggs of laying hens after oral administration. J Vet Pharmacol Ther 2012;35(1):67–72.

103. Bugyei K, Black WD, McEwen S. Pharmacokinetics of enrofloxacin given by the oral, intravenous and intramuscular routes in broiler chickens. Can J Vet Res 1999;63:193–200.

104. Sumano LH, Gutierrez OL, Zamora QM. Strategic administration of enrofloxacin in poultry to achieve higher maximal serum concentrations. Vet J 2003;165(2):143–8.

105. Turbahn A, Cortez De Jäckel S, Greuel E, et al. Dose response study of enrofloxacin against Riemerella anatipestifer septicaemia in Muscovy and Pekin ducklings. Avian Pathol 1997;26(4):791–802.

106. Garmyn A, Martel A, Froyman R, et al. Effect of multiple- and single-day enrofloxacin medications against dual experimental infection with avian pneumovi-
rus and in turkeys. Poult Sci 2009;88(10):2093–100.
107. Dimitrova DJ, Lashev LD, Yanev SG, et al. Pharmacokinetics of enrofloxacin in
turkeys. Res Vet Sci 2007;82:392–7.
108. Lashev LD, Dimitrova DJ, Milanova A, et al. Pharmacokinetics of enrofloxacin
and marbofloxacin in Japanese quails and common pheasants. Br Poult Sci
2015;55(2):255–61.
109. Haritova A, Dimitrova D, Dinev T, et al. Comparative pharmacokinetics of enrofloxacin, danofloxacin, and marbofloxacin after intravenous and oral administration in Japanese quail (Coturnix coturnix japonica). J Avian Med Surg 2013;
27(1):23–31.
110. Anadón A, Martínez-Larrañaga M, Díaz M, et al. Pharmacokinetic characteristics and tissue residues for marbofloxacin and its metabolite N-desmethyl-mar-
bofloxacin in broiler chickens. Am J Vet Res 2002;63(7):927–33, 115.
111. Haritova A, Rusenova N, Parvanov P, et al. Integration of pharmacokinetic and
pharmacodynamic indices of marbofloxacin in turkeys. Antimicrob Agents Che-
mother 2006;50(11):3779–85.
112. Best R. Breeding problems. In: Beynon PH, Forbes NA, Hartcourt-Brown NH,
editors. Manual of raptors, pigeons and waterfowl. Gloucester (United
Kingdom): British Small Animal Veterinary Association; 1996. p. 208–15.
113. Noonan B, Johnson P, de Matos R. Evaluation of egg-laying suppression effects
of the GnRH agonist deslorelin in domestic chickens. Proc Annu Conf Assoc
Avian Vet. Louisville (KY): AAV; 2012. p. 321.
114. Molter C, Fontenot D, Terrell S. Use of deslorelin acetate implants to mitigate
aggression in two adult male domestic turkeys (Meleagris gallopavo) and correlating plasma testosterone concentrations. J Avian Med Surg 2015;29(3):
224–30.
115. Petritz O, Sanchez-Migallon D, Paul-Murphy J. Evaluation of the efficacy and
safety of a single administration of 4.7-mg deslorelin acetate implants on egg
production and plasma sex hormones in Japanese quail (Coturnix coturnix
japonica). Am J Vet Res 2013;72(2):316–23.
116. Dickerman R, Wise T, Bahr J. Effect of ovarian regression and molt on plasma
concentrations of thymosin 4 in domestic chickens. Domest Anim Endocrinol
1992;9(4):297–304.
117. Burke W, Attia Y. Molting single comb White Leghorns with the use of Lupron
Depot formulation of leuprolide acetate. Poult Sci 1994;73:1226–32.
118. Petritz OA, Lierz M, Samour J. Advancements in Methods for Decreasing Reproductive Success. In: Speer BL, editor. Current Therapy in Avian Medicine and
Surgery. St louis (MO): ElSevier; 2016. p. 446–60.

Reproductive Disorders of Marsupials

Cathy A. Johnson-Delaney, DVM[a,1],
Angela M. Lennox, DVM, DABVP-Avian, Exotic Companion Mammal, DECZM-Small Mammals[b],*

KEYWORDS

• Marsupial • Reproductive disorders • Sugar glider • Opossum • Wallaby

KEY POINTS

• Marsupial reproduction differs from that of placental mammals, as the female gives birth to a fetus that develops outside of the uterus.
• Pouch infections are unique to marsupials and may jeopardize the development of the joey.
• Marsupial reproductive tract diseases include infectious and traumatic etiologies and are similar to those of placental mammals.
• Castration and ovario-vaginal-hysterectomy surgeries differ from those of placental mammals because of the marsupial anatomy, especially in the female; inattention to differences can lead to inadvertent ligation of the ureters.

Captive marsupials are occasionally presented to practitioners. Many owners are breeding marsupials such as sugar gliders, wallabies, and short-tailed opossums for the pet trade. Reproductive disorders, such as dystocia, found in placental mammals are not seen in marsupials. A brief discussion of the unique anatomy and physiology of the marsupial is necessary to evaluate reproductive health and disease.

The most commonly presented captive marsupials are the sugar glider (*Petaurus breviceps*), the Brazilian (short-tailed, laboratory, gray) opossum (*Monodelphis domestica*), and macropods including the Tammar or Dama wallaby (*Macropus eugenii*) and, more commonly, the Bennett's wallaby (*Macropus rufogriseus*). In North America, injured or orphaned Virginia opossums (*Didelphis virginiana*) are frequently brought into clinics or rehabilitation centers and occasionally kept as pets. Marsupial infants are called joeys. Sex determination is usually easy, even at a young age (**Fig. 1**).

The authors have nothing to disclose.
[a] Washington Ferret Rescue & Shelter, Kirkland, WA, USA; [b] Avian and Exotic Animal Clinic of Indianapolis, 9330 Waldemar Road, Indianapolis, IN 46268, USA
[1] Present address: 13813 65th Avenue W #7, Edmonds, WA 98026.
* Corresponding author.
E-mail address: birddr@aol.com

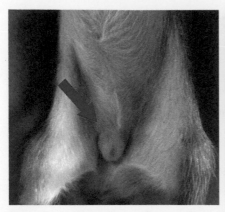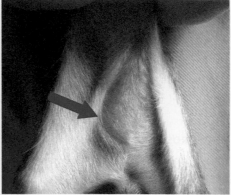

Fig. 1. Red arrows show infant Virginia opossum premature scrotal sac (*Left*) and pouch (*Right*).

REPRODUCTIVE ANATOMY AND PHYSIOLOGY

Marsupial reproductive anatomy and physiology is considerably different than that of placental mammals.[1] The gastrointestinal tract, urinary ducts, and genital ducts all open into a cloaca.[1,2]

Female Marsupials

The reproductive tract of the female marsupial is smaller than that of placental mammals. It consists of the ovaries, oviducts, and paired uterus bodies that form the proximal half and the 2 lateral and central (median) vaginal canals that form the distal half (**Fig. 2**). The 3 vaginal canals join and form a urogenital sinus that also contains the urethral opening before entrance into the cloaca. The ureters are contained within the vaginal canals unlike in placental mammals, where they arrive at the bladder from around the lateral aspect of the reproductive tract.

All marsupials except the potoroo (*Potorous* sp.) give birth through the median vaginal canal.[3,4] The reproductive tract of the sugar glider has been described in detail by Smith[5] and is similar to that of all marsupials, with differences primarily in sizes and relative dimensions. The ovaries lie against the medioventral side of the uterus, near the junction of the uterus and oviduct. The oviduct is convoluted with a voluminous

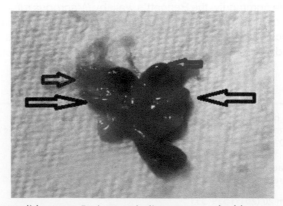

Fig. 2. Female sugar glider tract. Red arrow indicates ovary, the blue arrow indicates uterus body, and the black arrows indicate lateral vaginal canals.

funnel. Each uterus is a fusiform-shaped body that is elongated caudally into a narrow uterine neck. The necks of both uteri run parallel for about 3 mm and are ensheathed in a common tunic of connective tissue. Each uterine neck opens into the vaginal cul-de-sac of its own side at the os uteri that is situated ventrolaterally on the uterine papilla. A median septum between the right and left vaginal cul-de-sacs arises in the midline at the junction of the uterine papillae. In the sugar glider, the median canal is short and has long lateral canals. In opossums and macropods, the median canal and lateral canals are nearly equal in length. In all, the median vaginal canal from each uterus merges with the lateral vaginal canal. Posterior to the bladder, the 2 merged lateral and median vaginae and the urethra join to form the urogenital sinus, which may be long, relative to the anterior components of the system.[5]

Other unique features of the many female marsupials are marsupial bones and pouches (marsupium); however, not all have them (**Figs. 3** and **4**). The sugar glider does not have marsupial bones but does have a pouch. The short-tailed opossum has marsupial bones but no pouch and has a variable number of mammae arranged in a circle on the abdomen. The Virginia opossum has both marsupial bones and a pouch and 13 mammae; wallabies have marsupial bones and pouches with 2 pairs of mammae near the base of the pouch and can have milk with different compositions in each mammae to support joeys of different ages. In particular, the milk in the teat of a newborn wallaby is lower in fat and protein content than that of a teat used by and older joey. As the pouch young grows, the milk changes to suit the joey's needs.

As marsupial fetuses are expelled early in gestation, dystocia is virtually unknown. About 1 week before birth, the dam will fully clean the pouch, which contains a brown scaly secretion when there are no young. The fetus emerges from the urogenital opening into the cloaca fully enclosed in an amniotic sac. The fetus breaks free from the sac with its claws, usually in about 10 to 15 seconds, and then climbs from the cloacal opening up to the pouch or abdominal area and firmly attaches itself to a teat, which may take up to 5 minutes in most macropods (kangaroos and wallabies).[1] To aid the newborn joey, the dam will lick a path from the cloaca to the pouch entrance or abdominal mammae. The newly emerged joey has no visible external ears or eyes and is red in color.[6]

The dam usually has a postpartum estrus, during which breeding and fertilization occur.[2,3] If the joey currently in the pouch survives, the fertilized egg stops development in the blastocyst stage and remains unimplanted until the pouch young have either died or finished suckling and left the pouch. At this point, the blastocyst continues development, and the new joey is born in a few weeks. This phenomenon is known as fetal diapause.[3]

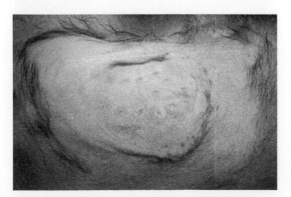

Fig. 3. Female Virginia opossum with pouch opened, exposing teats.

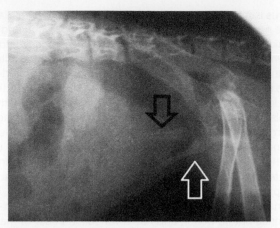

Fig. 4. Radiograph shows marsupial bones (*Black and white arrows*) in Virginia opossum.

Male Marsupials

The penis of the male is located in the ventral floor of the cloacal. It is bifid or forked, which owners often mistake for an abnormal structure or injury (**Fig. 5**). In the sugar glider, each half has a ventral groove from the base to the pointed tip.[5] The scrotum and testes are external and found proximal to the cloacal opening.[2,3] Spermatorrhea seems to be a normal condition in some marsupial males.[3] The paired testes and epididymides connect via the vasa deferentia to the prostatic portion of the urethra with a large disseminate prostate gland and one or more pairs of Cowper (bulbourethral) glands. The duct of each Cowper gland enters the urethra on the ventral surface near the crus penis. The sugar glider, has 2 pairs of multibulbed Cowper glands dorsal and lateral to the rectum.[5] The male marsupial reproductive system lacks seminal vesicles and coagulating glands. Methods for control of testicular temperatures in possums and gliders are uncertain; however, observation of male marsupials finds they may use scrotal licking and evaporative cooling to modify temperature of the scrotal pouch.[7] Male kangaroos have been observed pulling the scrotum up against the body wall in periods of high ambient temperature. Of interest, comparison between wild and captive male sugar gliders finds that captive males often have a marked

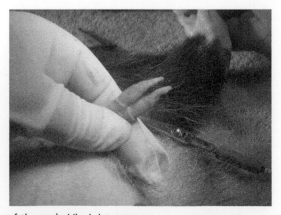

Fig. 5. Bifid penis of the male Virginia opossum.

reduction in the size of sex organs and glands.[3] Wild sugar gliders actively defend their territories, with continual hormonal stimulation. In addition, they normally urine and scent mark using secretions from the sex and cloacal glands. In captivity, the territory is small, and little territory defense or marking takes place, resulting in little stimulation of the sex organs or glands.

Both males and females possess paracloacal glands, which discharge a white, oily secretion that may be released when the animal is frightened or stressed. Secretions may also be deposited with urine and feces.[5] **Table 1** lists reproductive parameters for companion marsupial species.

REPRODUCTIVE DISORDERS

Spontaneous disease of the reproductive system in marsupials is uncommonly reported; however, the increase in numbers in the pet trade may increase overall incidence. **Table 2** lists reported reproductive disorders.

Pouch Eviction

Pouch eviction, or premature ejection of the joey, is a commonly described reproductive problem. This can occur when captive females clean the pouch excessively or become overexcited or stressed or when a yearling joey evicts the new joey. Accidental expulsions may occur secondary to stress owing to loss of tone in the wall of the pouch. If there is no pouch infection, the joey can be replaced. One technique is the use of a thin strip of surgical adhesive tape placed over the pouch entrance positioned so that the anterior and posterior lips of the pouch entrance are held together centrally.[3] The dam is then housed in a small, quiet, and dark area with minimal stimulation; ultimately she will remove the strip, but this may allow time for the problem to resolve.[3] If the joey is evicted repeatedly, another investigator suggested using 2 button sutures through the pouch that allow the dam to reach the joey and interior to clean but not fully open the pouch.[2] Continually evicted joeys may require foster care, which is challenging, depending on the stage of development.[2] Joeys without fur are particularly vulnerable to dehydration and hypothermia. Guidelines for temperatures for hand-reared joeys are unfurred, 32°C (89.6°F) with 70% humidity; and furred, 28°C (82.4°F). Moisture barrier–warmed gels or lotions (Keri Lotion; Bristol-Myers Squibb, Princeton, NJ) may help prevent dehydration of the unfurred joey.[12,13]

Pouch Infections

An infected pouch exhibits an odor, can be brown instead of the normal pink coloration, and can have a thick discharge (**Fig. 6**).[14] Various bacteria including *Pseudomonas aeruginosa* and yeasts have been cultured from infected pouches. There may also be mastitis. Diagnostics should include culture and sensitivity of the exudates.[15] Systemic antibiotics and treatment of the pouch itself should be done. The author cleans the pouch gently using cotton buds and a 2% chlorhexidine solution every 12 hours followed by a saline swabbing then drying with soft cotton until resolution. Silver sulfadiazine cream applied in the pouch has been used if no joeys are present. If young are present, as much exudate as possible should be removed without dislodging the joey using cotton buds and saline; main treatment consists of systemic antibiotics. If mastitis is present and the joey cannot nurse, it may be fostered or hand reared. Prevention of pouch infections and mastitis in breeders relies on optimal husbandry sanitation of environment and good hygiene of cage mates. In macropods, long-term use of antibiotic therapy seems to predispose development of pouch infection.[16]

Table 1
Reproductive parameters for selected marsupials

Reproductive Characteristics	Sugar Glider	Short Tailed Opossum	Virginia Opossum	Wallaby Tammar	Wallaby Bennett's
	Polyestrus Monogamous	Polygynandrous (Promiscuous)	Promiscuous	Promiscuous	Promiscuous
Sexual Maturity (mo)					
Male	12–14	4–5	6–8	24	18–24
Female	8–12			9	12–18
Breeding season	All year	All year in captivity	Seasonal-late winter through summer	Seasonal, January/February wild	Seasonal
Gestation (d)	16	14–15	12.5–13	25–28	30
Time in Pouch	70 d	No pouch	70 d	8–9 mo	7–8 mo
Birth Weight (mg)	190	100	130	460	460
Litter Size	2	4–14	Up to 21, only 13 can be suckled	1	1
Litters/y	2	Up to 5	1–3	1–2	1–2
Weaning Age	3–4 mo	3–4 wk	3 mo	28–36 wk	52 wk
Independent	17 wk	50 d	4.5–5 mo	11–12 mo	12–17 mo

Data from Refs. [1,3,8–11]

Table 2
Reproductive disorders

Species	Disorders
Captive Species (Sugar glider, short-tailed opossum, Virginia opossum, macropods-wallabies, kangaroos)	Failure-to-thrive joeys Mastitis Metritis Pouch eviction Pouch infection Vaginitis
Sugar glider	Infertility Penile mutilation/necrosis Prostatis

Short-tailed opossum	Female:
	    Endocrine alopecia caused by pituitary adenoma, prolactinemia
	    Endometritis
	    Mammary gland abscess
	    Mammary gland papillary cystadenoma
	    Ovarian cysts
	    Ovarian mineralization
	    Uterine cyst, hemorrhage, leiomyoma
	Male:
	    Accessory sex glands adenitis, cysts, hypertrophy
	    Hydrocele
	    Penile fibrosarcoma
	    Testicular atrophy, cyst, granuloma, necrosis

Virginia opossum	Cushingoid syndrome secondary to genital tract infection Endometritis Mammary carcinoma, hyperplasia Prostatitis Uterine prolapse

Macropods	Herpesvirus genitorurinary infection (infertility, lesions, ulcerations)
	Neoplasias:
	    Mammary adenocarcinoma, carcinoma
	    Ovarian stromal tumor
	    Pouch basal epithelioma
	    Sertoli cell tumor
	    Testicular seminoma

Brush-tailed phascogale, brown antechinus, dusky antechinus	Cytomegalovirus-related prostatitis

Data from Refs.[2,3,12–24]

Mastitis

Teats may be enlarged, erythemic, hardened, painful, and secreting an exudate rather than milk. The joey may also be ill or dead because of the infective exudate or starvation. A culture with sensitivity may be done from the exudate. The joey usually needs to be administered antibiotics and fostered or hand reared. Prognosis for the joey is poor if it is ill and nonfurred. The female should also be given analgesics and nonsteroidal anti-inflammatory drugs meloxicam (0.1–0.2 mg/kg subcutaneously or orally every 24 hours), and the pouch should be kept clean from the exudates by swabbing it out with saline or 2% chlorhexidine solution.

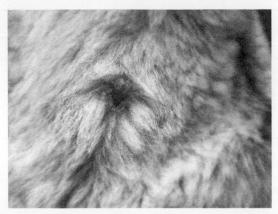

Fig. 6. Female sugar glider with brown discharge typical of a pouch infection.

Failure-to-Thrive Joeys

Pouch trauma, infection, dislodgement from a nipple, or presence of mastitis may result in development problems by the joeys. Affected joeys may need supportive care, including treatment of fluid deficits and antibiotics and be hand reared or fostered to a lactating female. Suggested fluid deficits are based those of on other mammals of similar weight. Antibiotics such as amoxicillin at 25 mg/kg orally every 12 hours have been used for sugar gliders, short-tailed opossums, and Virginia opossums. Enrofloxacin at 5 mg/kg orally every 24 hours has been used for macropods. These are extrapolated from dosages used in other mammalian species. The affected female should be treated accordingly; this often requires separation from an aggressive cage mate and improvement in the environment.

Female Reproductive Tract Infection

Ascending infections from the cloaca may cause vaginitis and metritis. There may be secondary peritonitis. The author has cultured *Staphylococcus aureus*, *Streptococcus* sp., *Escherichia coli*, and *Proteus* sp., although others are possible. The cloaca is the common opening for the digestive and urinary systems along with the reproductive tract. Infection may also result from tears made from an overly aggressive male during breeding. Along with antibiotics and analgesics, ovario-vaginal-hysterectomy may be required if medical therapy does not lead to resolution.

Species-Specific Conditions

Sugar glider

Infertility is commonly seen in certain lines of mosaic color mutations. Mosaic gliders have characteristic white patches on the body, feet or tail (https://www.google.com/?gws_rd%20=%20ssl&gws_rd=ssl#q=sugar+glider+mosaic). The trait is codominant to the standard wild-type coloration. Certainly lines of mosaics may produce sterile males.[15] The male is more likely affected. It is thought likely that it is linked to one of the genes associated with the color mutation. Infertility may also involve underlying medication conditions; obesity or inappropriate social situations may cause failure to breed in the females.

A common problem of sugar glider males is mutilation or necrosis of the penis.[15] Etiologies may include concurrent prostatitis or urinary tract infection, trauma, or self-mutilation syndrome in socially deprived or isolated captive males. Trauma may stem from aggressive cage mates, either male or female. Affected gliders present with varying degrees of necrosis, hemorrhage, and swelling. Pain may result in dysuria and bladder distention. In severe cases, septicemia and shock may result. Treatment includes supportive care and broad-spectrum antibiotics such as enrofloxacin (5 mg/kg orally every 12–24 hours) an analgesic such as buprenorphine (0.01–0.03 mg/kg subcutaneously every 12–24 hours) a nonsteroidal anti-inflammatory drug such as meloxicam (0.1–0.2 mg/kg subcutaneously or orally every 24 hours). Severe bladder distention can be temporarily addressed with cystocentesis, preferably under general anesthesia. Surgical removal of the necrotic portion of the bifid penis is performed, avoiding the urethral opening. If the entire penis is necrotic, urethrostomy may be required, which is especially difficult when tissue surrounding the urethra is inflamed. In some cases, surgery is delayed until the patient is stable and swelling is reduced. Castration seems to be preventive and indicated once the sugar glider is stabilized.

Prostatitis in intact males presents with hematuria, local pain, constipation, anorexia, and elevated rectal/cloacal temperature. Treatment includes broad-spectrum antibiotics, analgesics, anti-inflammatory medications, and supportive care.[17] Antihormonal medications such as bicalutamide (Casodex; AstraZeneca, Wilmington, DE, at 5 mg/kg orally every 24 hours) and leuprolide acetate, depot formulation (Lupron 30; Abbvie Inc, North Chicago, IL), may be useful in controlling hormonal stimulation to the prostate. Castration is recommended.

Brazilian, Laboratory, Gray, Short-Tailed Opossum (M domestica)

There are few gross and histologic lesions of the genital tract reported in *M domestica*. In females these include ovarian cyst, mineralized ovary, metritis, uterine cyst, endometritis, uterine hemorrhage, and uterine metaplasia. Mammary gland abscesses have also been found. In males, lesions include testicular atrophy, testicular granuloma, testicular cyst, edematous testicle, hydrocele, and necrotic testicle. There are also sporadic reports of adenitis, hypertrophy, or cysts in the accessory sex glands.[18]

Although uncommon, various neoplasia of the genital tract has been reported.[18] Neoplasms include uterine leiomyoma, mammary gland papillary cystadenoma, and penile fibrosarcoma. Of interest are reports of pituitary adenoma with prolactinemia.[19] These tumors are apparently similar to hemorrhagic adenomas found in Wistar rats.[19] Although noninvasive tumors are locally expansive and may compress adjacent neuroparenchyma, they stain strongly for prolactin. Affected animals present with patchy, endocrine alopecia (**Fig. 7**).[19]

Virginia Opossum (D virginiana)

Conditions reported in female Virginia opossums include uterine prolapse, endometritis, mastitis, mammary hyperplasia, and mammary adenocarcinoma.[2,20] In males, prostatitis presents with clinical signs of hematuria, local pain, constipation, anorexia, and elevated rectal/cloacal temperature.[2] Treatment includes broad-spectrum antibiotics, analgesics, anti-inflammatory medications, and supportive care. Antihormonal medications such as bicalutamide (Casodex at 5 mg/kg orally every 24 hours) and leuprolide acetate, depot formulation (Lupron 30), may be useful in controlling hormonal stimulation to the prostate. Castration is recommended.

An unusual Cushingoid syndrome secondary to genital tract infection in female Virginia opossums has been described.[21] Although clinical signs mimic true Cushing's disorder, a primary lesion in either the pituitary or adrenal glands has not been confirmed. Cases featured obese females, with a history of previous or current urinary tract infections and periodic mucoid discharge from the genitourinary opening. Affected animals have had previous trauma altering normal urinary patterns; they

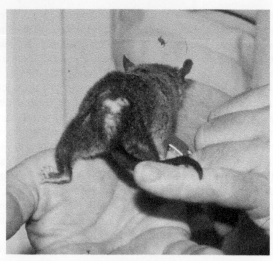

Fig. 7. Endocrine alopecia in a short-tailed opossum.

may have held urine longer than normal or incompletely evacuated the bladder. Clinical presentation included brown discoloration of the fur and slight thinning to full alopecia. All seemed to be slightly to moderately depressed and had variable anorexia and pelvic limb weakness. Many had neutrophilia with elevated left shift, and some were anemic. Urinalysis found high bacterial loads (various coliforms, *Staphylococcus* sp.), and antibiotics were selected based on culture and sensitivity results. Amoxicillin at 20 mg/kg orally every 12 hours and trimethoprim sulfa at 10 to 20 mg/kg every 12 to 24 hours are the most commonly used. Many animals responded to therapy but relapsed once antibiotics were discontinued. It was postulated that urinary tract infection can lead to metritis or vice versa. Treatment was complete ovario-vaginal-hysterectomy including the lateral canals. If the vaginal canals are left, they may continue to serve as a nidus to infection. Surgery was curative.[1,21]

Macropods: Tammar Wallaby (M eugenii); Bennett's Wallaby (M rufogriseus)

A herpesvirus has been linked with transient infertility, ulcerations, and lesions in the genitourinary area of Tammar wallabies living on Kangaroo Island, South Australia. Diagnosis was via serology and histopathology. There were no mortalities. Herpesviruses may also cause ocular/nasal discharge, lingual ulcers, depression, anorexia, and death in other wallaby species.[22] A Sertoli cell tumor was reported in an aged red kangaroo.[2] Neoplasias of the reproductive tract have been documented in several species of macropod and include ovarian stromal tumor, pouch basal cell epithelioma, mammary carcinoma with pulmonary and renal metastases, and testicular seminoma.[16]

Although bacterial diseases of the reproductive tract of macropods are poorly documented, antibiotics described for use in macropods include oxytetracycline (long acting, 20 mg/kg intramuscularly every 72 hours), clindamycin (unpalatable, 11 mg/kg orally every 12 hours), metronidazole (use benzoate for palatability, 20 mg/kg orally every 12 hours), enrofloxacin (5 mg/kg subcutaneously, 1 injection or orally every 24 hours), ceftiofur sodium (1–2 mg/kg intramuscularly or intravenously every 24 hours), gentamycin plus amoxicillin (4–7 mg/kg intramuscularly every 12 hours plus 10 mg/kg intramuscularly every 8 hours, respectively), and procaine penicillin/benzathine penicillin G (30 mg/kg intramuscularly every 48 hours).[16]

Other Marsupials

A cytomegalovirus-related prostatitis was reported in Australian dasyurid marsupials, *Phascogale tapoatafa* (brush-tailed phascogale), *Antechinus stuartii* (brown antechinus), and *Antechinus swainsonii* (dusky antechinus).[23,24] Lesions were most common in mature animals during breeding, times of stress, or in animals treated with high levels of corticosteroids. Venereal transmission was postulated. Affected dusky antechinus males succumbed and often died 2 to 3 weeks after breeding.

SURGERY OF THE REPRODUCTIVE TRACT OF MARSUPIALS

Anesthetic techniques are described elsewhere but should include premedication (an opioid and a sedative such as midazolam at minimum) and induction and maintenance with inhalant agents. Testicular and incisional blocks are easy to perform; the authors use 2 mg/kg each lidocaine and bupivacaine combined into a single syringe. In many cases, drugs must be diluted for accurate dosing in small patients (**Figs. 8** and **9B**).

Marsupial Castration

Castration is performed to reduce the natural odors of some species, in particular the sugar glider, to reduce social tension and for birth control.

Castration can be performed scrotally or prescrotally along the scrotal stalk. This distinction is often referred to by sugar glider breeders or enthusiasts as *pom on* or *pom off*, and some appear to have a preconceived preference for one technique over the other. However, in the authors' experience, both techniques are equally suitable for all marsupials if performed correctly.

For the prescrotal technique, an incision is made in the stalk midway between the scrotum and the abdominal wall. The spermatic cord is easily separated from the skin, clamped, ligated close to the body wall, and transected. The entire scrotal sac including the testes is removed. Subcuticular sutures can be used to close the incision. Alternatively, a radiosurgical unit or surgical laser can be used to simply ligate the stalk.

One author has seen opening of the suture site when the incision is made too close to the abdominal wall, possible caused by retraction of the remaining cremaster muscle.

For the scrotal technique, a single incision can be made into the scrotal sac and both testicles isolated and the spermatic cord ligated with suture or hemostatic slips. In sugar gliders, a single small hemostatic clip can be placed over the spermatic cords of both testes. The incision is then manually sealed without glue or suture (**Fig. 9**).

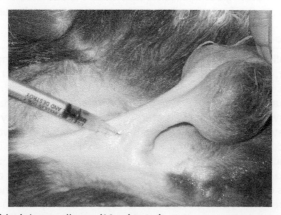

Fig. 8. Incisional block in a wallaroo (*M robustus*).

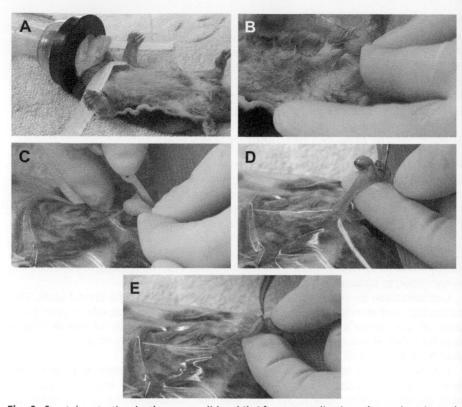

Fig. 9. Scrotal castration in the sugar glider. (*A*) After premedication, the patient is mask induced and placed in dorsal recumbency. (*B*) Lidocaine/bupivacaine testicular block is administered. (*C*) Note the use of transparent drapes to allow direct visual monitoring of the patient. A single incision is made into the scrotal sac. (*D*) Both testicles and spermatic ducts and vessels are isolated. (*E*) A single small hemostatic clip is used to ligate both. After ligation, the incision is opposed without suture or glue.

Techniques to prevent post castration mutilation include careful aseptic surgical technique, minimal use of sutures, clips or glue, and multimodal analgesia.[15,17,25,26]

Marsupial Ovario-Hysterectomy and Ovario-Vaginal-Hysterectomy

There are no confirmed health benefits associated with elective altering of female marsupials; however, the procedure may be performed therapeutically or for birth control in mixed groups.

As mentioned above, in females, most of the genital tract can be removed, but this is complicated by the position of the ureters. In obese animals, it may not be possible to isolate the ureters. If the ureters cannot be clearly isolated, the ovaries and uterus can be removed, leaving the central and lateral vaginal canals. In marsupials with pouches, the incision is made midline through the inner wall of the pouch. The mammae should be avoided. Ovarian vessels should be ligated and each ovary lifted. The uterus can be clamped as a pedicle at the junction with the vaginal canals if these will not be removed. The uterus is then ligated at the junction with the vaginal canals using a pedicle ligation. If the ureters can be isolated, then the vagina is clamped just proximally to where the bladder empties into the urogenital sinus. Careful blunt dissection is necessary to avoid tearing the ureters (**Fig. 10**). The abdominal incision should be closed, as in other mammals. Subcuticular sutures may prevent disruption of the suture line. Postoperative analgesics are indicated, as in other species.[1,15,17]

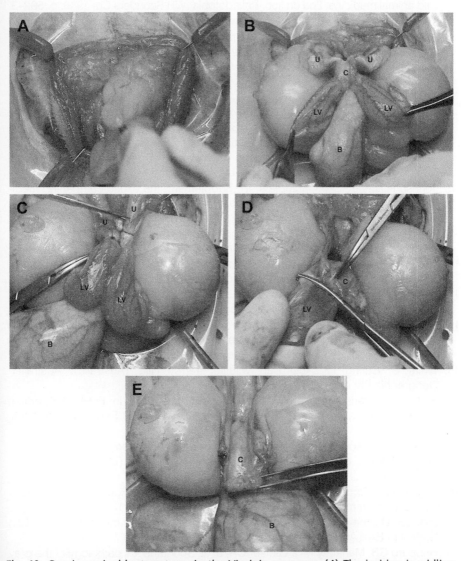

Fig. 10. Ovario-vaginal-hysterectomy in the Virginia opossum. (*A*) The incision is midline, directly into the skin of the pouch. In most patients, there is ample abdominal fat. (*B*) Surgical appearance of the reproductive tract. Note the bladder (*B*), the uterus (U) and the lateral vaginas (LV). The central vaginal canal (C) contains the openings of the ureters. (*C*) Ligation of both uterine horns (U). (*D*) Clamping for transection of the right lateral vagina (LV). (*E*) Finished procedure with removal of both uterine horns and lateral vaginas, leaving the central vaginal canal (C).

REFERENCES

1. Johnson-Delaney CA. Reproductive medicine of companion marsupials. Vet Clin North Am Exot Anim Pract 2002;5:537–53.
2. Wallach JD, Boever WJ. Diseases of exotic animals. Medical and surgical management. Philadelphia: WB Saunders Co; 1983.
3. Finnie EP. Reproduction. Monotremes and marsupials. In: Fowler ME, editor. Zoo & wild animal medicine. 2nd edition. Philadelphia: WB Saunders Co; 1986. p. 592–3.
4. Finnie EP. Anatomy. Monotremes and marsupials. In: Fowler ME, editor. Zoo & wild animal medicine. 2nd edition. Philadelphia: WB Saunders Co; 1986. p. 558–60.
5. Smith MJ. The reproductive system and paracloacal glands of *Petaurus breviceps* and *Gymnobelideus leadbeateri* (Marsupialia: Petauridae). In: Smith A, Hume I, editors. Possums and gliders. Chipping Norton (Australia): Surrey Beatty & Sons PtyLtd; 1996. p. 321–30.
6. Williams A, Williams R. Caring for kangaroos and wallabies. East Roseville (Australia): Kangaroo Press/Simon & Schuster Australia Pty. Ltd; 1999.
7. Temple-Smith PD. Reproductive structures and strategies in male possums and gliders. In: Smith A, Hume I, editors. Possums and gliders. Chipping Norton (Australia): Surrey Beatty & Sons Pty. Ltd.; 1996. p. 89–106.
8. Johnson-Delaney CA. Marsupials. In: Supplement, the exotic companion medicine handbook for veterinarians. Lake Worth (FL): ZEN Publishing (previously Wingers Publishing); 1997. p. 1–52.
9. Johnson R, Hemsley S. Gliders and possums. In: Vogelnest L, Woods R, editors. Medicine of Australian mammals. Collingswood (NJ): CSIRO; 2008. p. 395–427.
10. Fadem BH, Trupin GL, Maliniak E, et al. Care and breeding of the gray, short-tailed opossum (Monodelphis domestica). Lab Anim Sci 1982;32:405–9.
11. Kraus DB, Faden BH. Reproduction, development and physiology of the gray short-tailed opossum (Monodelphis domestica). Lab Anim Sci 1987;37:478–82.
12. George H. The care and handling of orphaned kangaroos. In: Hand SJ, editor. Care and handling of Australian native animals. Emergency care and captive management. Chipping Norton (Australia): Surrey Beatty & Sons Pty. Ltd; 1990. p. 123–41.
13. White S. Caring for Australian wildlife. Terrey Hills (Australia): Australian Geographic Pty Ltd; 1997.
14. Butler R. Bacterial diseases. Monotremes and marsupials. In: Fowler ME, editor. Zoo &wild animal medicine. 2nd edition. Philadelphia: WB Saunders Co; 1986. p. 572–6.
15. Ness RD, Johnson-Delaney CA. Sugar gliders. In: Quesenberry KE, Carpenter JW, editors. Ferrets, rabbits, and rodents. 3rd edition. St Louis (MO): Elsevier; 2012. p. 393–410.
16. Vogelnest L, Portas T. Macropods. In: Vogelnest L, Woods R, editors. Medicine of Australian mammals. Collingswood (NJ): CSIRO; 2008. p. 133–225.
17. Johnson-Delaney CA. Therapeutics of companion exotic marsupials. Vet Clin North Am Exot Anim Pract 2000;3:173–81.
18. Hubbard GB, Mahaney MC, Gleiser CA, et al. Spontaneous pathology of the gray shorttailed opossum (*Monodelphis domestica*). Lab Anim Sci 1997;47:19–26.
19. Kuehl-Kovarik MC, Ackermann MR, Hanson DL, et al. Spontaneous pituitary adenomas in the Brazilian gray short-tailed opossum (*Monodelphis domestica*). Vet Pathol 1994;31:377–9.
20. Gupta BN, Feldman DB. Carcinosarcoma in an opossum. J Am Vet Med Assoc 1973;163:586–8.

21. Henness AM. Cushingoid syndrome secondary to genital tract infection in the female opossum (D. virginiana). Possum Tales 1994;8(1–2):9–11.
22. Finnie EP. Viral diseases. Monotremes and marsupials. In: Fowler ME, editor. Zoo & wild animal medicine. 2nd edition. Philadelphia: WB Saunders Co; 1986. p. 576–7.
23. Barker IK, Carbonell PL, Bradley AJ. Cytomegalovirus infection of the prostate in the dasyurid marsupials, *Phascogale tapoatafa* and *Antechinus stuartii*. J Wildl Dis 1981;17:433–41.
24. Munday BL, Obendorf DL. Cytomegalic lesions in Australian marsupials. J Wildl Dis 1983;19:132–5.
25. Johnson SD. Orchiectomy of the mature sugar glider. Exot Pet Pract 1997;2:71.
26. Morges MA, Grant KR, MacPhail C, et al. A novel technique for orchiectomy and scrotal ablation in the sugar glider (PETAURUS BREVICEPS. J Zoo Wildl Med 2009;40:204–6.

Disorders of the Reproductive Tract of Rabbits

Frances Margaret Harcourt-Brown, BVSc, FRCVS

KEYWORDS

- Rabbit • Behavior • Reproduction • Reproductive disorders • Neutering

KEY POINTS

- The reproductive problems of rabbits kept for meat or fur production are different from those that are kept as pets.
- Knowledge of the normal anatomy of the reproductive tract is essential in the recognition and treatment of abnormalities.
- Pet rabbits that are not neutered suffer from a range of age-related conditions of the reproductive tract.
- Abdominal palpation and examination of the external genitalia are important parts of clinical examination.
- Although neutering is an important part of treatment, complications can arise from transecting the vagina.

INTRODUCTION

There is a difference in the reproductive problems of rabbits that are farmed for their meat or fur and those that are kept as pets (**Box 1**). A doe on a large-scale breeding farm has no individual value. She may be classified as 'old' after 14 litters, that is, when she is 2 to 3 years old and will be culled, rather than treated, if there are health or reproductive problems. In contrast, pet rabbits can live for up to 15 years and are not considered to be old until they are more than 8 years of age and individual health problems are investigated and treated.

Although there is a wealth of information from the rabbit farming industry about reproductive physiology and how to increase breeding performance, there is little information about reproductive disorders. Most information is obtained from surveys of health records or postmortem examination.[1,2] In contrast with breeding rabbits, there is plenty of information about reproductive diseases in pet rabbits. Basic reproductive data are listed in **Box 2**.

The author has nothing to disclose.
Crab Lane Vets, 30 Crab Lane, Bilton, Harrogate, North Yorkshire HG1 3BE, UK
E-mail address: frances@harcourt-brown.co.uk

Vet Clin Exot Anim 20 (2017) 555–587
http://dx.doi.org/10.1016/j.cvex.2016.11.010
1094-9194/17/Crown Copyright © 2016 Published by Elsevier Inc. All rights reserved.

Box 1
Reproductive disorders recorded in female rabbits

Breeding rabbits (disorders found during postmortem examination at the slaughterhouse[1] or on farm[2]).

Percentages are of total number of rabbits (with or without reproductive disorders) that were examined.

In these surveys, no abnormalities of the reproductive tract of males were reported. This was probably because the external genitalia were not examined during postmortem examination. Skin disorders affecting the genital orifice, such as Treponema cuniculi, were not reported either.

Extrauterine pregnancy (0.1%)

Mastitis (5%)

Mummified fetuses (<1%)

Metritis (2.6%)

Pyometra (6.5%)

Pregnancy toxemia (5%)

Uterine torsion in last week of pregnancy (7%)

Vaginal prolapse (4%)

Reproductive disorders of pet rabbits (disorders found during routine ovariohysterectomy, exploratory laparotomy or occasionally postmortem examination[17,20,21]):

Uterine adenocarcinoma (45%–49%)

Other uterine tumors (20%)

Endometrial hyperplasia (22%–40%)

Hydrometra or mucometra (12%)

Pyometra (2%)

Ovarian tumors (2%–7%)

Mammary gland tumors (7%)

Percentages are of rabbits with confirmed uterine disease

Comparison of these tables shows that uterine diseases that are most common in breeding does (pyometra, metritis, uterine torsion) are rare in pet rabbits whereas uterine conditions that are commonly diagnosed in pet rabbits (endometrial hyperplasia, uterine tumors) are not recorded in breeding does.

ANATOMY OF THE REPRODUCTIVE TRACT

Important clinical features of the female and male reproductive tracts are listed in **Box 3**.

Female Reproductive Tract

Both ovaries lie in the dorsal abdomen, close to the kidneys. They are elongated elliptical structures that, in a sexually mature female, contain multiple follicles at varying stages of development (**Fig. 1**). Each long uterine tube (Fallopian tube or oviduct) opens into a convoluted uterine horn that ends in a cervix. The term 'uterus duplex' is used to describe the uterus because the right and left uterine horns are separate structures and are, therefore, separate uteri. Some texts refer to the horns as the right

Box 2
Reproductive data
Descent of testicles through inguinal canal: Approximately 6 days
Descent of testicles into tunica vaginalis: Approximately 22 days
Descent of testicles into scrotum: 8 to 12 weeks
Age of puberty—male: 4 to 5 months
Age of puberty—female: 4 to 5 months

Age to neuter:
    From 3 months in males
    From 5 months in females (after puberty)

Interval between castration and infertility: up to 4 weeks
Gestation: 30 to 32 days

Pregnancy diagnosis:
    After 10 to 12 days by abdominal palpation
    After 11 days radiologically

Litter size: 4 to 10
Number of nipples: 8

and left uterus. There is no uterine body and the cervices from each uterine horn are attached to form a bicornuate cervix that separates the uterus from the vagina. The vagina is a long, flaccid structure that lies between the bladder and rectum with the ureters in close proximity. The urethra lies ventral to the vagina and opens into a large orifice in the vaginal floor about one-half way along its length. The orifice is at the level of the center of the pubic symphysis.[3] The part of the vagina that is distal to the urethral opening is sometimes called the urogenital sinus. It is attached to supporting musculature that can constrict and move the vagina and vulva during urination, mating, and parturition. The urogenital sinus opens into the vulva.

Mammary Glands

The mammary glands are distributed along the ventrolateral aspect of the abdomen and extend into the thoracic and inguinal regions. There are usually 8 nipples.

Placenta

The placenta of rabbits is discoid so maternofetal exchange takes place over a roughly circular area of the chorionic sac. It is hemodichorial, that is, there a direct connection between the chorion and maternal blood with 2 trophoblast layers.[4]

Male Reproductive Tract

The male reproductive tract is illustrated in **Fig. 2**. The sexually mature male has 2 external testicles that lie on either side of the penis in 2 relatively hairless scrotal sacs. The scrotal skin is thin and the caudal section of the epididymis can be seen through the thin skin of the scrotum at the caudal end of the scrotal sac where the epididymis is attached to the inner layer of the tunica vaginalis. The testicles enlarge with age and sexual maturity. The vas deferens and spermatic cord pass through the inguinal canal to the abdomen (**Fig. 3**). In the abdomen, the vas deferens loops over the ureter and enters an ejaculatory duct in the floor of the vesicular gland, which is located on the dorsal surface of the urethra at neck of the urinary bladder. The

> **Box 3**
> **Clinically important anatomic features of the reproductive tract**
>
> *The female reproductive tract*
>
> - The uterine tube (Fallopian tube, oviduct) is long, convoluted, and red. It could be mistaken for a blood vessel during ovariohysterectomy.
> - Two complete uteri are present in the rabbit (uterus duplex). Two uterovaginal canals are present, with no uterine body.
> - The vagina has an abundance of smooth muscle[3] and contractions of the vagina occur readily. They may be seen during ovariohysterectomy. These are normal.
> - The urethra opens into the vagina.
> - The vagina distends and fills with urine during micturition. This is normal but is an important consideration during ovariohysterectomy. If the vagina is transected, it is vital that the repair prevents leakage of urine into the abdomen, which can cause localized peritonitis and adhesion formation.
>
> *The male reproductive tract*
>
> - In rabbits (and rodents) the inguinal canal does not constrict after the testicle has descended into the scrotum. This allows abdominal contents to herniate through the inguinal ring after castration unless it is closed.
> - The cremaster muscle is well-developed in rabbits. This muscle is an extension of the internal oblique abdominal muscle that passes through the inguinal canal and attaches to the tunica vaginalis to enclose the testicle. The function of the cremaster is to retract the testicle from the scrotum. This happens readily.
> - The tunica vaginalis has a long (2 cm) tubular section between the inguinal ring and the cranial end of the testicle. Retracted testicles lie in this section and can be pulled into the scrotum during surgery.
> - The tunica vaginalis is a pouch of peritoneum that encloses the testicles and the spermatic cord. Placing a ligature around the tubular section of the vas deferens during castration seals the pouch and prevents herniation of the abdominal contents.
> - In the urethra, the opening into the vesicular gland is large enough to be inadvertently catheterized during catheterization of the urinary bladder.[5]

ejaculatory duct communicates with the dorsal urethra through an orifice close to the neck of the bladder. There is a clefted protuberance at this orifice (the colliculus seminalis) that controls the release of semen into the urethra. The other accessory glands are the proprostate, prostate, paraprostates, and bulbourethral glands. These glands lie at the neck of the bladder, deep within the pelvic cavity (see **Fig. 2**). They are not palpable and cannot be visualized surgically without splitting the pubic symphysis.[5]

Scent Glands

In both sexes, there are many scent glands associated with the reproductive tract that consist of:

- *Anal glands* that lie immediately adjacent to the lateral rectal wall.
- *Inguinal glands* situated deep in 2 pouches that are lateral to the cleft between the anus and either the vaginal or preputial opening. Each inguinal gland consists of a superficial, pale-colored spherical lobe an adjacent, deeper lying, dark

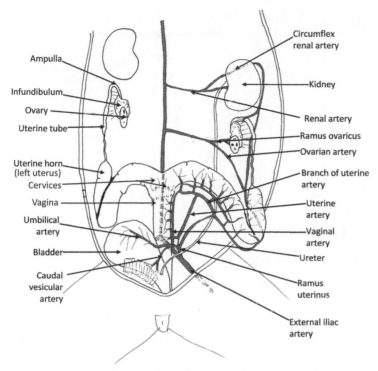

Fig. 1. Female reproductive tract. Ventral view of the female reproductive tract shows its arterial blood supply and the relationship with the bladder. (*Courtesy of* Frances Harcourt-Brown, BVSc, FRCVS, Harrogate, United Kingdom.)

brown lobe. The inguinal gland opens into the inguinal pouch through a pore that is found deep within the pouch.

- *Preputial glands* contain a whitish secretion. In the female these tiny glands form a necklacelike ring embedded in the vulval labia.[3]

REPRODUCTION IN RABBITS

Rabbits are well-known for their ability to reproduce quickly. The gestation period is 30 to 32 days and the average litter size is 4 to 10 (**Fig. 4**). Females are able to conceive within hours of giving birth so they can be lactating while they are pregnant. This means it is possible for a single female to give birth to more than 60 offspring each year. The rate of reproduction depends on the way the rabbit lives. Wild rabbits have a period of reproductive inactivity in the winter when the gonads in both males and females regress.[6] Rabbits in captivity breed all year round. In some systems of intensive production of meat rabbits, the young are weaned at 28 days and the mother gives birth to the next litter 3 days later.[7] This happens for the duration of the rabbit's adult life. Exhibition rabbits tend to have 2 to 3 litters a year and pet rabbits usually have none at all.

Ovulation and Sexual Receptivity

Rabbits are induced ovulators with no defined estrous cycle, although a cyclic rhythm in sexual receptivity exists. Mating stimulates ovulation approximately 10 hours post

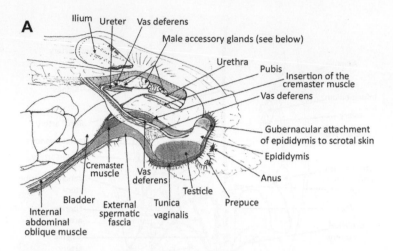

Male accessory glands

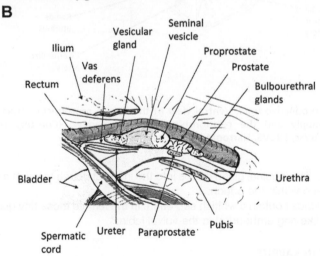

Fig. 2. Male reproductive tract. (*A*) Left lateral view of the male reproductive tract shows the course of the vas deferens and the relationship of the accessory glands with the urethra. (*B*). The male accessory glands are show in greater detail. (*Courtesy of* Frances Harcourt-Brown, BVSc, FRCVS, Harrogate, United Kingdom.)

coitus. Follicular development occurs in waves, with 5 to 10 follicles on each ovary at any one time. When the follicles reach maturity, they produce estrogens for about 12 to 14 days; if ovulation has not occurred during this period, the follicles then degenerate with a corresponding reduction in estrogen level and sexual receptivity. After 4 to 7 days, a new wave of follicles develops and the doe becomes receptive again. This means the doe has a cycle of 16 to 18 days with about 12 to 14 days of receptivity followed by a period of nonreceptivity for 2 to 4 days.[8] The appearance of the vulva alters according to the state of sexual receptivity. When the doe is nonreceptive, the vulva is pale pink and dry. During receptivity, the vulva becomes swollen, moist, and red, becoming darker until it is purple at the end of the receptive period (**Fig. 5**). If the doe is mated, the vulva returns to a light pink color in about 24 hours.

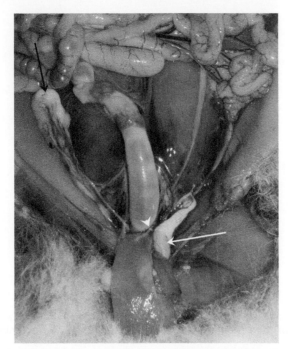

Fig. 3. Abdominal and descending testicle. This post mortem image of a young male wild rabbit shows the position of the testicles during the descent into the scrotum. The right testicle is in the abdomen (*black arrow*) and the left testicle (*white arrow*) in the inguinal canal. Note the relationship of the vas deferens with the ureter (*arrowhead*). Exteriorizing the bladder to reveal the ureters is often the easiest way to locate an abdominal testicle during exploratory surgery. (*Courtesy of* Frances Harcourt-Brown, BVSc, FRCVS, Harrogate, United Kingdom.)

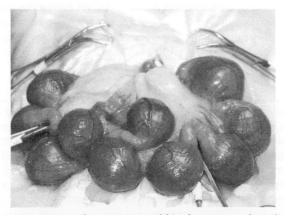

Fig. 4. Pregnant uterus. Uterus of a pregnant rabbit that was undergoing ovariohysterectomy. The length of gestation was about 12 to 14 days. Pregnancy diagnosis by abdominal palpation is easy in rabbits. The uterus is palpable in the caudoventral abdomen. (*Courtesy of* Frances Harcourt-Brown, BVSc, FRCVS, Harrogate, United Kingdom.)

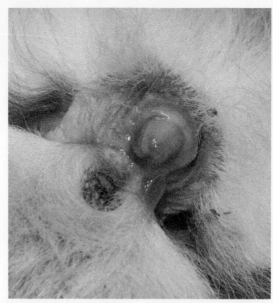

Fig. 5. Vulva of sexually receptive female. Color of the vulva in a sexually receptive female rabbit. (*Courtesy of* Frances Harcourt-Brown, BVSc, FRCVS, Harrogate, United Kingdom.)

Female rabbits become sexually receptive as soon as they have given birth but receptivity declines during lactation until after the young are weaned approximately 21 days later.[9]

Artificial Insemination

Artificial insemination is used in farmed rabbits, where a high reproductive rate increases profits but overheads are kept to a minimum. It allows a large number of does to be inseminated at 1 time regardless of their receptivity. Litters can be born in batches, which allows them to grow up together. Once a batch has gone for slaughter, the housing can be cleaned and disinfected before the next batch moves in. Because ovulation is induced by gonadotrophin-releasing hormone, synthetic analogues are given at the time of insemination, either by injection or by inclusion in the semen.[10] It is possible to inseminate 100 does per day with a 70% to 80% conception rate. This means 500 to 700 rabbits will be born within 2 days.[7]

Gestation

Some does remain sexually receptive during pregnancy and may continue to be mated by a male companion. Rarely, it leads to superfetation, which is the simultaneous occurrence of more than 1 stage of developing offspring in the same animal. During late pregnancy, the doe may be seen carrying bedding material into her chosen nesting site. Mammary gland development takes place in late pregnancy when the doe starts to prepare her nest by filling it with hay or other material before lining it with fur pulled from the hip, dewlap, and mammary glands (**Fig. 6**).

Parturition and Lactation

Parturition usually takes place in the morning. It is rapid with all the fetuses expelled in less than 30 minutes. The babies are born blind, without hair and helpless. After giving

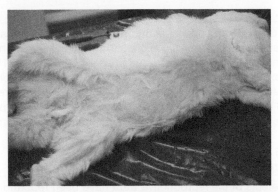

Fig. 6. Pulling hair out to make a nest. During late pregnancy and during pseudopregnancy, female rabbits will pull out the hair from the ventral abdomen and inner thighs to line their nest with. This also exposes the mammary glands and nipples for the young rabbits to suckle from. (*Courtesy of* Frances Harcourt-Brown, BVSc, FRCVS, Harrogate, United Kingdom.)

birth, maternal behavior is minimal and the babies are left alone in the nest for most of the time. The doe only returns to the nest for less than 10 minutes once or occasionally twice a day to feed them. In the absence of pregnancy, lactation takes place for approximately 5 weeks after parturition. If the rabbit is mated soon after birth, she is continually lactating.

Maternal Aggression

In the wild, finding a good place to dig a burrow to make a nest is an important factor in the survival of baby rabbits and females will fight over nesting sites.[11] Although nests may be predated, competing breeding females may also kill entire litters within the first 10 weeks of life. During late pregnancy and early lactation, female rabbits can become very aggressive as they protect their nesting site. In pet rabbits, this is often their cage or hutch and they may attack humans that handle them. The doe is particularly susceptible to disturbance in the first few days after parturition and may mutilate or even cannibalize the young if she is upset. The legs or ears may be bitten, or even removed (**Fig. 7**).

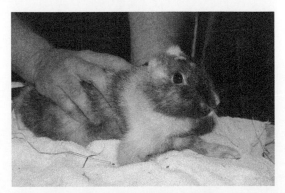

Fig. 7. Mutilated young rabbit. This young rabbit has no pinnae and is missing a foreleg. It was born in a breeding establishment where the conditions were bad. No nest boxes were provided so the does were stressed when they gave birth. The mother caused the injuries. This rabbit was one of many mutilated rabbits that were on the farm. (*Courtesy of* Frances Harcourt-Brown, BVSc, FRCVS, Harrogate, United Kingdom.)

Pseudopregnancy

Although the act of courtship, mounting, and mating stimulates ovulation, it may also take place in the absence of tactile stimuli. Visual contact, olfactory and auditory stimulation can also induce ovulation[12] and result in pseudopregnancy. This can be stimulated by the proximity of other rabbits or by the act of being mounted by another female or neutered male. Pseudopregnancy is shorter than true pregnancy, lasting approximately 16 to 18 days. During this period, the doe may show many of the signs of late pregnancy, such as aggression, fur pulling, and mammary gland development.

DISEASES OF THE FEMALE REPRODUCTIVE TRACT
Congenital Abnormalities

Developmental defects of the reproductive tract have been reported. These include:

- *Hermaphrodism*: a hermaphrodite wild rabbit has been described.[13]
- *Aplasia* of parts of the uterus (**Fig. 8**).[14,15]
- *Endometrial venous aneurysm* (**Fig. 9**)[16,17]: multiple blood-filled varices occur in the endometrium of some rabbits. These thin-walled blood vessels can rupture into the uterine lumen and cause intermittent hematuria or even fatal hemorrhage. They are considered to be a congenital defect.[17]

Ovarian Tumors

Ovarian tumors can occur in rabbits and are often "silent." The tumors may be incidental findings during ovariohysterectomy and can be seen in association with uterine adenocarcinoma. Clinical signs are often associated with hormonal imbalances or

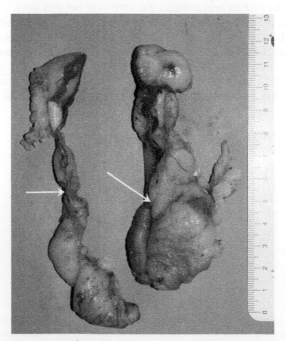

Fig. 8. Uterine aplasia. Uterus of a rabbit that was removed during routine ovariohysterectomy. There is segmental uterine dysplasia where parts of the uterus have failed to develop (*arrows*). (*Courtesy of* Frances Harcourt-Brown, BVSc, FRCVS, Harrogate, United Kingdom.)

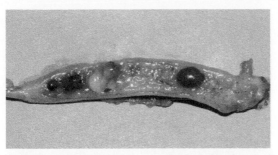

Fig. 9. Endometrial venous aneurysm. Internal surface of the uterus of a rabbit that was presented shocked and bleeding from the vulva. The rabbit died during ovariohysterectomy. There was a large blood clot in the other horn and evidence of multiple endometrial aneurysms in both uterine horns (right and left uteri). Cystic endometrial hyperplasia is also present. (*Courtesy of* Frances Harcourt-Brown, BVSc, FRCVS, Harrogate, United Kingdom.)

metastases to other sites. Several types of ovarian tumors occur ranging from benign luteoma (**Fig. 10**) to ovarian granulosa cell tumors and malignant adenocarcinomas.[18]

Endometrial Hyperplasia

Endometrial hyperplasia is characterized by thickening of the endometrium, cystic development of mucus-filled glands, and accumulation of mucus in the lumen of the uterus (**Fig. 11**). It is believed to result from prolonged estrogenic and progesteronic stimulation.[19] It usually occurs in rabbits greater than 3 years of age, although it has been reported in younger rabbits.[18] Although the uterus is thickened and may be palpable during clinical examination, most cases are asymptomatic and the condition is discovered as an incidental finding during ovariohysterectomy. A serosanguinous discharge may be noticed by observant owners. It is not clear if there is an association between endometrial hyperplasia and uterine adenocarcinomas.

Uterine Tumors

Uterine adenocarcinoma is the most common neoplasm encountered in rabbits, although it is not recorded in postmortem surveys of does that are used for intensive

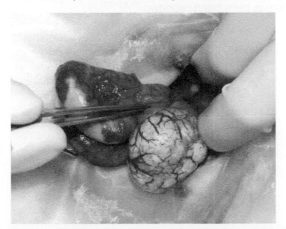

Fig. 10. Ovarian luteoma. An ovarian tumor that was removed during ovariohysterectomy. There is also necrosis of the uterine wall. The rabbit was undergoing surgery because of her aggressive and agitated behavior. Recovery was uneventful. (*Courtesy of* Frances Harcourt-Brown, BVSc, FRCVS, Harrogate, United Kingdom.)

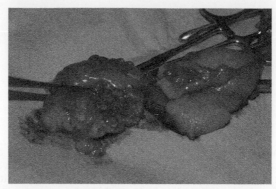

Fig. 11. Cystic endometrial hyperplasia. The internal surface of the uterus of a 4-year-old rabbit that was undergoing ovariohysterectomy because a palpably enlarged, sausage-shaped uterus was detected during clinical examination. (*Courtesy of* Frances Harcourt-Brown, BVSc, FRCVS, Harrogate, United Kingdom.)

meat production. A survey of 849 nonbreeding female laboratory rabbits revealed that 4.2% had uterine tumors by 3 years of age and 75% had uterine tumors by the time they were 7 years old. The tumors were detected by abdominal palpation and confirmed by biopsy or autopsy.[20] This incidence is reflected in the pet rabbit population where the tumors are often discovered during routine neutering. Uterine adenocarcinomas are often multicentric and can involve both horns of the uterus, appearing as globular polypoid structures that project into the uterus (**Fig. 12**). As the condition advances, the tumors enlarge and coalesce so that large portions of the uterus are affected and they become progressively more palpable. They may contain large areas of hemorrhage, necrosis, or calcification. Metastasis is slow and occurs via local spread into the peritoneum and other abdominal organs, such as the liver, or by hematogenous spread to distant sites, such as the lung, brain, skin, or bones (**Figs. 13** and **14**). Not all uterine tumors are adenocarcinomas. Malignant mixed Mullerian tumor,[21] carcinosarcoma, adenoma, metastasis from ovarian tumors, leiomyoma, and leiomyosarcomas have been reported.[18,21-23]

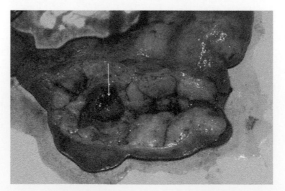

Fig. 12. Uterine adenocarcinoma. Typical appearance of a uterine adenocarcinoma. There are multicentric enlargements of the uterine wall. The internal surface is ulcerated and bleeding. There is a large blood clot over a necrotic area of tumor (*arrow*). (*Courtesy of* Frances Harcourt-Brown, BVSc, FRCVS, Harrogate, United Kingdom.)

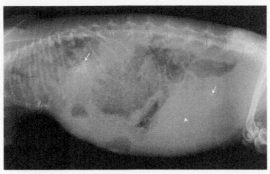

Fig. 13. Radiograph of rabbit with a metastasized tumor. Lateral radiograph of a rabbit that was presented with dyspnea. A large mass can be seen in the ventral abdomen (*arrowhead*). The nipples are prominent. There is calcification in the area of the mass and the liver (*arrow*). Metastases are evident in the lungs. (*Courtesy of* Frances Harcourt-Brown, BVSc, FRCVS, Harrogate, United Kingdom.)

Hydrometra and Mucometra

Hydrometra is defined as the accumulation of watery fluid in the uterus. The fluid is mucoid in the case of mucometra. These conditions are encountered occasionally in rabbits[24,25] and the etiology is not understood. Clinically, abdominal distension is

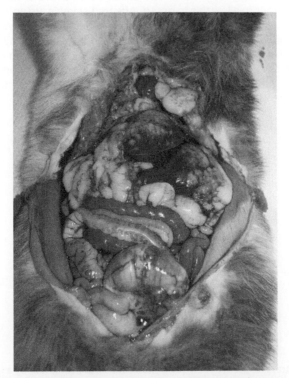

Fig. 14. Postmortem examination of a rabbit with a metastasized tumor. Postmortem picture of a rabbit that was presented dying. There was blood in the abdominal cavity. There is a large uterine tumor and metastasized tumors in the liver and lungs. (*Courtesy of* Frances Harcourt-Brown, BVSc, FRCVS, Harrogate, United Kingdom.)

the most striking feature. Surgically, the size and weight of the uterus can be impressive (**Fig. 15**). The uterus can make up one-quarter of the rabbit's body weight.[26] It is easily detected on ultrasound examination.

Pyometra

Pyometra can occur in pet rabbits, but is more common in breeding does from colonies of rabbits than in animals kept as pets. Pyometra has been cited as a manifestation of pasteurellosis.[17] It may be seen in association with other suppurative infections in the genital tract, such as in the ovary, uterine tube, or uterine wall (see **Fig. 10**). Abscesses may be present. Affected rabbits are lethargic and inappetant, with a purulent vaginal discharge, abdominal distension, and a palpable abdominal mass. Abdominal palpation can rupture the uterus. Ultrasound examination is indicated for these cases. Surgery is the only option, but can be difficult owing to the risk of rupturing the uterus and the difficulty in breaking down any adhesions to adjacent organs.

Vaginal Prolapse and/or Bladder Eversion

Although it is rare, vaginal prolapse can occur in rabbits.[27,28] It is usually seen within a few days of giving birth, although there is a report of the condition in 8 closely related females, suggesting a genetic predisposition.[27] There are also reports of bladder eversion and prolapse through the urethra. The orifice between the urethra and vagina is large enough in rabbits to allow this to occur. Affected animals are anorexic and straining with a soft tissue mass protruding from the vulva. Surgery is always indicated even for vaginal prolapse. Replacing the vagina and performing an ovariohysterectomy can be successful if the prolapse has been recognized before too much dehiscence has occurred. Bladder eversion carries a poor prognosis, although cystopexy in conjunction with partial cystotomy can be successful. The prolapsed bladder is replaced gently and any necrotic areas removed.

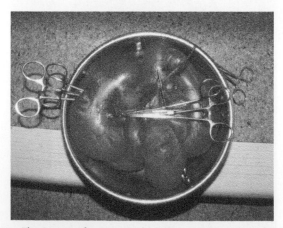

Fig. 15. Hydrometra. The uterus of a young rabbit that was brought in by a rescue center for routine ovariohysterectomy. The rabbit was thin with a pendulous abdomen and ravenous appetite. The rabbit weighed 4.2 kg before surgery. The uterus weighed 1 kg. The rabbit made a full recovery after surgery. (*Courtesy of* Frances Harcourt-Brown, BVSc, FRCVS, Harrogate, United Kingdom.)

Complications of Pregnancy

Fetal resorption

Fetal death before 21 days of gestation results in fetal resorption.[29] It occurs during periods of poor nutrition or stress. Viable fetal units may be seen alongside resorbing ones (**Fig. 16**).

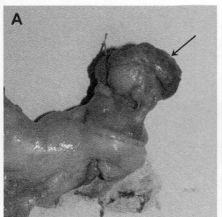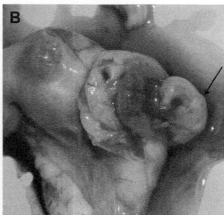

Fig. 16. Fetal resorption. Two fetal units from the same uterus that was removed during routine ovariohysterectomy. A disparity in size of the fetal units could be seen. The smaller unit was filled with degenerative tissue (*A, arrow*) and the larger unit contained an embryo (*B, arrow*). (*Courtesy of* Frances Harcourt-Brown, BVSc, FRCVS, Harrogate, United Kingdom.)

Abortion

Abortion occurs if there is death of the fetus after 21 days.[29] There are several potential causes including infectious disease. A survey of pathogens in the reproductive tract of farmed rabbits showed the presence of Chlamydia, spp. *Escherichia coli, Leptospira interrogans, myxomatosis, Mycoplasma spp., Staphylococcus aureus, Pasteurella multocida, Salmonella spp.*, and *Toxoplasma gondii* on farms where abortions had occurred.[30] Abortion can also be a sign of listeriosis in breeding establishments. Adult nonpregnant males and females are normally resistant to *Listeria monocytogenes*, but the organism has a predilection for the gravid uterus in late pregnancy. Abortions, still-births, and death of the dam may occur. The organism can be recovered from the uterine wall, placenta, and fetuses.[17] Other causes of abortion include herpes virus[31] and vitamin E deficiency.[32]

Dystocia

Dystocia is rare in rabbits but, as in other species, it can happen if there is a malpresentation, single large fetus, or uterine inertia. Signs of dystocia include a bloody or brown vaginal discharge and straining. The fetuses can be felt during abdominal palpation. Radiography will confirm pregnancy. Sedation and analgesia is indicated before attempting vaginal delivery by transabdominal manipulation.[33] Oxytocin (1-3 U) can be used if uterine inertia is suspected. Calcium borogluconate 10% (5–10 mL per rabbit) can also be given orally[29] or subcutaneously. Ultrasound examination can be performed to assess the uterus and surrounding structures, and to confirm fetal viability or death. Caesarean section is indicated if attempts at vaginal delivery fail. The success of the procedure depends on how long the rabbit has been in labor (**Fig. 17**).

Extrauterine Pregnancy

Extrauterine pregnancy occurs in domestic rabbits.[34] It is thought to be the result of a traumatic event or weakness in the uterine wall that allows a fetus to be released into the abdominal cavity (**Fig. 18**). The condition may be an incidental finding during ovariohysterectomy or if an abdominal mass is palpated.

Uterine torsion

Uterine torsion is most common in multiparous rabbits. It is recorded as a cause of death in surveys of culled or dying breeding does.[35] There are also isolated reports in laboratory rabbits[36,37] and anecdotal reports in pet rabbits. Affected rabbits are presented dead or dying from shock (**Fig. 19**).

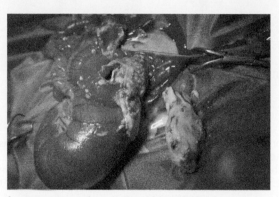

Fig. 17. Dead fetus from exteriorized uterus in a rabbit. The owner was unaware that the rabbit shown in the picture was pregnant. Anorexia was the presenting sign. Abdominal radiography showed the presence of fetuses and large amounts of abdominal gas. Exploratory laparotomy showed the presence of decomposing fetuses and pus in the uterus. The rabbit died later during surgery. (*Courtesy of* Frances Harcourt-Brown, BVSc, FRCVS, Harrogate, United Kingdom.)

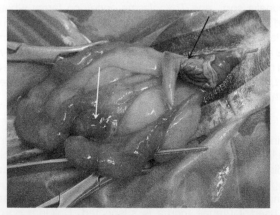

Fig. 18. Extrauterine pregnancy in a rabbit. The uterus of a rabbit that was undergoing routine ovariohysterectomy. A perforation was found in the right uterine horn (*right uterus*) near the cervix (*white arrow*) and a dead fetus was in the abdominal cavity. Its leg can be seen in the photograph (*black arrow*). The rabbit made an uneventful recovery after ovariohysterectomy and removal of the fetus. (*Courtesy of* Frances Harcourt-Brown, BVSc, FRCVS, Harrogate, United Kingdom.)

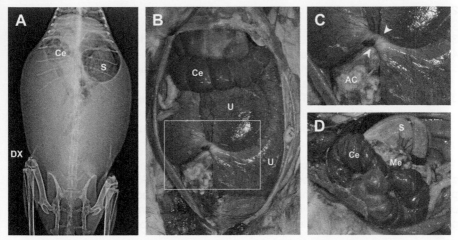

Fig. 19. Radiography (*A*) and dissection (*B–D*) in a 6-year-old entire female rabbit presented with dyspnea. (*A*) Radiography revealed indistinct abdominal mass of soft tissue opacity. The cecum (C) is pushed cranially close to the stomach (S). (*B–D*) On postmortem examination, both uteri (U) were markedly distended with fluid. Torsion of the left uterus and the presence of uterine neoplasia was obvious. (*C*) Detailed view of a marked area from the image (*B*). Uterine torsion of more than 360° (*arrows*) and uterine adenocarcinoma (AC). The tumor had macroscopic metastases (me) in the abdominal wall, liver, and stomach. (*Courtesy of* Vladimir Jekl, Brno, Czech Republic.)

Mammary Gland Problems

- *Mammary gland development* and milk secretion can occur in pseudopregnant females. It is also a sign that there may be uterine problems, such as endometrial hyperplasia or adenocarcinoma in mature entire females. Rabbit mammary gland tissue is sensitive to prolactin and it is possible to encounter mammary gland development and lactation even in spayed females, in spayed females in association with pituitary adenomas.[17] One reported case had a mammary gland adenocarcinoma.[38]
- *Mastitis* is relatively common in breeding does, but rare in pet rabbits unless they have come from a breeder. Acute cases can show pyrexia and painful, enlarged, and discolored mammary glands. Abscesses can develop in the mammary tissue. Surgery may be required in addition to systemic antibiotics. Necrotic tissue may need to be removed.
- *Mammary gland tumors* occur. They can range in malignancy from benign cysts to carcinomas. A survey of mammary gland tumors from 109 pet rabbits found that 12% were benign.[39]

PREVENTION AND TREATMENT OF UTERINE PROBLEMS

Although ovariectomy in rabbits less than 1 year of age may prevent uterine disease later is life,[40] ovariohysterectomy is the only treatment for existing uterine disease. The surgical technique is described and illustrated in several texts.[26,41]

Postspay Adhesions and Granulomas

Postspay adhesions and granulomas occur readily in rabbits because:

1. Rabbits readily form adhesions between abdominal viscera. They are used as laboratory models for the problem in humans.[42]

2. Granuloma formation and calcification in any area of devitalized tissue also occurs readily (**Fig. 20**).
3. Inflammation and foreign body reaction to catgut is marked in rabbits.[43]
4. The vagina fills with urine during micturition and applies pressure on a vaginal repair. Any leakage of urine will cause a local (or even) generalized peritonitis that stimulates adhesion and granuloma formation.
5. The vagina is not sterile. The main constituents of the vaginal and cervical micro-flora are coagulase-negative staphylococci, micrococci, and nonfermentative bacilli, mainly pseudomonas.[10] The cervices act as a natural barrier between the nonsterile vagina and the sterile uterus.

Where to place the cervical ligature during ovariohysterectomy is an important consideration in preventing postoperative complications. Some authors recommend placing the ligature across the vagina and removing as much of the vaginal body as possible in the belief that it will prevent reflux of urine and infection.[44] In this author's opinion, vaginectomy has the potential to cause many complications. There are a

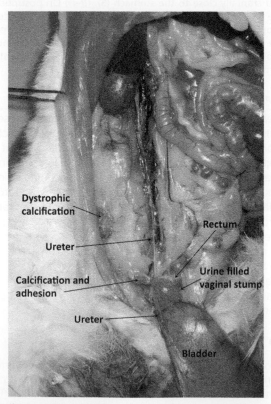

Fig. 20. Post spay adhesion. Dissection of a 4-year-old neutered rabbit that was euthanized because of posterior paresis. The calcified adhesion from a vaginectomy was an incidental finding. The image shows the vaginal remnant filled with urine. The ureter and rectum are in close proximity. It was fortunate that these structures were not involved in the adhesion formation. (*Courtesy of* Frances Harcourt-Brown, BVSc, FRCVS, Harrogate, United Kingdom.)

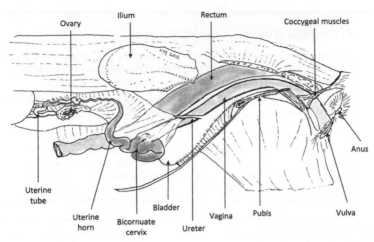

Fig. 21. Lateral view of the female reproductive tract. The lateral view of the female reproductive tract shows the relationship of the vagina with the bladder, ureter, and rectum. (*Courtesy of* Frances Harcourt-Brown, BVSc, FRCVS, Harrogate, United Kingdom.)

number of important neighboring structures (**Fig. 21**). Adhesions that involve the ureters, colon, or bladder can cause strictures, hydronephrosis, and other problems.[45] The author has seen many of these problems causing a variety of clinical signs, ranging from intermittent colic to urinary incontinence or death from peritonitis, acute renal failure, or intestinal obstruction (**Box 4**). These complications can be avoided by tying off the uterine horns at the cervix rather than transecting the vagina. It is easy to tie off each horn individually before encircling the both cervices and tightening the ligature (**Fig. 22**). This ligature lies securely and takes advantage of the natural barrier that the cervix forms between the commensal infections of the vagina and the sterile uterus. After neutering, the cervix and vagina regress to be small structures (**Fig. 23**).

Partial vaginectomy is indicated in rabbits with uterine tumors or other pathology that extends to the cervix. In these cases, it is important to remove any vestige of uterine tissue and to ensure that the vaginal stump is oversewn securely to prevent urine leakage and adhesion formation (**Fig. 24**).

DISEASES OF THE MALE REPRODUCTIVE TRACT
Testicular Problems

Testicular problems are usually treated by castration and several techniques are described in various textbooks, articles, and websites. This author prefers a mixed open and closed technique that is quick and easy. The scrotum is incised toward the caudal end and the testicle is exteriorized and pulled out. Applying tension to the testicle stretches the attachments so they can be sectioned with scissors before identifying, ligating, and sectioning the testicular blood vessels. These retract into the tubular section of the tunica vaginalis and the ligature can be seen through the thin tissue. A ligature is then placed around the tunica vaginalis after making sure the ligated blood vessels are enclosed. This ligature closes the inguinal canal. The testicle is removed and the skin edges pulled together. No sutures are required.

Box 4
Clinical signs of disorders of the female reproductive tract

- Palpable abdominal masses: This may be the most obvious sign of uterine disease that is encountered during clinical examination. Palpation of the caudoventral abdomen is always recommended even if the rabbit is meant to be neutered.

- Vaginal discharge: May be serosanguinous, purulent, or hemorrhagic. Bleeding from the vulva may be sudden and severe, and is always significant.

- Visible vaginal prolapse.

- Hematuria: Normal urine is rabbits can vary in color from yellow to orange, brown, or red, so it is important to differentiate normal urine from hematuria. Blood in the urine can come from the uterus because it mixes with urine in the vagina before it is voided. Close observation may show more blood at the end of urination. Blood clots are highly suggestive of uterine disease. Hematuria owing to bladder disease is usually associated with dysuria.

- Abdominal distension: Abdominal distension can be caused by pregnancy and some uterine disorders. In rabbits, abdominal fat deposits can be large and it is not always easy to differentiate fluid from fat. Hydrometra or ascites owing to metastasized tumors can cause abdominal distension.

- Abnormal appearance of vulva: Hormonal stimulation results in vulvar enlargement and a deep red-purple appearance of the mucosa. This may be marked in rabbits with ovarian tumors.

- Mammary gland development: Mammary gland development and prominent nipples may be seen in rabbits with uterine and/or ovarian tumors. Sometimes milk can be expressed from the nipples. There is an association with uterine neoplasia and mammary gland tumors or cysts.

- Urinary incontinence: This can be owing to an enlarged uterus pressing on the bladder or adhesions affecting the function of the internal urethral sphincter.

- Behavioral changes: The can include lethargy, aggression, or increased sexual behavior.

- Regenerative anemia: This can be a feature of chronic blood loss from the uterus.

- Nonspecific signs of ill health: Uneaten cecotrophs, inappetence, and weight loss may be seen in associated with uterine tumors. This may be owing to abdominal discomfort or metastasis.

- Dyspnea or other signs of metastatic disease: The lungs are a common site for metastasis of uterine adenocarcinomas. Sudden-onset dyspnea in a mature entire female is suspicious. Radiography is diagnostic (see **Fig. 12**). Metastasis to other organs such as the liver and bones can occur (see **Fig. 13**) and can lead to pathologic fractures.

If a reproductive disorder is suspected, further diagnostic techniques such as radiography or ultrasound examination are indicated. In many cases, surgery is required both to diagnose and treat the condition by removing the uterus and ovaries.

Infection

Infected fight wounds can affect the testicles. Epididymitis and orchitis can occur in breeding rabbits and is attributed predominantly to pasteurellosis. It also occurs with myxomatosis. Male rabbits that recover may have decreased libido and fertility.[46]

Absent testicles

In some mature rabbits, one or both testicles cannot be palpated in the scrotum or inguinal canal. This can be owing to previous surgical removal, fighting, or cryptorchidism.

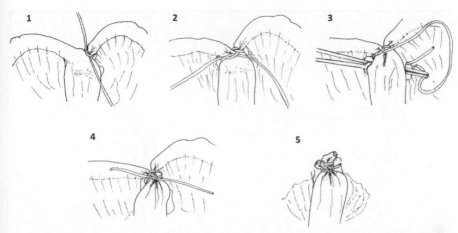

Fig. 22. Cervical ligature. The cervices can be tied off without the need for a transfixing ligature or oversewing by using the illustrated method. Each horn is tied off individually before taking the suture material around the cervix and tightening it. The ligature is secure and prevents leakage of urine from the vagina. Small size suture material (eg, 4-0 polyglactin 910) is recommended to prevent tissue reaction around the ligature. (*Courtesy of* Frances Harcourt-Brown BVSc FRCVS, Harrogate, United Kingdom.)

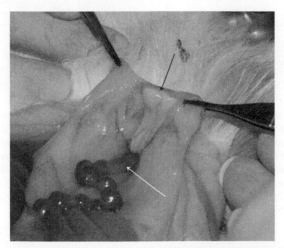

Fig. 23. Appearance of cervical stump years after placing cervical ligature. Examination of the cervical stump is recommended during any postmortem examination of a neutered female rabbit. This image shows the cervical remnant (*black arrow*) of a rabbit that was spayed by the author some years previously. There are no adhesions to either the rectum (*white arrow*) or bladder. (*Courtesy of* Frances Harcourt-Brown, BVSc, FRCVS, Harrogate, United Kingdom.)

Cryptorchidism
Cryptorchidism is the failure of the testicle to descend into the scrotum and there are 3 types:

1. The testicle is in the abdomen, in which case there is no evagination of the peritoneum to form the tunica vaginalis and the scrotal sac does not develop
2. The testicle is partially descended through the inguinal ring

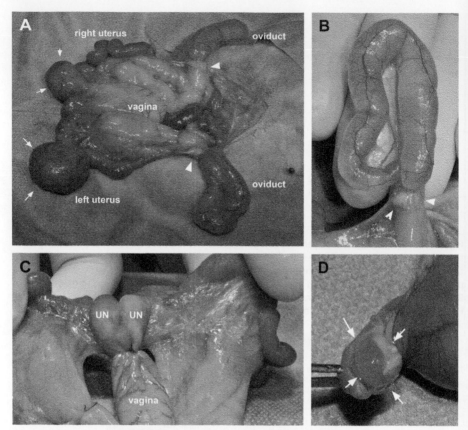

Fig. 24. Ovariohysterectomy and partial vaginectomy in a 4.5-year-old entire female rabbit (*A–D*). (*A*) Bilateral uterine adenocarcinoma (*arrows*) and distension of both uterine tubes (*oviducts*) with fluid. The ovaries are pointed with *arrowheads*. (*B*) Enlarged view of the right uterine tube (*oviduct*) that was dilated with fluid and had cystic hyperplasia. It was associated with high blood estrogen levels. (*C*) The vagina was ligated with a transfixing ligature below the vaginal end of the cervices ("high vaginectomy)". (*D*) Detailed view of the uterus showing with cystic hyperplastic changes (*arrows*). (*Courtesy of* Vladimir Jekl, Brno, Czech Republic.)

3. The testicle has descended through the inguinal ring, but has not descended into the scrotum. This can occur in young rabbits.

    Retained testicles in cryptorchid rabbits are small unless they are neoplastic.

Retracted testicles

The well-developed cremaster muscle is an extension of the internal oblique muscle that inserts on the tunica vaginalis (see **Fig. 2**). It allows rabbits to retract the testicle into the tubular section of the tunica vaginalis that is in the groin. The caudal tip of the testicle is just palpable. In most cases, it can be pushed into the scrotum by applying gentle pressure to the inguinal region. This is also possible in young rabbits that have no descended testicles in the scrotum. A suggested approach to the rabbit with absent testicles is shown in **Box 5**.

Box 5
Suggested approach to a rabbit with absent testicles in the scrotum

Absent testicles are owing to

1. Previous surgical removal of one or both testicles.

2. Fighting rabbits will bite the scrotum and even remove part or all of the testicle.

3. Retracted testicles—owing to stress, fear, severe illness, or malnutrition.

4. Cryptorchidism.

It is important to establish whether the rabbit has a testicle or not and there are some observations that can help:

Examine the penis: Mature males with testicles are easily aroused. The penis of an entire male is long and curved in comparison with a neutered male (**Figs. 33** and **34**) and an immature male. If the penis becomes erect during examination, this suggests the rabbit is entire, so the rabbit is probably cryptorchid, or possibly an aged rabbit with an adrenal tumor.

Clip the fur and examine the inguinal area: The inguinal skin of a cryptorchid is smooth on the side of the absent testicle because a scrotal sac has never developed. If the testicle is retracted or has been removed, the empty scrotum persists, either as a wrinkled empty structure (retracted testicle) or as a fold of skin (after castration).

Examine the scrotum: Scars suggest that the testicle has been damaged or removed as the result of a fight. Subsequent surgical exploration may show remnants of a testicle or its surrounding structures.

Testicular tumors

Tumors of the testicle can occur in aged entire males. Sometimes they are very large before they are noticed by the owner (**Fig. 25**). Benign interstitial cell tumors and gonadoblastoma are reported.[47–50] Clinical signs may not be obvious and it often the

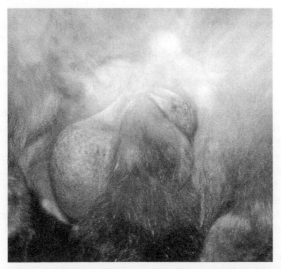

Fig. 25. Testicular tumor. Testicular tumors can develop in aged entire males. Owners are often unaware of them until they become large. Most are benign and surgical removal is curative. (*Courtesy of* Frances Harcourt-Brown, BVSc, FRCVS, Harrogate, United Kingdom.)

presence of a large testicle that alerts the owner to a problem. Urine scalding and dysuria may be present if the tumor is so large that it distorts the genitalia and diverts the stream of urine during urination. Melanomas of the scrotal skin can occur with varying degrees of malignancy (**Fig. 26**).

Testicular torsion

Torsion of a testicle can occur in uncastrated males of any age. It is a painful condition and sudden-onset depression and anorexia may be the presenting signs. The affected testicle is sore and tense. Its position in the scrotal sac is abnormal.[26]

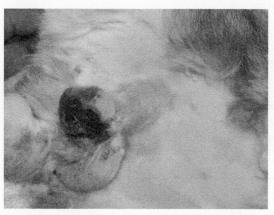

Fig. 26. Scrotal melanoma. A highly malignant melanoma originating from the scrotal skin. The tumor had already metastasized to the lungs. (*Courtesy of* Frances Harcourt-Brown, BVSc, FRCVS, Harrogate, United Kingdom.)

Other Problems of the Male Reproductive Tract

Inguinal hernias

Inguinal hernias containing part, or all, of the bladder are encountered occasionally in rabbits (**Fig. 27**). In any species, inguinal hernias may be indirect or direct.[51] Indirect hernias occur when the abdominal contents herniate into the tunica vaginalis. Direct hernias occur when a separate peritoneal evagination develops so the abdominal contents are contained in a pocket within the tunica vaginalis. Both types occur in rabbits. Inguinal hernias are nearly always found in aged entire male rabbits, but the condition has been reported in a young female.[52] The hernia is nearly always found on the left, presumably because the large cecum occupies the right inguinal area of the abdomen. In the early stages, a palpable swelling in the inguinal region may be detected by the owner. In the later stages, dysuria may be the presenting sign because, once part of or the entire bladder has passed through the inguinal canal, sediment accumulates in the herniated part of the bladder, which cannot empty properly. In severe cases, partial or complete ureteral obstruction can occur. Surgical repair is usually straightforward (**Fig. 28**), but the testicle needs to be removed so the inguinal canal can be closed after excising the tunica vaginalis and the sac that contained the bladder.

Urethral stenosis

Some aged male rabbits develop progressive problems with urination. They strain and often grunt as they urinate and can only dribble a few drops of urine at a time. Buildup of sludge in the bladder is a complication. Catheterization is difficult or impossible,

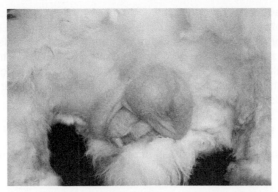

Fig. 27. Typical appearance of an Inguinal hernia in a 7-year-old entire male Dwarf Lop. Inguinal hernias usually occur in entire male rabbits. In rabbits, hernias are often on the left and contain part of the bladder. (*Courtesy of* Frances Harcourt-Brown, BVSc, FRCVS, Harrogate, United Kingdom.)

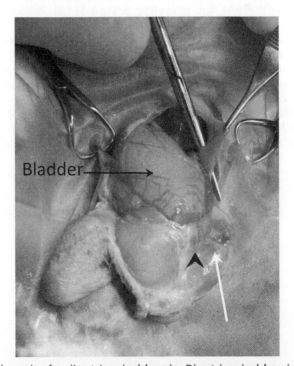

Fig. 28. Surgical repair of a direct inguinal hernia. Direct inguinal hernias occur when a separate peritoneal evagination develops to form a sac within the tunica vaginalis in the inguinal canal. In this rabbit (also shown in **Fig. 27**), a direct hernial sac (*black arrowhead*) can be seen as a separate structure from the tunica vaginalis (*white arrow*). The bladder has herniated into the sac, which has developed between the muscle layers at the origin of the cremaster. In the picture, the tips of the scissors show the path of the inguinal canal. A direct hernia that forms between muscle layers is easy to repair because the muscles can be stitched to close the defect once the bladder has been replaced in the abdomen. Removal of the testicle and closure of the inguinal canal is also necessary. (*Courtesy of* Frances Harcourt-Brown, BVSc, FRCVS, Harrogate, United Kingdom.)

even from the bladder during cystotomy. Diseases of the male accessory glands are reported rarely, although there is a report of seminal vesiculitis in 3 entire male rabbits.[53] This author has also encountered problems in castrated males. Radiography can indicate a urethral stenosis. Exploratory surgery is indicated although it difficult to visualize the glands because they are deep in the pelvis (see **Fig. 2**). Ultrasound or computed tomography scanning may yield more information as the normal appearance of the glands has been published.[54]

PROBLEMS WITH EXTERNAL GENITALIA IN BOTH SEXES

Problems with the external genitalia can occur in both male and female rabbits.

Infections

Treponematosis

Treponematosis (*Treponema paraluis-cuniculi*) is transmitted sexually in rabbits and is more common in breeding colonies than individual pets. Vertical transmission can take place, with young rabbits being infected during the passage through the birth canal of an infected dam. The disease is characterized by crusty lesions on the mucocutaneous junctions of the nose, lips, or eyelids, or the external genitalia.[55] The prepuce of males and the vulva in females are the usual sites of infection in breeding animals and the lesions can extend to the anus and into the surrounding skin (**Fig. 29**). Untreated lesions may resolve or persist indefinitely. The disease has a long incubation period. Studies on outbreaks have suggested a period of 10 to 16 weeks and subclinical infections can occur. In pet rabbits, the disease is most common in juvenile animals, but it is occasionally encountered in an adult pet rabbit that has been kept on its own. Latent infection can flare up in stressful situations. Theoretically, positive diagnosis can be made by examination of material scraped from the lesion or skin, biopsy but special silver staining techniques are required. Without a laboratory at hand, the

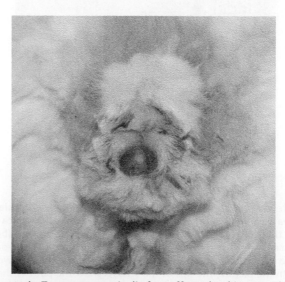

Fig. 29. Treponematosis. *Treponema cuniculi* often affects the skin around the genital opening and anus. The lesions are crusty and nonprogressive. There are often lesions on the nose or lips as well. In this case, the skin around the anus is affected. (*Courtesy of* Frances Harcourt-Brown, BVSc, FRCVS, Harrogate, United Kingdom.)

organism is seldom encountered and the diagnosis is presumptive. There is a serologic test, but lesions can occur before the development of positive serology so false-negative results may occur in early infections. Rabbits can remain seropositive after lesions have resolved, so false-positive results can also occur. Response to treatment is often the easiest way of establishing the diagnosis. In most cases, *Treponema cuniculi* responds dramatically to antibiotics, although it is not sensitive to all of them. It is very responsive to penicillin and the treatment of choice used is 3 injections of long-acting procaine penicillin (40 mg/kg) at weekly intervals.[56] Enrofloxacin is ineffective.

Myxomatosis

Myxomatosis is caused by a Leporipox virus. The severity of infection depends on the virulence of the virus and the immune status of the rabbit. The most common route of infection is through an insect bite. Replication of the virus takes place at the inoculation site and in the regional lymph node. It is followed by cell-associated viremia and generalized infection throughout the body. The disease starts with a skin lesion, which typically develops 4 to 5 days after inoculation of the virus and enlarges up to 3 cm in diameter 9 to 10 days after infection. The rabbit is viremic, with virus replication taking place throughout the lymphoid system. The eyelids become thickened and eventually the eyes are completely closed by the ninth day with a semipurulent ocular discharge. Secondary swellings develop throughout the body, typically on the nares, lips, eyelids, and base of the ears and on the external genitalia and anus (**Fig. 30**). Initially, there is hyperemia followed by soft swellings that enlarge, harden, and become crusty. The lesions then become necrotic and the skin may die. Eventually (if the rabbit survives) the necrotic tissue falls away and the skin heals, although there may be some deformity. It takes 6 to 8 weeks for the lesions to regress. If the rabbit can survive this period, it may recover but many cases do not. Death from secondary bacterial infection owing to severe

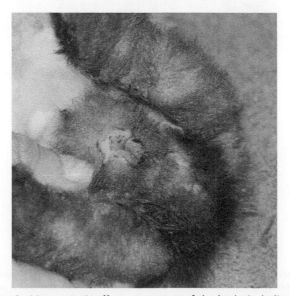

Fig. 30. Myxomatosis. Myxomatosis affects may parts of the body, including the genitalia. It causes inflammation followed by edema and nodule formation. There are also lesions on the eyelids and nares. (*Courtesy of* Frances Harcourt-Brown, BVSc, FRCVS, Harrogate, United Kingdom.)

immunosuppression can occur at any time. In male rabbits that recover, inflammation of the testicles makes them infertile for up to 12 months. There is no specific treatment for myxomatosis. Supportive care is necessary.

INFECTED SKIN FOLDS

Female and castrated male rabbits can develop large skin flaps cover the genital opening. The skin fold under the flap becomes infected and causes urethritis and urine scalding. Surgical removal of the skin flaps is indicated.[57] In aged males, the scrotum can become pendulous and result in a skin infection beneath it that may extend to the genitalia (**Fig. 31**). Scrotal ablation is needed for these cases.[26]

Preputial Adhesion

In some castrated male rabbits, especially obese ones, the penis can become adherent to the prepuce. If these rabbits develop urinary incontinence, the genital orifice and prepuce easily become inflamed and sore, which can exacerbate the adhesions and scarring so that urine is directed down the inside of 1 thigh. Occasionally, the preputial opening in some males becomes so stenotic (phimosis) that the rabbit can only dribble urine rather than direct a jet of urine away from the inside of the legs or under the tail (**Fig. 32**).

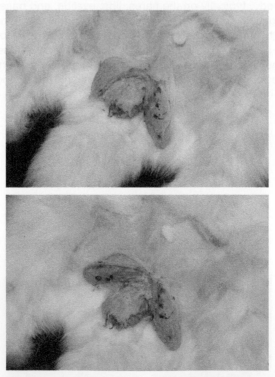

Fig. 31. Pendulous scrotum. Aged entire male rabbits often develop a pendulous scrotum. The rabbit is unable to groom and clean the skin under the scrotum and it becomes infected and inflamed. Urine scalding and uneaten cecotrophs are common complications. Scrotal ablation and castration is very effective in resolving the problem. (*Courtesy of* Frances Harcourt-Brown, BVSc, FRCVS, Harrogate, United Kingdom.)

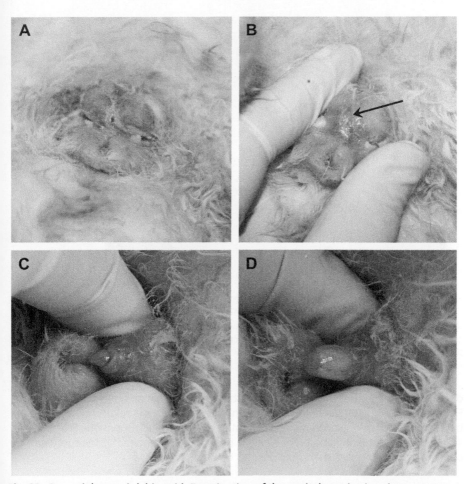

Fig. 32. Preputial stenosis (phimosis). Examination of the genital opening is an important part of clinical examination of incontinent rabbits (*A*). Chronic inflammation can cause preputial adhesions and stenosis of the urethral opening. In this case the urethral opening was tiny (*arrow* in *B*). General anesthesia is initially necessary to extrude the penis and break down the adhesions (*C* and *D*). The owner can be taught how to repeat the procedure on a daily basis. Lubrication with a petroleum jelly–based products (eg, some eye ointments) can be helpful. (*Courtesy of* Frances Harcourt-Brown, BVSc, FRCVS, Harrogate, United Kingdom.)

Genital Deformity

Scarring or deformity of the external genitalia can result in alterations in urine flow and urine scalding. Scarring may be the results of fight wounds or skin loss owing to fly-strike (**Fig. 33**). Deviation of the tail can occur as an age-related change that deforms the external genitalia.

Hypersexuality

Hormone production from hyperplastic or neoplastic adrenal glands can occur in rabbits and is manifested by behavioral changes. Unusually aggressive or sexual behavior, especially in older animals, is highly suggestive. Examples include mounting or chasing other pets and humans, biting, scratching, and urine spraying. Ultrasound examination of the adrenal glands is indicated although some cases may be pituitary

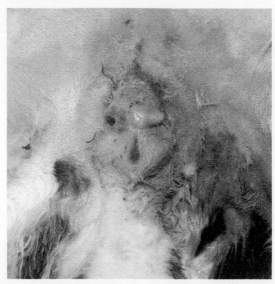

Fig. 33. Deformed prepuce. Examination of the genitalia may show deviation in the direction of urine flow. In this rabbit, scarring of the prepuce had pulled the penis to the left so the rabbit was forced to urinate down the inside of the left leg. Surgery was performed to correct the condition, but was only partial successful because there was a limited amount of skin. (*Courtesy of* Frances Harcourt-Brown, BVSc, FRCVS, Harrogate, United Kingdom.)

dependent. A test dose of 1.5 mg/kg of subcutaneous delmadinone acetate (Tardak, Pfizer, New York, NY) can be helpful in confirming a hormone-related problem. If the behavior recurs, the injection may be repeated or a deslorelin (Suprelorin [Virbac, UK], 4.7 mg/rabbit) implant placed. These have been used in rabbits.[58–60] Surgery can be considered for adrenal tumors, but can be challenging.[61]

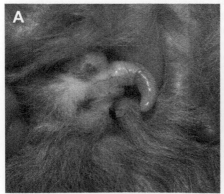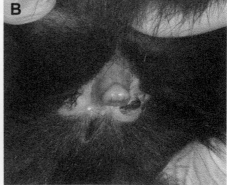

Fig. 34. Appearance of the penis in entire and castrated male rabbits. Castration changes the shape of the penis. It is long, curved, and erectile in an entire male (*A*) in contrast with the short, flaccid penis of a castrated male (*B*). In some cases, extrusion of the penis will evert the tip to expose the urethra (*B*). This is clinically insignificant. (*Courtesy of* Frances Harcourt-Brown, BVSc, FRCVS, Harrogate, United Kingdom.)

REFERENCES

1. Rosell JMM, de la Fuente LFF. Causes of mortality in breeding rabbits. Prev Vet Med 2016;127:56–63.
2. Rosell JM, de la FLF, Badiola JI, et al. Study of urgent visits to commercial rabbit farms in Spain and Portugal during 1997-2007. World Rabbit Sci 2010;17(3): 127–36.
3. Martinez-Gomez M, Luclo RA, Carro M, et al. Striated muscles and scent glands associated with the vaginal tract of the rabbit. Anat Rec 1997;247(4):486–95.
4. Furukawa S, Kuroda Y, Sugiyama A. A comparison of the histological structure of the placenta in experimental animals. J Toxicol Pathol 2014;27:11–8.
5. Uthamanthil R, Hachem R. Urinary catheterization of male rabbits: a new technique and a review of urogenital anatomy. J Am Assoc Lab Anim Sci 2013; 52(2):180–5.
6. Gonçalves H, Alves PC, Rocha A. Seasonal variation in the reproductive activity of the wild rabbit (Oryctolagus cuniculus algirus) in a Mediterranean ecosystem. Wildl Res 2002;29(2):165–73.
7. McNitt JI, Lukefahr SD, Cheeke PR, et al. Rabbit management. In: Rabbit production. 9th edition. Oxford (United Kingdom): CABI; 2013. p. 42–64.
8. Patton NM. Colony husbandry. In: Manning PJ, Ringler DH, Newcomer CE, editors. The biology of the laboratory rabbit. 2nd edition. San Diego (CA): Academic Press; 1994. p. 27–45.
9. Marongiu ML, Dimauro C. Preliminary study on factors influencing rabbit doe reproductive efficiency: effect of parity, day of mating, and suckling on ovarian status and estrogen levels at day 6 of pregnancy. Can J Vet Res 2013;77:126–30.
10. Dal Bosco A, Rebollar PG, Boiti C, et al. Ovulation induction in rabbit does: current knowledge and perspectives. Anim Reprod Sci 2011;129:106–17.
11. Rödel HG, Starkloff A, Bautista A, et al. Infanticide and maternal offspring defence in European rabbits under natural breeding conditions. Ethology 2008; 114(1):22–31.
12. Ola I, Oyegbade M. Buck effect on rabbit oestrous: vulva colour, vaginal lumen cells and ovarian follicle populations. World Rabbit Sci 2012;20(2):71–9.
13. Sheppard EM. The reproductive system of a pregnant hermaphrodite rabbit (Oryctolagus cuniculus). J Anat 1943;77(4):288–93.
14. Sladakovic I, Guzman DSM, Petritz OA, et al. Unilateral cervical and segmental uterine horn aplasia with endometrial hyperplasia, mucometra, and endometritis in a domestic rabbit (oryctolagus cuniculus). J Exot Pet Med 2015;24(1):98–104.
15. Thode HP, Johnston MS. Probable congenital uterine developmental abnormalities in two domestic rabbits. Vet Rec 2009;164(8):242–4.
16. Bray MV, Weir EC, Brownstein DG, et al. Endometrial venous aneurysms in three New Zealand white rabbits. Lab Anim Sci 1992;42(4):360–2.
17. Percy DH, Barthold SW. Rabbit. In: Pathology of laboratory rodents and rabbits. 3rd edition. Oxford (United Kingdom): Blackwell; 2007. p. 253–308.
18. Walter B, Poth T, Bohmer E, et al. Uterine disorders in 59 rabbits. Vet Rec 2010; 166(8):230–3.
19. Vinci A, Bacci B, Benazzi C, et al. Progesterone receptor expression and proliferative activity in uterine tumours of pet rabbits. J Comp Pathol 2010;142(4): 323–7.
20. Greene HSN. Uterine adenomata in the rabbit III. Susceptibility as a function of constitutional factors. J Exp Med 1941;73(2):273–92.

21. Zadravec M, Gombač M, Račnik J, et al. Uterine heterologous malignant mixed Müllerian tumor in a dwarf rabbit (Oryctolagus cuniculus). J Vet Diagn Invest 2012;24(2):418–22.

22. Künzel F, Grinninger P, Shibly S, et al. Uterine disorders in 50 pet rabbits. J Am Anim Hosp Assoc 2015;51(1):8–14.

23. Saito K, Nakanishi M, Hasegawa A. Uterine disorders diagnosed by ventrotomy in 47 rabbits. J Vet Med Sci 2002;64(6):495–7.

24. Morrell JM. Hydrometra in the rabbit. Vet Rec 1989;125(12):325.

25. Bray MV, Gaertner DJ, Brownstein DG, et al. Hydrometra in a New Zealand white rabbit. Lab Anim Sci 1991;41(6):628–9.

26. Harcourt-Brown FM. Neutering. In: Harcourt-Brown F, Chitty J, editors. BSAVA manual of rabbit surgery, dentistry and imaging. Gloucester (United Kingdom): BSAVA; 2013. p. 138–56.

27. Becha B, Unnikrishnan M, Harshan H. Chronic postpartum vaginal prolapse in a rabbit doe. J Vet Anim Sci 2006;42:84.

28. Klaphake E, Paul-Murphy J. Disorders of the reproductive and urinary systems. In: Quesenberry KE, Carpenter JW, editors. Ferrets, rabbits and rodents: clinical medicine and surgery. 3rd edition. St Louis (MO): Elsevier; 2012. p. 217–31.

29. Van Herck H, Hesp AP, Versluis A, et al. Prolapsus vaginae in the IIIVO/JU rabbit. Lab Anim 1989;23(4):333–6.

30. Boucher S, Gracia E, Villa A, et al. Pathogens in the reproductive tract of farm rabbits. Vet Rec 2001;149:677–8.

31. Jin L, Valentine B a, Baker RJ, et al. An outbreak of fatal herpesvirus infection in domestic rabbits in Alaska. Vet Pathol 2008;45(3):369–74.

32. Yamini S, Stein S. Abortion, stillbirth, neonatal death, and nutritional myodegeneration in a rabbit breeding colony. J Am Vet Med Assoc 1989;194(4):561–2.

33. Dickie E. Dystocia in a rabbit (Oryctolagus cuniculus). Can Vet J 2011;52(1):80–3.

34. Bergdall VK, Dysko RC. Metabolic, traumatic, mycotic and miscellaneous diseases. In: Manning PJ, Ringler DH, Newcomer CE, editors. The biology of the laboratory rabbit. 2nd edition. San Diego (CA): Academic Press; 1994. p. 336–51.

35. Rosell JM, de la Fuente LF. Culling and mortality in breeding rabbits. Prev Vet Med 2009;88(2):120–7.

36. Sebesteny A. A case of torsion of the uterus in a rabbit. Lab Anim Sci 1972;6:357–8.

37. Hobbs BA, Parker RF. Uterine torsion associated with either hydrometra or endometritis in two rabbits. Lab Anim Sci 1990;40(5):535–6.

38. Sikowski P, Trybus J, Cline JM, et al. Cystic mammary adenocarcinoma associated with a prolactin-secreting pituitary adenoma in a New Zealand white rabbit (Oryctolagus cuniculus). Comp Med 2008;58(3):297–300.

39. Baum B, Hewicker-Trautwein M. Classification and epidemiology of mammary tumours in pet rabbits (Oryctolagus cuniculus). J Comp Pathol 2015;152(4):291–8.

40. Divers SJ. Clinical technique: endoscopic oophorectomy in the rabbit (Oryctolagus cuniculus): the future of preventative sterilizations. J Exot Pet Med 2010;19(3):231–7.

41. Richardson C, Flecknell P. Routine neutering of rabbits and rodents. Pract 2006;28(2):70–9.

42. Wiseman DM, Gravagna P, Bayon Y, et al. Collagen membrane/fleece composite film reduces adhesions in the presence of bleeding in a rabbit uterine horn model. Fertil Steril 2001;76(1):175–80.

43. Wainstein M, Anderson J, Elder JS. Comparison of effects of suture materials on wound healing in a rabbit pyeloplasty model. Urology 1997;49(2):261–4.
44. Capello V, Lennox A. Gross and surgical anatomy of the reproductive tract of selected exotic pet mammals. Proc Am Exot Mamm Vet Conf San Antonio 2006;2(1):19–28.
45. Guzman DSM, Graham JE, Keller K, et al. Colonic obstruction following ovario-hysterectomy in rabbits: 3 cases. J Exot Pet Med 2015;24(1):112–9.
46. Fountain S, Holland M, Hinds LA, et al. Interstitial orchitis with impaired steroido-genesis and spermatogenesis in the testes of rabbits infected with an attenuated strain of myxoma. J Reprod Fertil 1960;110:161–9.
47. Roccabianca P, Ghisleni G, Scanzianri E. Simultaneous seminoma and interstitial cell tumour in a rabbit with a previous cutaneous basal cell tumour. J Comp Pathol 1999;121(1):95–9.
48. Marino F, Ferrara G, Rapisarda G, et al. Reinke's crystals in an interstitial cell tumour of a rabbit (Oryctolagus cuniculus). Reprod Domest Anim 2003;38(5):421–2.
49. Veeramachaneni DN, Vandewoude S. Interstitial cell tumour and germ cell tumour with carcinoma in situ in rabbit testes. Int J Androl 1999;22(2):97–101.
50. Suzuki M, Ozaki M, Ano N, et al. Testicular gonadoblastoma in two pet domestic rabbits (Oryctolagus cuniculus domesticus). J Vet Diagn Invest 2011;23(5):1028–32.
51. Thas I, Harcourt-Brown F. Six cases of inguinal urinary bladder herniation in entire male domestic rabbits. J Small Anim Pract 2013;54(12):662–6.
52. Grunkemeyer VL, Sura PA, Baron ML, et al. Surgical repair of an inguinal hernia-tion of the urinary bladder in an intact female domestic rabbit (Oryctolagus cuni-culus). J Exot Pet Med 2010;19(3):249–54.
53. Ardiaca M, Bonvehi C, Cuesta M, et al. Seminal vesiculitis in three pet rabbits (Or-yctolagus cuniculus). J Am Anim Hosp Assoc 2016;52(5):335–40.
54. Dimitrov R. Anatomical imaging analysis of the prostate gland in rabbit (Orycto-lagus cuniculus). Rev Med Vet 2013;164(5):245–51.
55. Saito K, Hasegawa A. Clinical features of skin lesions in rabbit syphilis: a retro-spective study of 63 cases (1999-2003). J Vet Med Sci 2004;66(10):1247–9.
56. Harcourt-Brown FM. Skin diseases. In: Textbook of rabbit medicine. 1st edition. Oxford (United Kingdom): Butterworth Heinemann; 2001. p. 224–48.
57. Melillo A. Removal of perineal and other skin folds. In: Harcourt-Brown F, Chitty J, editors. BSAVA Manual of rabbit surgery, dentistry and imaging. Gloucester (United Kingdom): BSAVA; 2013. p. 274–83.
58. Arlt S, Spankowski S, Kaufmann T, et al. Fertility control in a male rabbit using a deslorelin implant. A case report. World Rabbit Sci 2010;18(3):179–82.
59. Goericke-Pesch S, Groeger G, Wehrend A. The effects of a slow release GnRH agonist implant on male rabbits. Anim Reprod Sci 2015;152:83–9.
60. Geyer A, Daub L, Otzdorff C, et al. Reversible estrous cycle suppression in prepubertal female rabbits treated with slow-release deslorelin implants. Therio-genology 2015;85(2):282–7.
61. Lennox AM. Surgical treatment of adrenocortical disease. In: Harcourt-Brown FM, Chitty J, editors. BSAVA manual of rabbit surgery, dentistry and imaging. Glou-cester (United Kingdom): BSAVA; 2013. p. 269–73.

Reproductive Disorders in Pet Rodents

Jaume Martorell, DVM, PhD, DECZM (small mammal)

KEYWORDS

- Rodent • Rat • Mouse • Hamster • Gerbil • Reproductive disorder
- Mammary gland

KEY POINTS

- Reproductive disorders are very common presentations in rodents; some of them can be an emergency, such as hemorrhagic vaginal discharge.
- Ovarian tumors are common in rats and mice; however, the prevalence of these tumors seems to be strain related.
- Although ovarian cysts are described in all small rodents, gerbils are more prone to this disorder, especially in animals older than 2 years of age.
- Uterine disorders are common in rodents. Pyometra and neoplasia are the most common problems, and ovariohysterectomy is the best treatment.
- Rats can easily develop mammary gland tumors, especially fibroadenomas; because they have an extensive mammary tissue, these tumors rapidly grow and are enlarged masses.

REPRODUCTIVE DISORDERS IN PET RODENTS

The rodent order encompasses 5 phylogenetic suborders (based on Systema Naturae 200):

1. *Hystricomorpha*: relatives to guinea pigs and similar species, including chinchillas, degus, coypus, capybaras, porcupines, dassie rats, cane rats, African mole rats, agoutis, and pakas
2. *Myomorpha*: relatives to mice, including rats, hamsters, gerbils, kangaroo rats, kangaroo mice and dormice
3. *Anomaluromorpha*: such as springhaas and scaly-tailed squirrels
4. *Sciuravida*: relatives to gundis
5. *Sciuromorpha*: relatives to squirrels, including chipmunks, prairie dogs, marmots, and beavers

Disclosure Statement: The author has nothing to disclose.
Departament de Medicina I Cirurgia Animals, Facultat de Veterinaria, Universitat Autònoma de Barcelona, Travessera dels Turons, Bellaterra 08193, Spain
E-mail address: jaumemiquel.martorell@uab.cat

Vet Clin Exot Anim 20 (2017) 589–608
http://dx.doi.org/10.1016/j.cvex.2016.11.015
1094-9194/17/© 2016 Elsevier Inc. All rights reserved.

The range of species sold as pets is increasing. Among them, the most common species kept as pets are guinea pigs, chinchillas, rats, hamsters, gerbils, squirrels, prairie dogs, degus, and mice. The intent of this article is to describe common reproductive diseases affecting small rodents, especially rats, mice, hamsters, gerbils, and others species, such as squirrels and prairie dogs. Unfortunately, literature is scarce in the last two species.

ANATOMY OF SMALL RODENTS

Small rodents have several reproductive anatomic features in common. Males and females can be easily identified. However, the sex identification can be more challenging in very young animals. Males have more distance between the genital papilla and the anus than females (**Fig. 1**). Females have a pair of small and nodular ovaries found in the fat caudal to the kidneys. The uterus is bicornuate, consisting of 2 uterine horns and a short uterine body that terminates at the vagina, except in rats. The rat uterus is duplex; it comprises 2 uterine horns that join together and open into the vagina via 2 separate cervices. The vagina and the urethral orifices are completely separate. A clinician can easily differentiate discharge of reproductive tract origin from one of the urinary tract.[1–3]

Adult male rodents possess a pair of testicles of a proportionately large size. The inguinal canal remains open throughout the life of the animal, like in rabbits and other rodents; the testes pass from the abdomen to the scrotum but can be retracted. A pair

A MALE   **B** FEMALE

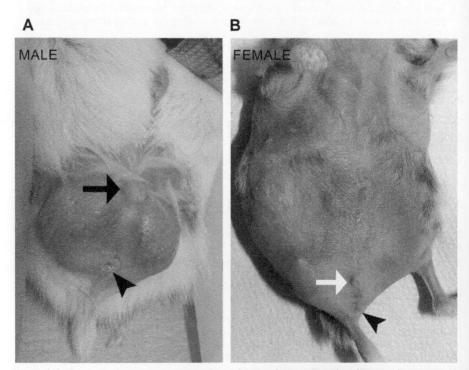

Fig. 1. (*A*) The male hamster anatomy. Dorsal recumbency. See the distance between the prepuce (*black arrow*) and the anus (*black arrowhead*) and the testicles. (*B*) The female hamster anatomy. Dorsal recumbency. See the short distance between the genital papilla (*white arrow*) and the anus (*black arrowhead*). (*Courtesy of* Jaume Martorell, Spain.)

of seminal vesicles and coagulating glands (also called anterior prostate) can be found dorsal and lateral to the urinary bladder, and the prostate is located caudally in the pelvis; other accessory sex glands are the bulbourethral glands and the ampullary glands (glands of the ductus deferens). Most rodents have preputial glands, but these are not present in male gerbils. Male rats possess an os penis.[4–6]

Rats and mice have large and extensive mammary tissues. Rats possess 12 mammary glands: 3 cranial pairs (cervical, cranial thoracic, and caudal thoracic glands), which can extend from the axillary space to the costal arc and the shoulders, and 3 pairs located caudally (abdominal, cranial inguinal, and caudal inguinal), which can extend caudally to the inguinal region. Female rats have one nipple per mammary gland, whereas males do not possess nipples. The female mouse has 5 pairs of nipples and mammary glands: 3 thoracic and 2 inguinal glands. They are embedded in the mammary fat pad, which is a thick layer of adipose tissue. Female hamsters have 6 to 7 pairs of nipples, whereas gerbils and squirrels have 4. However, variation in numbers can be seen. Male rats have 6 pairs of mammary glands; mice and hamsters have 4 pairs of mammary glands with no grossly observable nipples. In gerbils, squirrels, and prairie dogs, mammary gland descriptions are confusing; but in general, it can be consider that female prairie dogs have 5 pairs of mammary glands and female gerbils and squirrels possess 4 pairs. Male gerbils and squirrels have 4 pairs of mammary glands. In all of them, the nipples are not grossly observable.[2,3,7]

Normal reproductive data are shown in **Table 1**.

Many reproductive diseases have been described in rodents. Clinical signs include apathy, hyporexia, anorexia, abdominal distension, subcutaneous masses with or without ulcerated skin, vaginal discharge (mucus, pus, or hemorrhage), and vaginal/uterine prolapse.[8] Minimal blood analyses are needed, especially when hemorrhage is present, in order to decide the best treatment. All animals require specific treatment (medicine or surgery) based on the cause of the disease, but patients should first be stabilized. Clinicians should consider the administration of fluids, analgesic, antibiotics, or any medication in order to give support to the animal. Especial care should be taken if patients need to undergo surgery.

DISEASES OF FEMALE RODENTS
Diseases of the Ovary

Ovarian cysts
Cystic ovaries have been described in all small rodents.[6,9] Many drugs have been used to induce ovarian cysts in laboratory rats, such as letrozole, an aromatase

Table 1
Reproductive data of rats, mice, hamsters, gerbils, squirrels, and prairie dogs

Value	Rats	Mice	Hamsters	Gerbils	Prairie Dogs
Life span (y)	2–3	1–3	1.5–3.0	2–3	8–10
Male maturation (mo)	1	1.5	2	2–4	2–3
Female maturation (mo)	1.0–1.5	1.5	1.5	2–3	2–3
Estrogen cycle length (d)	4–5	4–5	4–5	4–7	2–3 (January–April)
Estrus (h)	9–20	9–20	8–26	12–18	Up to 24
Gestation (d)	21–23	19–21	15–18	23–26	34–37
Pups per litter (number)	6–13	7–11	5–10	3–8	2–10
Weaning age (d)	20–22	18–21	19–21	21–28	6–7

inhibitor.[10] These drugs are not commonly used in pet rodents. Probably there are other mechanisms to develop ovarian cysts. The female rats' estrous cycle is sensitive to hours of light. Exposure to constant light for 3 days can induce a persistent estrus; with such exposure, these rats have been found to develop hyperestrogenism with polycystic ovaries and endometrial hypertrophy.[11] This presentation is not often seen in pet rats.

Cystic ovaries have been described as a common occurrence in laboratory gerbils, pet gerbils older than 2 years, and hamsters.[11–13] They are easily palpated and can be unilateral or bilateral. In many cases, ovarian neoplasia is involved as well.[9] Many animals are present with symmetric alopecia (if the cyst secretes estrogens), abdominal distension, and dyspnea. Ultrasonography can be very useful to confirm the diagnosis (**Fig. 2**).

A definitive diagnosis will require ovariectomy/ovariohysterectomy along with a histopathologic examination of the affected tissues.[6] Some investigators recommend performing a complete drainage of ovarian cysts before ovariohysterectomy to facilitate the surgery; the slow reduction of the fluid volume contained in the cysts would prevent postsurgical shock.[12] The author prefers to do a blunt dissection of the ovary; after a good exposition, the ovarian tissue is taken gently out of the abdominal cavity and finally removed. If it is necessary, the skin and muscular incision can be enlarged.

Another alternative treatment to surgery is percutaneous ultrasound-guided cyst drainage, but this procedure is not recommended because cysts often refill with fluid after drainage.[14] The use of a gonadotropin-releasing hormone agonist, such as leuprolide acetate or deslorelin acetate, has been suggested to treat ovarian cysts and the clinical signs in the guinea pig; however, they can only be useful if they are follicular cysts.[14] A new investigation revealed that the size of the ovarian cysts in all guinea pigs of the study did not vary significantly during the treatment with deslorelin acetate.[15] Further studies are needed to investigate the efficacy of these treatments in other rodents.

Ovarian neoplasia

Rats are prone to tumors and are an excellent ovarian carcinoma rodent model. There are some studies about spontaneous tumors in laboratory Sprague-Dawley rats, with

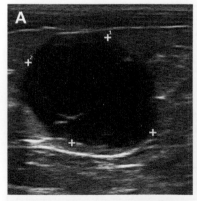
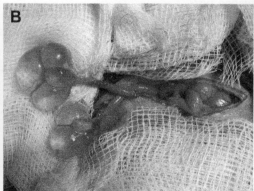

Fig. 2. Ovarian cysts in a gerbil. (*A*) On abdominal ultrasound examination, a round anechoic structure (between calipers) with posterior enhancement can be observed. (*B*) Photograph taken during an ovariohysterectomy in a gerbil. Right and left ovarian cysts can be observed. (*Courtesy of* Jaume Martorell, Spain.)

the tubular ovarian adenoma seen the most commonly.[16,17] In one study, 116 out of 5903 rats had this type of tumor. Approximately 74% of all ovarian tumors were of this type. It usually affected 1.9- to 2.3-year-old rats, whereby the tumor was grossly evident and appeared as a firm, lobulated mass with a unilateral, and occasionally bilateral, presentation. Other ovarian tumors described in this study were granulosa cell tumors (11.0%), thecal cell tumors (6.0%), malignant granulosa cell tumors (4.5%), ovarian mesotheliomas (2.0%), tubular adenocarcinomas (1.3%), papillary cystadenomas (1.3%), papillary cystadenocarcinomas (0.7%), and Sertoli cell tumors (0.7%).[16] Other tumors reported are sertoliform tubular adenomas, polycystic sex cord/stromal tumors, and lipoid cell tumors.[17] Another study of spontaneous neoplasm in Wistar rats showed that 74% of all neoplasms were in endocrine and reproductive systems; however, ovarian neoplasms represented only 2% (ovarian granulosa cell tumor).[18]

Mice commonly develop ovarian tumors.[19] Similar to rats, mice are a rodent carcinogenesis model. However, there are very few studies of spontaneous neoplasms without inducers. Tillman and colleagues[20] (2000) did a study in 631 untreated CBA/ J mice; 51 of the female mice had neoplastic lesions. Ovary tumors were found in 15.68% of cases. The mean age of the female mice was 94 weeks. Tumors of the ovary included tubulostromal adenomas (12.0%), benign granulosa cell tumors (3.0%), tubulostromal adenocarcinomas (0.34%), and benign mixed sex cord stromal tumors (0.34%).[20]

Ovarian tumors of the golden hamster are uncommon and are usually benign.[21] Unilateral granulosa cell or thecal cell tumors of the ovary are the most common reproductive system tumors in the hamster.[19]

In a study performed by Kondo and colleagues[22] (2008) on 85 hamsters, none of them had ovarian tumors.

The neoplastic incidence in gerbils more than 2 years of age is high, from 8.4% to 26.5%. Ovarian tumors are the most common (**Fig. 3**). They include granulosa, thecal and luteal cell tumors, dysgerminomas, and teratomas.[12,19]

Ultrasonography can help in the diagnosis of the disease (**Fig. 4**). The definitive treatment of ovarian disease is ovariectomy. A dorsal approach to the ovary has been recommended in rodents; it diminishes the gastrointestinal tract manipulation.[23] Ovariectomized rats had a lower incidence of mammary and pituitary tumors than intact rats with a greater rate of survival (day 630); however, they had a greater predisposition to osteopenia as well.[24] The author recommends performing ovariohysterectomy in rats older than 6 months, although the lesion is located in the ovary.

Diseases of the Uterus

Pyometra, mucometra, metritis, and endometritis

Although the literature states that pyometra is rare in small rodents, the number of cases seen by the author is increasing every year (**Fig. 5**). The role of progesterone in the etiopathogenesis of pyometra in rodents is not known. A study about the pathogenicity of anaerobic bacteria in a rat pyometra model showed that the growth of bacteria, such as *Prevotella bivia* end *Escherichia coli*, was promoted by estrogen but not by progesterone.[25] On the other hand, some strains of rats are less sensitive to estrogen's effects; Sprague-Dawley rats did not developed pyometra after estrogen administration.[26] *Mycoplasma pulmonis* is a pathogenic bacterium of the respiratory tract of rats and mice. It causes respiratory tract infections, but some strains of rats and mice are highly susceptible to genital disease.[5,11,13] In such cases, purulent endometritis, pyometra, and perioophoritis can be observed. In mice, some presentations include infertility, reduced fertility, and early abortions.[13] Mousepox virus can cause

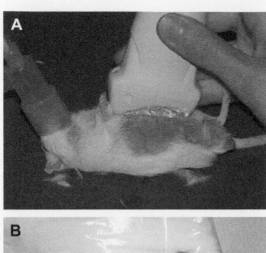

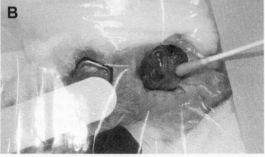

Fig. 3. A gerbil with an ovarian granulosa cell tumor. (*A*) Abdominal ultrasonography. (*B*) A laparotomy in a gerbil; the ovarian granulosa cell tumor is exposed. (*Courtesy of* Jaume Martorell, Spain.)

high mortality among adult mice, whereby many tissues can be affected; inclusion bodies, inflammation, and erosion have been observed in various mucosal regions.[27] For example, *Pasteurella pneumotropica* can colonize the vagina and the uterus without disease, whereas the litter can be infected.[27]

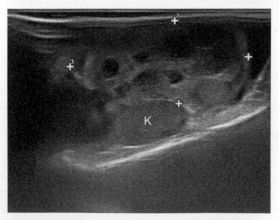

Fig. 4. Ultrasonographic image of a gerbil with an ovarian granulosa cell tumor. An irregular mass showing areas of medium echogenicity and hypoechoic areas. The mass is close to the kidney (K). (*Courtesy of* Adrian Melero, Spain.)

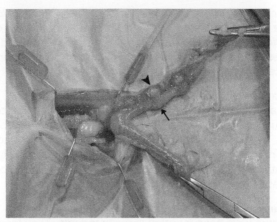

Fig. 5. A laparotomy in a rat with a pyometra. The right uterus is enlarged (*arrow*), and some abscess attached to the serosa can be observed (*arrowhead*). (*Courtesy of* Jaume Martorell, Spain.)

Pyometra has been observed in clinically ill hamsters[3,9] and gerbils.[28] Care must be taken not to misinterpret pus from a pyometra with the normal postovulatory white discharge of female hamsters that occurs at the end of the estrous cycle.[29]

Pyometra may be seen in chipmunks; affected animals may present with vulval discharge that is sometimes tinged with blood, anorexia, lethargy, and polydipsia. Metritis may be seen shortly after parturition, with females presenting as collapsed and weakened with a swollen abdomen and signs of peritonitis.[13]

Ultrasonography and cytology could help to confirm the diagnosis of a pyometra (**Fig. 6**); the definitive treatment is an ovariohysterectomy.[29] A detailed description on how to perform this surgery in rodents can be found in the literature.[9] Pisu and colleagues[30] (2012) described a case of pyometra in a golden hamster that was successfully treated with 2 doses of aglepristone combined with antibiotics. In dogs, aglepristone is an alternative to surgical treatment or it can be administered before surgery in order to improve the general condition of patients.[31]

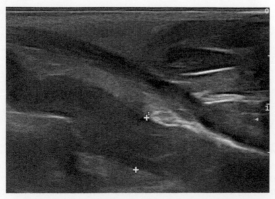

Fig. 6. Abdominal ultrasound of a rat with pyometra. The uterus is distended and full of hypoechoic to anechoic content (*between calipers*). (*Courtesy of* Jaume Martorell, Spain.)

Mucometra is common in some strains of mice, including BALA/c, B6, and DBA. Vaginal septa are often a frequent occurrence in some inbred lines of mice.[32] Some mice have imperforated vaginas, caused by the retained fluid produced during the estrous cycles, resulting in uterine and vaginal distension. This syndrome is inherited as a complex recessive genetic defect.[27,32]

Cystic endometrial hyperplasia

Cystic endometrial hyperplasia (CEH) can be associated with aging but also with hormonal changes, usually high estrogens levels. CEH may occur in obesity, polycystic ovary syndrome, estrogen-producing tumors, and estrogen replacement therapy. CEH is a common finding in aged female rodents (**Fig. 7**), especially in mice. It may be associated with secondary *Klebsiella oxytoca* pyometra.[27] In laboratory rodents, CHE has been described in hermaphrodite mice.[33]

Tumors of the uterus

Tumors of the uterus have been reported in many rodents. They tend to be benign in rats and malignant in hamsters and gerbils.[19]

Benign endometrial stromal tumors occur in up to 66% of some strains of rats older than 21 months; these are more common in virgin rats than in breeding females.[9] Endometrial stromal polyps represented 9.6% of the neoplasms in female Wistar rats.[18]

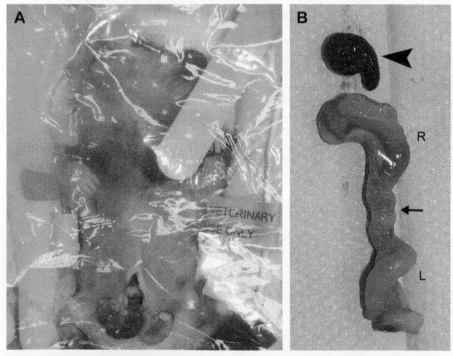

Fig. 7. A hamster with a uterine hemorrhage secondary to a chronic cystic endometrial hyperplasia. (*A*) Photograph taken during the surgery; uterus is exposed. Right uterine horn is dark and full of blood. (*B*) The uterus after the ovariohysterectomy. The clot from the right horn (R) was removed (*arrowhead*). The cervix (*arrow*) and the left horn are shown (L). (*Courtesy of* Jaume Martorell, Spain.)

Histiocytic sarcomas are common in aged B6 and SJL mice. They affect tissues such as the liver, spleen, uterus, vagina, kidney, lung, and ovaries.[27] In CBA/J mice, uterus neoplasia represented less the 1.5% of the neoplasms in females; they were leiomyosarcoma, stromal sarcoma, and adenocarcinoma (**Figs. 8** and **9**).[20]

In Syrian and Chinese hamsters, uterine adenocarcinoma is the most common uterine tumor (**Fig. 10**).[9] They usually affect animals older than 1.9 years. The process presents with vaginal hemorrhagic discharge.[19] These tumors can metastasize. Surgical treatment is recommended; however, the tumor can be spread by implantation of malignant cells during surgery. Other reproductive tract tumors described in hamsters are endometrial polyps, leiomyomas, leiomyosarcomas, cervical carcinomas, and squamous papillomas of the vagina.[19] In the study from Kondo and colleagues[22] (2008), only one of the 85 hamsters had a reproductive neoplasm: uterine leiomyosarcoma (excluding the mammary gland).

Adenocarcinoma of the oviduct, uterus, and leiomyoma has also been described in gerbils.[19]

Any cause of uterine or vaginal disease can predispose to a tissue prolapse. Patients usually present with abdominal distention, and abdominal viscera are displaced cranially because of the presence of enlarged reproductive organs (see **Fig. 9**). Radiology and ultrasonography are very useful in the diagnosis of the uterine diseases, especially when the uterus appears distended or enlarged.

Dystocia

Clinical signs of dystocia include vaginal discharge (bloody, green, or brown in color), abdominal swelling, or an impacted fetus protruding from the vulva.[28] Some species

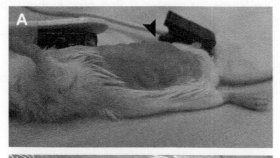
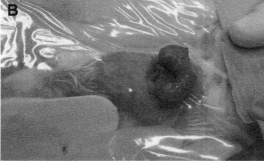

Fig. 8. A mouse with a uterine leiomyosarcoma. (*A*) The preparation for the surgical procedure. Abdominal distension is noticed (*arrowhead*). (*B*) Uterus is exposed; an enlargement of the uterus can be observed due to a uterine leiomyosarcoma. (*Courtesy of* Jaume Martorell, Spain.)

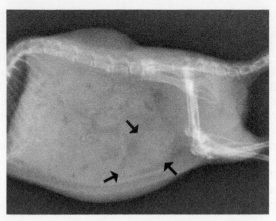

Fig. 9. Radiographs of the mouse in **Fig. 8** with a uterine leiomyosarcoma. An irregular mass displacing the rest of abdominal viscera can be observed (*arrows*). (*Courtesy of* Jaume Martorell, Spain.)

are prone to cannibalism, such as hamsters, mice, and rats.[28] Disturbing the female during parturition, close observation, like an excessive worrying owner, or newborn handling can be contraindicated because it may predispose to this behavior,[28] especially in the hamster[29]; low environmental temperatures, lean diets, and low body weight can contribute to cannibalism as well. In gerbils, cannibalism can occur when the size of the litter is very small, no suitable nesting area is found, animals are disturbed, or the female has mastitis.[28] Parturition in these species is usually completed within 1 to 2 hours.[28]

Dystocias are uncommon in rats, mice,[13] and the other species treated in this article.[8,28]

If it occurs, the procedure to follow can be extrapolated from other species recommendations. The surgical treatment of a hysterotomy is the most recommended, but

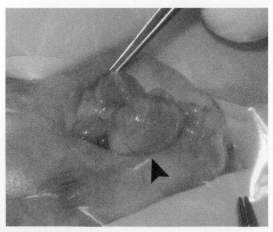

Fig. 10. A hamster with a uterine adenocarcinoma (*arrowhead*). (*Courtesy of* Jaume Martorell, Spain.)

an ovariohysterectomy would be the best definitive treatment after removing the fetus or fetuses.

One case of caesarean section has been described in a gerbil.[34] Male and female gerbils have a sebaceous gland located midventrally on the abdomen near the umbilicus; the skin incision should be made paramedially to avoid the gland and undermine the skin to expose the linea alba.[9]

Mammary Gland Diseases

Mastitis

Rats and mice are the mastitis rodent model. In rats, one mammary gland is usually affected. It can be ulcerated (**Fig. 11**). *P pneumotropica* and *Staphylococcus aureus* are most commonly cultured in laboratory rats.[35,36] Predisposing factors are dirty environments, abrasive material bedding, inappropriate size and equipment cage, biting puppies, and mammary impaction.

Mastitis in hamsters is common; streptococcal and coliform mastitis have been described in the golden hamster.[37,38]

Mastitis is uncommon in chipmunks; but bacteria, such as *E coli, Klebsiella* spp, and *Staphylococcus* spp, have been isolated.[13]

Treatment of the mastitis is based on the culture and antibiotic sensitivity; however, fluoroquinolones or sulfamides can be used as a first-choice antibiotic. All these patients should be treated with analgesics and supported treatment.

Tumors of the mammary gland

Mammary tumors are a very common neoplasm of rats.[5] Although they occur more frequently in females, they can also occur in males. In rats, most mammary tumors are benign fibroadenomas; adenocarcinomas can appear but are uncommon. The incidence increases with age, especially after 18 months of age; however, the growth rate of these tumors is slow.[5] The study of Walsh and Poteracki[18] (1994) observed that

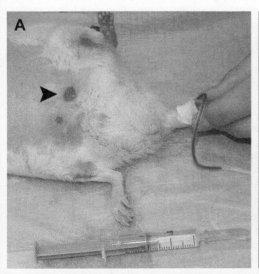
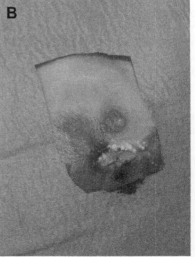

Fig. 11. (*A*) An ulcerated inguinal mammary gland (*arrowhead*) secondary to infection in a rat. (*B*) The surgery of a rat with a mastitis and abscess. A lateral skin incision was made to the ulcer; purulent material is going out of the mammary gland abscess. (*Courtesy of* Jaume Martorell, Spain.)

mammary tumors were the second most common neoplasm in Wistar rats; mammary fibroadenoma represented 25.3% of neoplasm in females and 1.0% in males and mammary adenocarcinoma 13.1% in females and 1.0% in males.[18] Mammary adenoma is included in the group of the neoplasms affecting less than 7% of the studied animals.[18]

As in previous descriptions,[6,24] it had been observed that spaying rats at 3 to 6 months of age had a protective effect against the formation of mammary tumors[24,39] and the development of pituitary tumors.[23] Increased incidence of mammary gland tumors is observed in rats with pituitary tumors, but the relation between them is difficult to determine.[5] There is a relationship between behavior, hormones, and mammary tumor development. Neophobic females (less exploratory behavior) develop palpable tumors earlier than neophilic females (more exploratory behavior).[40]

In mice, mammary gland tumors are very common as well.[19] In contrast to rats, 90% of mouse cases are malignant adenocarcinoma and fibrosarcoma[6]; they usually metastasize to the lung.[19] The tumor incidence depends on the mouse strain. Tillman and colleagues[20] (2000) reported only 3% of mammary gland neoplasms in CBA/J mice, with adenocarcinoma as the most common. Some strains of mice can carry the mouse mammary tumor virus endogenously, a retrovirus. This virus predisposes the development of mammary gland adenocarcinoma. In mice, the prognosis is poor.[27] Furthermore, there is a relationship between the coat color and the spontaneous mammary tumor development in mice; mammary tumors occur significantly earlier in yellow mice than in nonyellow mice but with similar malignancy.[41]

Mammary gland tumors have been described in hamsters, particularly the Russian hamster. Although they seemed to be uncommon,[19] in posterior reports, mammary gland tumors were the most common integumentary tumor in the hamster. They represented 20% of neoplasia cases, especially in the Russian hamster; 9 out of 15 animals had adenomas and 6 had adenocarcinoma mammary gland tumors; they were between 18 and 32 months old, and only 2 hamsters were male.[22]

There are no descriptions about mammary gland tumors in gerbils in the literature.[42]

Mammary gland tumor reports are scarce in squirrels; however, one tumor resembling a malignant mixed mammary tumor was diagnosed in a gray squirrel.[43] They have been described in pet chipmunks as well. They are usually benign, with fibroadenomas the most commonly reported.[44] A case of a mammary gland adenocarcinoma with distant metastases in the lung and abdominal cavity has been described in an 8-year-old chipmunk. One of the abdominal metastatic masses compressed the ureter, causing a hydronephrosis.[45]

Mammary gland tumors can be very large and depending on the location can interfere with normal displacement, gate, and the ability to hold the food with the extremities, especially in rats and mice (**Figs. 12** and **13**). The mammary tissue extends from the axilla until the shoulders and from the inguinal area caudally. Mammary gland infection or abscesses can be associated with these tumors (**Figs. 14** and **15**). In hamsters, gerbils, and squirrels, mammary tissue is confined to the ventral thorax and abdomen; when the gland enlarges, the skin over it can sometimes ulcerate. Fine-needle aspiration cytology can help the diagnosis. An imaging study of the thorax and the abdomen will be needed to check metastases. Surgery to remove the affected mammary glands along with castration/spaying is the best treatment option. In rats, these tumors are firm and unattached to other structures, making removal easy via blunt dissection. However, tumors are likely to affect another mammary gland[11]; in contrast, in mice the tumors are highly vascular and infiltrative and the rate of recurrence is high.[19,29] In small animals, chemotherapy is administered as a treatment protocol, including the oral administration of a tyrosine kinase inhibitor,

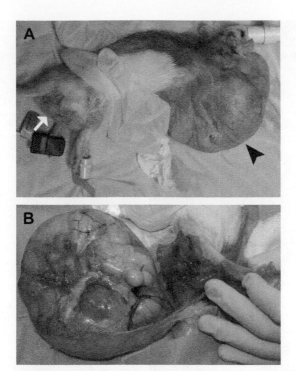

Fig. 12. A female rat with 2 mammary gland fibroadenomas. (*A*) The axillar fibroadenoma was very enlarged (*arrowhead*); it involved the right rear limb. The inguinal fibroadenoma was ulcerated caudally (*white arrow*). (*B*) The mass after blunt dissection; the limb could be completely separated from the mass. (*Courtesy of* Jaume Martorell, Spain.)

such as toceranib, and nonsteroidal antiinflammatory drugs, such as meloxicam. Dosages for rodents are usually extrapolated from other species' recommendations. Ovariectomy or ovariohysterectomy at a young age reduces the incidence of mammary tumors.

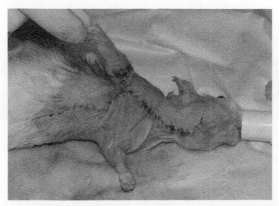

Fig. 13. The rat of **Fig. 12** after removal of the axillary fibroadenoma. (*Courtesy of* Jaume Martorell, Spain.)

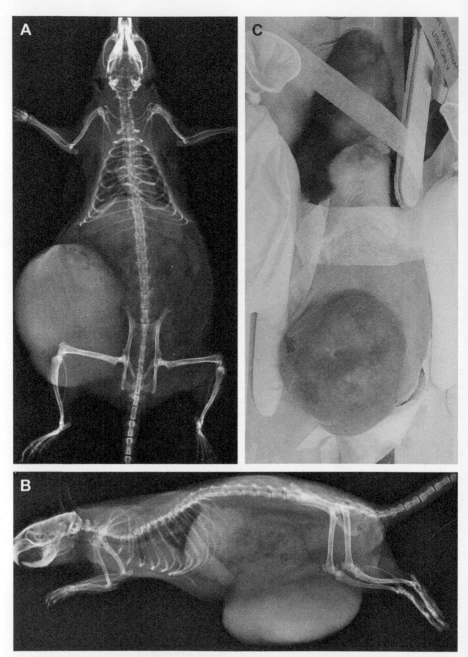

Fig. 14. (*A*) Ventrodorsal abdominal radiograph of a female rat with an inguinal mass. (*B*) Lateral abdominal radiographs of the same rat. (*C*) The rat with an inguinal mass before the surgery. (*Courtesy of* Jaume Martorell, Spain.)

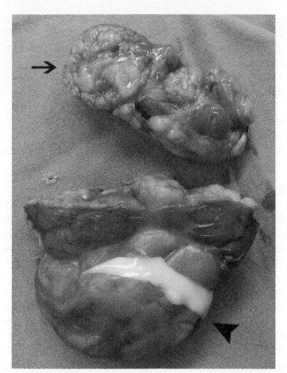

Fig. 15. The inguinal mass of the rat of **Fig. 14**. The mass was transected. It was composed of a mammary fibroadenoma (*arrow*) and a mammary gland abscess (*arrowhead*). (*Courtesy of Jaume Martorell, Spain.*)

DISEASES OF MALE RODENTS
Urethral Plugs

Urethral plugs have been described in male rats, gerbils, golden hamsters, mice, and guinea pigs as a normal finding.[46] In fact, the presence of these plugs is correlated with good health.[47] One study describes that all healthy adult male rats surveyed presented with urethral plugs. Urethral plugs are composed of proteins I to V excreted by the seminal vesicles or vesicular gland mixed with vesiculase from the coagulating glands. The amino acid composition of the seminal vesicles' content and the urethral plug are very similar to the content of the copulatory vaginal plug in female rodents.[47]

If retro-ejaculation occurs, the plugs can be seen in the urinary bladder. They should not be mistaken with uroliths. Furthermore, the plug can cause a urethral obstruction in rats and mice.[6,46] The animals can present with dysuria and stranguria. Hydronephrosis secondary to an occlusive urethral plug has been suspected in mice.[48]

A routine orchidectomy is recommended at a young age, at 3 months old. Orchidectomy causes an involution of the penis and the male accessory sex glands along with a decrease in the size of the urethral plug, eliminating the risk of an obstruction.[9,46]

Diseases of the Testicles

Orchitis and epididymitis
Kilham rat virus is a DNA virus of the family Parvoviridae; laboratory and wild rats are the natural hosts. The virus is shed in the urine, feces, milk, and nasal secretions. The disease is usually subclinical; but affected animals can present with scrotal cyanosis

and hemorrhage, abdominal swelling, and dehydration. Pregnant rats may increase the number of reabsorbed fetuses. Histopathology reveals hemorrhagic infarction with thrombosis in the central nervous system, testes, and epididymis along with multifocal liver necrosis. Diagnosis is made by serologic assay or immunocytochemistry on affected tissue.[5] *Streptococcus pneumoniae* can cause orchitis in rats; other lesions include fibrinopurulent bronchopneumonia, pleuritic, pericarditis, peritonitis, and meningitis.[5]

Infectious or inflammatory processes affecting the testicles seem to be underreported in other rodents. A case of unilateral orchidectomy and scrotal ablation for recurrent testicular abscess was described in a 1.5-year-old male pet golden Syrian hamster.[49]

Testicle neoplasia

The incidence of testicular neoplasia varies between strains and colonies of rats. The most common reproductive tumor and third most common tumor overall is the testicular interstitial cell tumor (Leydig cell tumor). These tumors are usually benign, can be bilateral, and have been associated with hypercalcemia. There is a high incidence of interstitial cell tumors in strains such as Fischer 344 and ACI/N rats.[5,19] However this kind of tumor represented a low percentage of neoplasms in Wistar rats.[18]

In mice, testicular interstitial cell tumors are the most common[19]; however, testicular tumors were not observed in CBA/J mice.[20] These data suggest that the development of neoplasms is strain related. Prostatic diseases in mice are very uncommon. Only one case of prostatic adenocarcinoma has been reported in mice.[19]

Male reproductive tumors are infrequent in hamsters.[19] Reports of testicular and secondary sex glands in hamster are seminomas, adenoma of the rete testis, prostatic adenocarcinoma, bulbourethral gland adenoma and cystadenocarcinoma, and epididymal adenoma and adenocarcinoma.[50]

The prevalence of tumors in gerbils older than 2 years is high. Tumors of the testicles and the secondary sexual glands of male gerbils include seminoma, teratoma, and prostatic adenoma.[6,19,51]

The recommended treatment of any testicular disease usually includes an orchiectomy (**Fig. 16**).

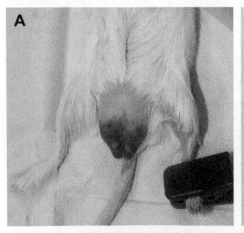 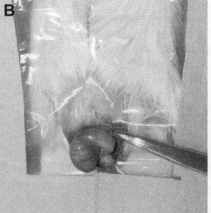

Fig. 16. An orchidectomy in an adult male gerbil. (*A*) Animal is prepared to perform the scrotal orchidectomy. (*B*) Photograph taken during the orchidectomy. A skin incision was made on the left scrotum. The left testicle is observed. (*Courtesy of* Jaume Martorell, Spain.)

Table 2
The most common reproductive tract disease in rats, mice, hamsters, gerbils, and squirrels

Organ/Species	Rats	Mice	Hamsters	Gerbils	Squirrels
Ovary	Tubular ovarian adenoma Granulosa cell tumor	Tubulostromal ovarian adenomas	Ovarian cysts	Ovarian cysts and granulosa, thecal, and luteal ovarian cell tumors	Uncommon
Uterus	Pyometra Benign endometrial stromal tumor	Pyometra Cystic endometrial hyperplasia	Pyometra Uterine adenocarcinoma	Pyometra	Pyometra
Mammary gland	Fibroma, fibroadenoma	Adenocarcinoma and fibrosarcoma	Adenoma and adenocarcinoma	Uncommon	Fibroadenomas
Testicle	Interstitial cell tumor	Interstitial cell tumor	Uncommon	Uncommon	Uncommon

SUMMARY

In summary, reproductive disorders are common in small rodents. The most common reproductive tract diseases in rodents are shown in **Table 2**. Many clinical presentations have been described related to rodents' reproductive disease. Unspecific clinical signs include apathy and anorexia; specific clinical signs are abdominal distension, subcutaneous masses with or without ulcerated skin, vaginal discharge (mucus, pus, or hemorrhage), and vaginal/uterine prolapse. A fast diagnosis and treatment can help to increase the survival rate of patients. Inflammatory, infectious, and neoplastic processes are very common in small rodents. Radiographs and ultrasound will help identify ovarian and uterine abnormalities in females and testicular, accessory sexual gland diseases in males, and cutaneous masses in both sexes. Fine-needle aspiration cytology or a biopsy will help to confirm the diagnosis. In many cases, the definitive treatment requires a surgery. Ovariectomy, ovariohysterectomy, castration, and mass excision are the most common procedures.

REFERENCES

1. Miedel EL, Hankenson FC. Biology and diseases of hamsters. In: Fox J, Anderson L, Loew F, et al, editors. Laboratory animal medicine. 2nd edition. Elsevier Inc; 2015. p. 209–45.

2. Otto G, Franklin C, Clifford C. Biology and diseases of rats. In: Fox J, Anderson L, Loew F, et al, editors. Laboratory animal medicine. 2nd edition. Elsevier Inc; 2015. p. 151–207.

3. Lennox AM, Bauck L. Basic anatomy, physiology, husbandry, and clinical techniques. In: Quesenberry K, Carpenter J, editors. Ferrets, rabbits, and rodents: clinical medicine and surgery. 3rd edition. Elsevier; 2012. p. 339–53.

4. Banzato T, Bellini L, Contiero B, et al. Abdominal anatomic features and reference values determined by use of ultrasonography in healthy common rats (Rattus norvegicus). Am J Vet Res 2014;75:67–76.

5. Sharp P, LaRegina M. The laboratory rat. In: Suckow M, editor. A volume in the laboratory animal pocket reference series. CRC Press LL; 1998. p. 1–167.

6. Sayers I, Smith S. Mice, rats, hamsters and gerbils. In: Meredith A, Johnson-Delaney C, editors. BSAVA Manual of exotic pet. Fifth. British Small Animal Veterinary Association; 2010. p. 1–27.

7. Tully TN. Mice and rats. In: Mitchell MA, Tully TN, editors. Manual of exotic pet practice. Elsevier Inc; 2009. p. 326–44.

8. McLaughlin A, Strunk A. Common emergencies in small rodents, hedgehogs, and sugar gliders. Vet Clin North Am Exot Anim Pract 2016;19:465–99.

9. Bennett RA. Soft tissue surgery. In: Ferrets, rabbits and rodents: clinical medicine and surgery. 3rd edition. Elsevier; 2012. p. 326–37.

10. Gozukara IO, Pınar N, Ozcan O, et al. Effect of colchicine on polycystic ovary syndrome: an experimental study. Arch Gynecol Obstet 2016;293:675–80.

11. Percy DH, Barthold SW. Rats. In: Percy DH, Barthold SW, editors. Pathology of laboratory rodents and rabbits. 3rd edition. Ames (IA): Blackwell Publishing; 2007. p. 125–77.

12. Lewis W. Cystic ovaries in gerbils. Exot DVM 2003;5:12–3.

13. Girling SJ. Common diseases of small mammals. In: Girlgling S, editor. Veterinary nursing of exotics pets. 2nd edition. Willey-Blackwell; 2013. p. 59–90.

14. Bean AD. Ovarian cysts in the guinea pig (Cavia porcellus). Vet Clin North Am Exot Anim Pract 2013;16:757–76.

15. Schuetzenhofer G, Goericke-Pesch S, Wehrend A. Effects of deslorelin implants on ovarian cysts in guinea pigs. Schweiz Arch Tierheilkd 2011;153:416–7.
16. Gregson R, Lewis D, Abbott D. Spontaneous ovarian neoplasms of the laboratory rat. Vet Pathol 1984;21:292–9.
17. Lewis DJ. Ovarian neoplasia in the Sprague-Dawley rat. Environ Health Perspect 1987;73:77–90.
18. Walsh K, Poteracki J. Spontaneous neoplasms in control Wistar rats. Fundam Appl Toxicol 1994;22:65–72.
19. Greenacre CB. Spontaneous tumors of small mammals. Vet Clin North Am Exot Anim Pract 2004;7:627–51, vi.
20. Tillman T, Kamino K, Mohr U. Incidence and spectrum of spontaneous neoplasms in male and female CBA/J mice. Exp Toxicol Pathol 2000;52:221–5.
21. Heatley JJ, Harris MC. Hamsters and gerbils. In: Mitchell MA, Tully TN, editors. Manual of exotic pet practice. Elsevier Inc.; 2009. p. 406–32.
22. Kondo H, Onuma M, Shibuya H, et al. Spontaneous tumors in domestic hamsters. Vet Pathol 2008;680:674–80.
23. Stout Steele M, Bennett RA. Clinical technique: dorsal ovariectomy in rodents. J Exot Pet Med 2011;20:222–6.
24. Hotchkiss C. Effect of surgical removal of subcutaneous tumors on survival of rats. J Am Vet Med Assoc 1995;206:1575–9.
25. Mikamo H, Kawazoe K, Izumi K, et al. Studies on the pathogenicity of anaerobes, especially Prevotella bivia, in a rat pyometra model. Infect Dis Obstet Gynecol 1998;6:61–5.
26. Brossia LJ, Roberts CS, Lopez JT, et al. Interstrain differences in the development of pyometra after estrogen treatment of rats. J Am Assoc Lab Anim Sci 2009;48:517–20.
27. Percy DH, Barthold SW. Mouse. In: Percy DH, Barthold SW, editors. Pathology of laboratory rodents and rabbits. 3rd edition. Ames (IA): Blackwell Publishing; 2007. p. 3–124.
28. Jackson P. Dystocia in other species. In: Jackson PG, editor. Handbook of veterinary obstetrics. 2nd edition. Elsevier Inc; 2004. p. 167–72.
29. Brown C, Donnelly TM. Disease problems of small rodents. In: Quesenberry K, Carpenter james W, editors. Ferrets, rabbits and rodents clinical medicine and surgery. 3rd edition. Elsevier; 2012. p. 354–72.
30. Pisu MC, Andolfatto A, Veronesi MC. Pyometra in a six-month-old nulliparous golden hamster (Mesocricetus auratus) treated with aglepristone. Vet Q 2012;32:179–81.
31. Gogny A, Fiéni F. Aglepristone: a review on its clinical use in animals. Theriogenology 2016;85:555–66.
32. Ginty I, Hoogstraten-Miller S. Perineal swelling in a mouse. Lab Anim (NY) 2008;37:196–9.
33. McIntyre A, La Perle KM. Hermaphroditism in 3 chimeric mice. Vet Pathol 2007;44:249–52.
34. Mighell J, Baker A. Caesarean section in a gerbil. Vet Rec 1990;126:441.
35. Hong C, Ediger R. Chronic necrotizing mastitis in rats caused by Pasteurella pneumotropica. Lab Anim Sci 1978;28:317–20.
36. Kunstytl I, Ernst H, Lenz W. Granulomatous dermatitis and mastitis in two SPF rats associated with a slowly growing Staphylococcus aureus-a case report. Lab Anim 1995;29:177–9.
37. Frisk C, Wagner JE, Owens DR. Streptococcal mastitis in golden hamsters. Lab Anim Sci 1976;26:97.

38. Huerkamp M, Dillehey DL. Coliform mastitis in a golden Syrian hamster. Lab Anim Sci 1990;40:325–7.
39. Planas-Silva MD, Rutherford TM, Stone MC. Prevention of age-related spontaneous mammary tumors in outbred rats by late ovariectomy. Cancer Detect Prev 2008;32:65–71.
40. Cavigelli SA, Yee JR, McClintock MK. Infant temperament predicts life span in female rats that develop spontaneous tumors. Horm Behav 2006;50:454–62.
41. Little C. The relation of coat color to the spontaneous incidence of mammary tumors in mice. J Exp Med 1934;59:229–50.
42. Rowe S, Simmons J, Ringler D, et al. Spontaneous neoplasms in aging gerbillinae: a summary of forty four neoplasms. Vet Pathol 1974;11:38–51.
43. Shivaprasad H, Sundberg J, Ely R. Malignant mixed (carcinosarcoma) mammary tumor in a gray squirrel. Vet Pathol 1984;21:115–7.
44. Johnson-Delaney C. Chipmunks and prairie dogs. In: Meredith A, Johnson-Delaney C, editors. BSAVA Manual of exotic pet. 5th edition. British Small Animal Veterinary Association; 2010. p. 63–75.
45. Oohashi E, Kangawa A, Kobayashi Y. Mammary adenocarcinoma in a chipmunk (Tamias sibiricus). J Vet Med Sci 2009;71:677–9.
46. Lejnieks DV. Urethral plug in a rat (Rattus norvegicus). J Exot Pet Med 2007;16:183–5.
47. Kunstýr I, Küpper W, Weisser H, et al. Urethral plug–a new secondary male sex characteristic in rat and other rodents. Lab Anim 1982;16:151–5.
48. Ninomiya H, Inomata T, Ogihara K. Obstructive uropathy and hydronephrosis in male KK-Ay mice: a report of cases. J Vet Med Sci 1999;61:53–7.
49. Johns J, George R, Anoopkumar T, et al. Unilateral orchidectomy and scrotal ablation for recurrent testicular abscess in a hamster. Int J Adv Res 2014;2:654–5.
50. Strandberg J. Neoplastic diseases. In: Van Hoosier G, McPerson C, editors. Laboratory hamster. 1st edition. Academic Press, Inc; 1987. p. 157–68.
51. Vincent AL, Ash LR. Further observations on spontaneous neoplasms in the Mongolian gerbil, Meriones unguiculatus. Lab Anim Sci 1978;28:297–300.

Reproductive Medicine in Guinea Pigs, Chinchillas and Degus

Leonie Kondert, Dr med vet,
Jörg Mayer, Dr med vet, MSc, DABVP (ECM), DECZM (Small Mammal), DACZM*

KEYWORDS

• Guinea pigs • Chinchillas • Degus • Reproductive medicine

KEY POINTS

- In-depth knowledge of the anatomy and physiology of the reproductive tract of hystrico-morph rodents is important, as they are commonly presented as exotic pets in veterinary practice.
- Careful assessment and choosing the right anesthesia protocol is the key stone to a successful outcome of surgery. Procedures like spays and neuters, C-sections or mastectomies can be performed on a routine basis.
- Performing in depth diagnostics is helpful in making the decision, if a reproductive problem can be managed medically or needs surgical intervention.

INTRODUCTION

Guinea pigs, chinchillas, and degus are hystricomorph rodents originating from South America. A moderate climate and grassland vegetation have significantly influenced their development.[1,2] Nowadays they are commonly presented as exotic pets in veterinary practice. A lot of data has been generated from their traditional use as laboratory animals.[1,3] However, after purchasing or acquiring a rodent in a pet store, most clients do not consider seeing a veterinarian for a wellness examination right away.[4] Preventive medicine is an area in which veterinarians have to provide a better client educational experience in the future. Objectively, anesthetic procedures in small mammals can be challenging and can be associated with the risk of complications,[5,6] which may be why a lot of small rodents are intact.[7] A recent study evaluating common diseases in guinea pigs shows that problems with the genital system are the third most common reason for presentation at a veterinary clinic.[8] In the degu, reproductive problems are the fifth most common reason for seeing a veterinarian.[9] This article

Disclosure: The authors have nothing to disclose.
Department of Small Animal Medicine and Surgery, College of Veterinary Medicine, University of Georgia, 2200 College Station Road, Athens, GA 30602, USA
* Corresponding author.
E-mail address: mayerj@uga.edu

Vet Clin Exot Anim 20 (2017) 609–628
http://dx.doi.org/10.1016/j.cvex.2016.11.014
1094-9194/17/© 2016 Elsevier Inc. All rights reserved.
vetexotic.theclinics.com

provides a short review of common diseases of the reproductive system of the 3 species, including diagnostics and treatment.

Originating from South America these small rodents share several features when it comes to reproduction. These features include the following[1,10,11]:

- Hystricomorph rodents are characterized by long gestation periods and estrus cycles (**Table 1**).
- Females have a vaginal closure membrane that resolves in healthy animals during estrus and parturition.
- A copulatory plug, a solid waxy mass, formed by coagulated ejaculate and sloughed vaginal epithelium can be found in the vagina after copulation.
- Males do not have a true scrotum; their testes are situated in a parascrotal sac inguinally or intra-abdominally.
- Their offspring are born with open eyes and are fully furred.

Guinea Pigs (Cavia Aperea f. Porcellus)

Reproductive behavior, or age of first conception, occurs at an average age of 2 months in female and 3 months in male guinea pigs.[10,11,17] Guinea pigs are polyestrous, their cycle is 15 to 17 days long, and they breed all year round with spontaneous ovulation.[11,18] Length of gestation is described to be between 59 and 72 days. On average they give birth to 2 to 4 cavies (**Fig. 1**). The birthing process should last no longer than 15 to 40 minutes. Guinea pigs have a unique form of gonadotrophin-releasing hormone (GnRH) that is different from mammalian GnRH. Guinea pig GnRH (GpGnRH) is the major neuropeptide in the guinea pig brain and it is characterized by a weaker binding affinity to GnRH receptors. Therefore, gpGnRh has a markedly lower activity to stimulate luteinizing hormone release.[19]

Male guinea pigs are characterized by their special reproductive anatomy. Like other hystricomorph rodents they have a prescrotal sac instead of a true scrotum. The open inguinal canal enables their testes to be intra-abdominal, inguinal, or located in the prescrotal sac. Their prominent testes are located bilaterally of the anus in connection with a large fat body. Their penis is stabilized by an os penis, which is situated dorsal to their urethra. The glans penis is spiculated (with little spikes on the surface) ventrally. Sebaceous glands are found bilaterally in the fold of perineal skin located next to the penis.[30]

Table 1
Gestation periods of hystricomorph rodents (including guinea pigs, chinchillas, and degus) compared with other small mammals

Species	Gestation Period (d)
Guinea pig (*Cavia aperea f. porcellus*)	59–72[11]
Chinchilla (*Chinchilla lanigera*)	105–120[12]
Degu (*Octodon degus*)	90[1]
Ferret (*Mustela putorius furo*)	41–43[13]
Black tailed prairie dog (*Cynomys ludovicianus*)	34–37[14]
Sugar glider (*Petaurus breviceps*)	15–17[15]
Golden hamster (*Mesocricetus auratus*)	15–18[16]
Gerbil (*Meriones unguiculatus*)	23–26[16]
White mouse (*Mus musculus*)	19–21[16]
Rat (*Rattus norvegicus*)	21–23[16]

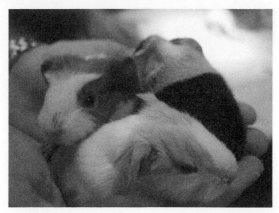

Fig. 1. A litter of guinea pig pups just a few hours after birth, which is typical for a precocial species. They can also consume solid food on the same day they are born.

SPAY AND NEUTER

Clients should be educated when presenting their pets for their annual health examination that spaying or neutering their guinea pigs can help with fertility management and behavioral problems, and prevent development of reproductive disease. Several different techniques can be used. In the boar, a scrotal or abdominal approach is described. There is a significantly lower risk of wound infections in guinea pigs neutered via an abdominal approach.[21] In females, ovariohysterectomy can be performed via a standard abdominal approach. The laparoscopic technique is found more commonly nowadays because it provides the advantages of a less invasive approach and smaller incisions. With this technique the ovaries are removed bilaterally. Prevention of uterine disorders cannot be guaranteed after the procedure.

CYSTS OF THE RETE OVARII

Ovarian cystic disease has a high incidence in intact female guinea pigs and is the most common disease of the reproductive tract.[8,22,23] Published percentages on prevalence vary from 58% to 100% and depend on study population, sample size, and diagnostic tests. The affected sows are, on average, 3 months to 5 years old.[24] Clinical symptoms include weight loss, abdominal distension, anorexia, depression, and nonpruritic symmetric alopecia of the flank region[22,23] (**Fig. 2**). In addition, cystic endometrial disease can be present in some of the females with ovarian cystic disease (**Fig. 3**). Some cavies are clinically asymptomatic, if the cysts are not hormonally active or detected when they are at a small size.[8] Diagnostics include abdominal palpation, radiographs, and abdominal ultrasonography (**Fig. 4**). Ultrasonography is the most accurate noninvasive diagnostic tool used for the differentiation of ovarian cysts, trichobezoars, or abdominal neoplasms.[25] Granulosa cell tumors are rare in guinea pigs but should always be on the list for the differential diagnosis.[23] Additional blood work to check on increased estradiol levels can be considered. Ovariohysterectomy is the treatment of choice for ovarian cystic disease. Ultrasonography-guided fine-needle aspiration of cyst fluid is commonly performed. However, the fluid reaccumulates within a few days to weeks.[17] A publication by Erwingmann and Gloeckner[26] in 2005 mentioned that, if the cyst ruptures during the aspiration process, no negative consequences are observed. However, a more recent unpublished study by Kohutova[27] in 2016 described severe

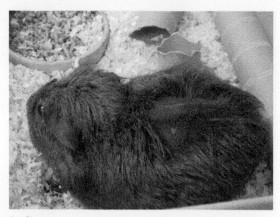

Fig. 2. Ovarian cystic disease.

complications, including the death of 10 guinea pigs, caused by hormonal overload. Ovarian hormone levels in cystic fluid are commonly 3 to 10 times higher than in plasma/serum.

Preferably, treatment should be performed with GnRH injections, if a surgical approach is declined. GnRH injections at a dose of 0.020 mg per animal every 14 days are effective in the author's (JM) experience. In general, the treatment prognosis for ovarian cystic disease is considered good. The author (JM) has tried deslorelin implants without a significant effect and no longer recommends trying this treatment approach. This observation was also mentioned in a published study in which it was noted that the size of the ovarian cysts in 11 guinea pigs did not vary significantly during the treatment (**Fig. 5**).[28]

NEOPLASMS OF THE REPRODUCTIVE TRACT

Neoplasms of the reproductive tract have been described as another common disease of the reproductive tract in guinea pigs.[8] Uterine leiomyomas are the most

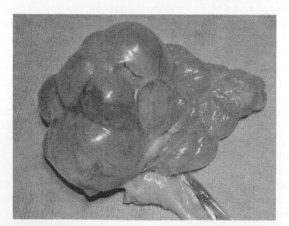

Fig. 3. The right ovary of a 5-year-old guinea pig with multiple cysts. The size of the ovary was 8 × 6 × 5 cm. Large cysts can also act as space-occupying masses. Histopathologic examination determined these to be rete ovarii cysts. (*Courtesy of* Vladimir Jekl, DVM, PhD, DipECZM, Brno, Czech Republic.)

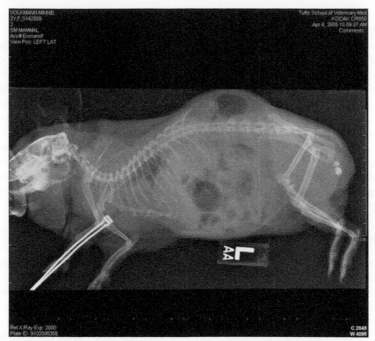

Fig. 4. This lateral whole-body radiograph is from a female guinea pig with ovarian cysts. Note how these can be difficult (if not impossible) to see on plain radiographs. An abdominal ultrasonography examination is the diagnostic method of choice in suspect cases. Also, note the caudally located uroliths, which can often be missed if the radiographs are collimated down or if the animal is restrained with lead gloves.

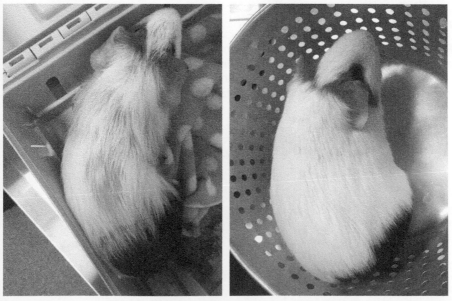

Fig. 5. Note the alopecia over the back (*left image*) caused by ovarian problems. The same animals a few weeks after successful therapy with 2 GnRH injections 10 days apart; note the improved hair coat (*right side*).

common neoplasm described to be associated with the reproductive tract in female guinea pigs (**Fig. 6**).[29,30]

A strong correlation between the occurrence of leiomyomas and a hormonally active cystic rete ovarii has been recognized.[23] However, the frequency of ovarian cysts is significantly higher than that of reproductive tumors. The cause of this phenomenon might be that many ovarian cysts are not hormonally active and do not have a negative impact on the uterine tissues. The neoplasms mainly consist of smooth muscle and fibrous connective tissue and are located in the uterine body or horn. Long-term high levels of estrogen seem to have a strong influence on their development.[31] Clinical symptoms can include hemorrhagic vaginal discharge or they can be asymptomatic. With abdominal palpation, neoplastic changes in the uterus can be detected. However, an abdominal ultrasonography examination is the tool of choice to diagnose changes of the reproductive tract (**Fig. 7**). Ovariohysterectomy via a ventral midline approach is the treatment of choice for neoplasms of the reproductive tract.

MAMMARY GLAND TUMORS

In a recently published study by Mikanova and colleagues,[8] diagnosis of mammary gland tumors occurred in 13 cases out of 1000 guinea pigs presented at an exotic pet clinic. Both male and female guinea pigs can be affected, although the prevalence is significantly higher in older age groups and males.[8,32] Several studies report that a large percentage of mammary tumors are benign.[33] Fibroadenomas, adenocarcinomas,[34] fibrosarcomas, tubulopapillary carcinomas, and solid carcinomas are described.[35] Surgical intervention is always advised. For prognosis and staging, thoracic radiographs and histopathology should be performed. One of the authors (JM) has removed multiple mammary adenocarcinomas from male guinea pigs that did not spread or show characteristics of malignancy after surgery. Prognosis seems to be guarded for these cases (**Fig. 8**).

PREGNANCY TOXEMIA

Pregnancy toxemia can be caused by a metabolic disorder mainly effecting obese sows, or by hemodynamic problems and uteroplacental ischemia.

The metabolic form is more common and develops from late pregnancy to early lactation. It is caused by starvation, dietary changes, environmental factors, and

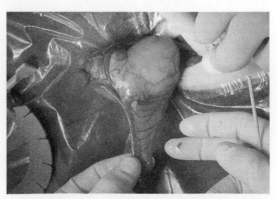

Fig. 6. A uterine leiomyoma in an elderly female guinea pig. There is often a close affiliation with the urinary bladder.

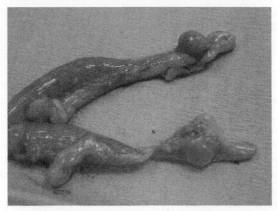

Fig. 7. Typical image of removed uterine tracts with bilateral cysts on the ovaries from a guinea pig.

stress. The sow is commonly presented as anorectic, dehydrated, and in severe cases laterally recumbent and dyspneic. Hypoglycemia (<60 mg/dL) can lead to convulsions and death. Performance of blood work and blood gas analysis is highly recommended. The hematologic changes include ketosis, hypoglycemia, and acidosis. Urine analysis can also be performed. Affected animals show proteinuria, ketonuria, and a pH of 5 to 6 (normal pH = 9).[33,36] Radiographs and abdominal ultrasonography show hepatic enlargement and gas-filled gastrointestinal tract. Treatment with intravenous fluids and glucose is essential. Feeding a high-caloric critical care rodent food, which contains readily available carbohydrates (Lafeber Emerald Herbivore Nutritional Care), every 2 to 3 hours is crucial.[37] After the patient is stable enough, a gradual change to a diet containing a larger amount of fiber is recommended. Pregnancy toxemia has a guarded to grave prognosis. Extensive client education about the needs of gravid sows is the best way to prevent the development of this disease.

The other form of pregnancy toxemia is caused by severe compression of the large blood vessels by the gravid uterus. Preeclampsia develops in late pregnancy. Ischemia of the uterus results in uterine necrosis, hypertension, proteinuria, and increased creatinine levels. If the condition is suspected, confirmation via blood

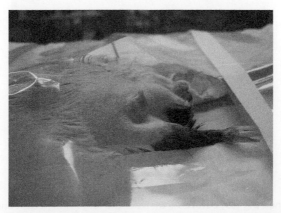

Fig. 8. Adenocarcinoma in a male guinea pig. Note the significant swelling of the teat.

work, radiographs, and abdominal ultrasonography is indicated. Emergency cesarean section must be performed immediately if confirmed.[38]

DYSTOCIA

Dystocia is seen in gravid females with large litter sizes, caused by female exhaustion or abnormally sized puppies.[8] Two cases of ectopic pregnancy were described as a rare reason for dystocia.[3] Under physiologic conditions the pubic symphysis is disconnected, to increase the width of the birth canal by up to 3 cm.[33] One of the authors (JM) has seen multiple events of older nulliparous females giving birth without any complications (**Fig. 9**). Whether breeding a female for the first time after the symphysis pubis has established results in dystocia is controversial. Predisposing factors for dystocia include obesity, hypovitaminosis C, abnormally large fetuses, uterine inertia, or mechanical obstruction.[34,39] Clients should be educated that continuous straining for 20 minutes or unproductive contractions for more than 2 hours is abnormal.[20] Bloody or green-brown vaginal discharge can be found in severe cases. Diagnostics include radiography to evaluate the size of the birth canal in relation to pup size and for exclusion of any mechanical obstruction. Abdominal ultrasonography is highly recommended to evaluate the heath of the young and the reproductive organs of the sow. Stabilization of the female in emergency situations includes treatment with warmed intravenous or intraosseous fluids (at 5–10 mL/kg/h), pain management (buprenorphine 0.01–0.05 mg/kg subcutaneously, intramuscularly, or intravenously 6–12 hours), thermoregulatory support, and providing a stress free environment.[40] First-line treatment, if uterine inertia is suspected, should include treatment with 5 to 10 mL of calcium gluconate in a 10% solution by mouth[41] and glucose 50% boluses 0.25 to 2 mL intravenously or by mouth.[37] If the patient does not respond with contractions, oxytocin (0.2–3 IU/kg subcutaneously with fluids) can be applied.[42] The authors

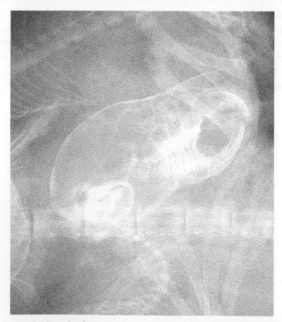

Fig. 9. A fetal guinea pig just before birth. Note the large skull, but it still passes through the pelvic canal.

advise against intramuscular injections of oxytocin/because of the potential for violent uterine contractions. If the drug is given by the subcutaneous route, the uptake might be slower, which might lead to a more natural and slower onset of uterine contractions.

When conservative treatment is not effective or in cases in which the pubic symphysis is less than 25 mm dilated, cesarean section should be performed.[33] Correction of electrolyte and fluid imbalances is crucial to the patient's stability during ovariohysterectomy.[43] The patient's owner should always be informed about the risk of anesthetic complications in an emergency situation.[7] An anesthetic protocol should be chosen according to the American Society of Anesthesiologists (ASA) standard. Premedication can be performed with an injectable combination of midazolam (1–2 mg/kg intramuscularly) and butorphanol (0.2–0.5 mg/kg intravenously or subcutaneously).[29] Premedication with fentanyl (5–20 µg/kg intravenously) provides another good option. Preoxygenation followed by mask induction and maintenance can be performed with sevoflurane or isoflorane.[33]

After the patient is prepared for surgery the abdomen is accessed via a ventral midline approach. Cesarean section can be performed, depending on the sow's condition. Because of the severe risks of surgery and anesthesia, the prognosis is guarded to poor (**Table 2**).

ENDOMETRITIS/PYOMETRA

Pyometra generally develops a few weeks after estrus or after delivery. Ovarian cysts can cause cystic endometrial hyperplasia, mucometra, or endometritis. Uterine infections can be caused by *Salmonella enterica*. Rare cases of infections caused by *Listeria monocytogenes* are described.[33] Under laboratory conditions it has been shown that infection with *Chlamydia caviae* can cause endometritis or salpingitis in the guinea pig (**Fig. 10**).[44] Clinical signs are depression, reduced food intake, purulent vaginal discharge, and hunched posture. Diagnostics include blood work, vaginal cytology, radiography, and abdominal ultrasonography.[45] If the female is not a breeding animal, ovariohysterectomy is the treatment of choice. In cases in which the patient's owner insists on breeding the animal in the future, treatment with aglepristone (10 mg/kg,

Table 2
Analgetic, sedative, and antiinflammatory drugs in small rodents[42]

	Dose	Caution
Buprenorphine	0.01–0.05 mg/kg SC, IM, or IV q 6–12 h	Do not combine with butorphanol, because of partial antagonistic effects
Butorphanol	0.1–0.5 mg/kg IV or SC q 2–4 h; lower dosages may be more effective because of ceiling effect	Use with caution in patients with impairment of liver or renal function, or CNS signs
Fentanyl	5–20 µg/kg IV bolus (lasts up to 60 min)	Respiratory and CNS depression can occur
Meloxicam	0.2–1 mg/kg PO or SC q 24–48 h	GI adverse effects may occur, do not combine with corticosteroids
Midazolam	1–2 mg/kg IM	—

Abbreviations: CNS, central nervous system; IM, intramuscularly; IV, intravenously; GI, gastrointestinal; PO, by mouth; q, every; SC, subcutaneously.
Data from Hawkins MG, Graham JE. Emergency and Critical Care of Rodents. Vet Clin North Am Exot Anim Pract 2007;10:501–31.

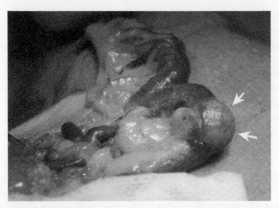

Fig. 10. Ovariohysterectomy in a 4.5-year-old guinea pig. The image shows unilateral (*right*) uterine adenocarcinoma (*arrows*) and distension of both uterine horns with blood. (*Courtesy of* Vladimir Jekl, DVM, PhD, DipECZM, Brno, Czech Republic.)

subcutaneously on day 1, 2, and 8) and enrofloxacin (5–10 mg by mouth or intramuscularly every 12 hours) can be performed.[46,47]

MASTITIS

Guinea pigs have a single pair of inguinal mammary glands without a common blood supply.[10] Predisposing factors for a mammary gland infection are large litter sizes of nursing pups, unsanitary cage conditions, or secondary infections (mammary gland tumors, infection of the urogenital tract). Clinical symptoms include painful, warm, and swollen mammary glands that are red to cyanotic in appearance. The milk contains a high level of neutrophils, and traces of blood can be found. Associated pathogens are *Escherichia coli*, *Pasteurella*, *Klebsiella*, *Staphylococcus*, *Streptococcus*, or *Pseudomonas* spp.[33] To prevent systemic illness of the sow or her puppies, antibiotic treatment is indicated (**Table 3**). Culture and sensitivity testing is highly recommended. Weaning of the young cavies prevents them from getting infected, and helps the mammary gland to recover. Hot compresses with mallow leaf (*Malva folium*) have local anti-inflammatory effects and can ease the sow's discomfort. The infected milk should be stripped out.[20] The prognosis depends on the severity of the infection and can range from good to grave.

ABORTION

Abortion can be observed in cases of dystocia resulting in fetal death. When more than 1 animal is affected, an infectious cause should always be suspected. Oral inoculation with *Campylobacter jejuni* can lead to fetoplacental infection resulting in abortion.[49] Other pathogens like *Salmonella* spp or *Listeria monocytogenes* can cause miscarriage as well.[33]

VAGINAL/UTERINE PROLAPSE

Vaginal or uterine prolapse can occur after parturition. In several genetic mouse models a spontaneous prolapse is described.[50] Clinical symptoms include straining and prolapsed vaginal or uterine tissue in varying condition. Diagnosis is based on clinical symptoms. If the tissue is healthy, lavage and lubricate it before reinserting with gentle digital manipulation. The authors like to perform vaginal closure to maintain reduction by placing 2 to 3 horizontal mattress sutures or similar.[43] Treatment with nonsteroidal antiinflammatory drugs (meloxicam 0.5–1 mg/kg by mouth or subcutaneously) is recommended to decrease swelling. Bathing the affected area in hypertonic saline solution can aid in decreasing the swelling. To prevent toxemia after replacement, ovariohysterectomy should be performed.[51] Prognosis of these cases depends on the severity and timeliness of correction, but it is usually guarded to poor (**Fig. 11**).

Chinchillas (Chinchilla lanigera)

Chinchillas, which originate from the Andes region in South America, are seasonal polyestrous animals.[11] Kept as pets, females give birth twice a year and births occur throughout the year, with peaks in spring and summer.[52] Females have a duplex uterus with 2 cervices.[53] They have 3 pairs of mammary glands[10]; 1 is located in the inguinal region, the other 2 pairs are located laterally on the thorax.[11,54] Males have testes that are located lateral to their penis and no true scrotum. Male chinchillas have an os penis. Reproductive behavior starts at an average age of 4 to 5 months in large females and 7 to 8 months in males.[12] Copulatory plugs can be found in the vagina after mating, similar to other hystrocomorphs.[55] Gestation length is 111 days on average and females usually give birth to 2 kits (**Fig. 12**).[11,52]

SEXUAL DIFFERENTIATION

Sexual differentiation can be challenging in young animals but it can easily be learned. In rodents, the distance between the urogenital opening and the anus is measured, and males have a greater distance than females.[56]

ESTRUS DIAGNOSTICS

Estrus lasts from 12 to 48 hours in female chinchillas. Diagnosis can be made by clinical presentation (swelling of the vulva, vaginal secretion, toleration of the male) or by vaginal cytology. Vaginal cytology is an easily accessible and cost-efficient tool, which is very useful in the clinical setting. A vaginal smear is performed with a small cotton swab. Staining can be performed with a special Papanicolaou stain, or with more easily accessible Diff-Quick stain. As a general rule, small, round cells with a large

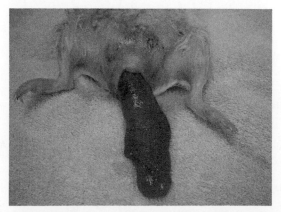

Fig. 11. Uterine prolapse presented after birthing episode. The prolapse was replaced and the animal recovered normally from the event.

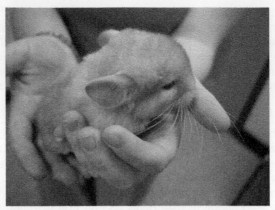

Fig. 12. This chinchilla is a few days old. As with guinea pigs, the kits are precocial; they are born fully furred, with well-developed sensory and locomotor abilities.

nucleus are found when the animal is in anestrus. When epithelial cells get larger, with a small nucleus and irregular-shaped edges, the female is in estrus (**Fig. 13**).

Cytologically, the vaginal epithelium consists of basal, parabasal, and intermediate cells during anestrus, correlating with high progesterone levels. Analyses of fecal progesterone levels can be used as a supportive diagnostic tool. Superficial or cornuated epithelial cells are seen when estrogen levels are high during estrus. In metestrus, a high level of neutrophils is observed.

FETAL RESORPTION/ABORTIONS

Multiple factors can cause an early termination of pregnancy. Poor nutrition, environmental factors (humidity, temperature), and social stress are the most common reasons for a miscarriage.[52] Their comfort zone is 18°C (65°F) to 27°C (80°F). Exposure to cold temperatures is tolerated better than heat. Humidity should be around 30% to 40%.

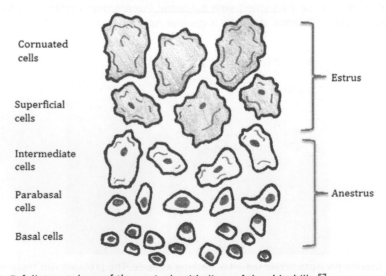

Fig. 13. Exfoliate cytology of the vaginal epithelium of the chinchilla.[57]

Infections with *Salmonella* spp, *Pseudomonas*, or *Listeria* spp can cause pathologic vaginal secretions followed by miscarriage.[18,33] The genetic lethal factor as a cause of abortion comes into effect when 2 albino or velvet chinchillas are bred. Fetal resorption during pregnancy is a common problem in chinchillas.[58] If bloody vaginal discharge or dead fetuses are observed, the patient's owner should be advised to bring the pet in for radiographs or abdominal ultrasonography to determine pregnancy. Treatment is usually not suggested, but a single dose of oxytocin (0.2–3 IU/kg subcutaneously with fluids) is beneficial to ensure expulsion of all uterine contents[37] (see the earlier comments for guinea pigs). Although oxytocin is US Food and Drug Administration approved for intramuscular or intravenous use, the authors believe that a subcutaneous application prevents a fast onset of violent contractions in chinchillas.

ENDOMETRITIS AND PYOMETRA

Infection of the endometrium can occur after parturition. Difficulties during labor, unsanitary conditions, or placental retention (toxemia) can be the underlying cause. Clinical symptoms include purulent vaginal discharge, increased body temperature, anorexia, and decreased milk production.[59] Palpation, radiography, and abdominal ultrasonography should be used to exclude fetal retention. Treatment with a single dose of oxytocin (0.2–3 IU/kg subcutaneously with fluids) is recommended.[12,37,47] Sensitivity and culture testing are recommended before using systemic antibiotics. Treatment with aglepristone can be beneficial (for treatment plan and dosing, see earlier discussion). In cases of unsuccessful treatment, surgical intervention is indicated (**Fig. 14**).

CYSTIC ENDOMETRIAL HYPERPLASIA

Cystic endometrial hyperplasia is described as an important differential diagnosis when females (older than 4 years) are presented with intermittent blood-stained fur around the perineum. As described in other species, animals with this condition are usually nulliparous and sexually intact. Diagnostics include urine analysis, urine culture (because urinary tract infection can have similar signs), abdominal radiographs, and/or

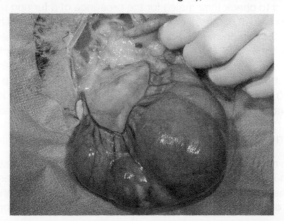

Fig. 14. Ovariohysterectomy in a 7-year-old chinchilla showing distension of the right uterus with pus. The histopathology revealed the presence of the cystic endometrial hyperplasia and chronic purulent endometritis. Bacteriology confirmed the presence of *E coli*. The final diagnosis was cystic endometrial hyperplasia and pyometra associated with *E coli* infection.

ultrasonography. Ovariohysterectomy, followed by pathohistologic analyses, is the treatment of choice.[60]

DYSTOCIA

Dystocia in chinchillas is rarely observed.[20,52] Fetal malpresentation and abnormal fetal size are the main reasons for problems during labor. Uterine inertia and even uterine torsion have been described. Diagnostics and treatment are similar to the guinea pig (discussed earlier). Cesarean section should be performed if the sow is in labor for more than 4 hours without producing any kits and is not responding to conservative treatment.[47]

UTERINE OR VAGINAL PROLAPSE

A spontaneous vaginal or uterine prolapse can occur in chinchillas as well. The patient is presented straining, and prolapsed vaginal or uterine tissue in varying condition is observed. If the tissue is healthy, treatment is similar to the guinea pig (discussed earlier). If the protruding tissue is necrotic, ovariohysterectomy is the only option. Prognosis of these cases depends on the severity and timeliness of correction, but it is usually guarded to poor.

NEOPLASM OF THE REPRODUCTIVE TRACT

Chinchillas rarely have tumors of the reproductive tract. None of the reports described any occurrence of metastasis. The described tumors were reported to be leiomyosarcomas and leiomyomas.[61]

FUR RING AND PARAPHIMOSIS

Fur rings are very common in male chinchillas. Frequent grooming in the perianal region may be a sign that they have paraphimosis caused by a fur ring. The condition is characterized by a ring of fur in the prepuce encircling the penis. If this ring of hair is undetected, it can prevent the penis from retracting into the prepuce. The owners should be advised to check their males for the presence of a fur ring regularly. Clinical symptoms can be mild, if detected early. The fur ring can be removed manually or clippers can be used for detachment. Severe damage can lead to penis necrosis or can be lethal in cases of total blockage of the urethra.[20,47,58] Cooling or applying hypertonic glucose solution can help decrease penile swelling and a water-soluble lubricant can be used to retract the penis into the prepuce. Treat the patient with pain medications (buprenorphine 0.01–0.05 mg intramuscularly, subcutaneously, or intravenously 6–12 hours), especially in severe cases in which surgical intervention is indicated (**Fig. 15**).

BALANOPOSTHITIS AND PREPUTIAL ABSCESSES

An accumulation of fur or smegma can lead to an infection of prepuce and glans penis. An infection with *Pseudomonas aeruginosa* can contribute to progression of the disease. Flushing the prepuce with diluted chlorhexidine solution and lancing abscesses is the treatment of choice. If phimosis is present, surgical intervention is indicated.[10]

Degus (Octodon degus)

Degus originate from the western Andes in South America. Males are usually 10% larger than females. They reach puberty at an age of 12 to 16 weeks in females and 16 weeks in males. Forming of breeding pairs is not recommended until they are

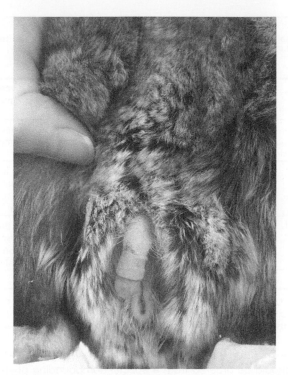

Fig. 15. Checking for the presence of a fur ring should always be performed during the routine clinical examination.

6 months old and have their full body size. Therefore, they are the slowest maturing hystricomorph rodents discussed in this article. Breeding pairs should consist of 1 male and 2 females.[62,63] Duration of gestation is approximately 90 days and females give birth to an average of 5 young.[1,9]

SEXUAL DIFFERENTIATION

The best way to differentiate the sexes is by measuring the distance between urethra and anus, which is shorter in females. In male degus, testes are in the inguinal canal or are intra-abdominal, similar to other rodents. The penis, stabilized by an os penis, is situated cranial to the perianal circle. The ventral spiculated glans penis is characterized by 2 openings: the dorsal urinary meatus and the ventral intromittent sac.[64]

DYSTOCIA

This condition is rarely observed in degus. Commonly caused by abnormal fetal size, dystocia is the most common reproductive disease in female degus.[9] Diagnosis and treatment are similar to those in other hystricomorph rodents (for further details, see the comments on guinea pigs).

HEMOMETRA/PYOMETRA

Bloody or purulent discharge can be seen mostly postpartum.[9] Causes and diagnostics are similar to those in other rodent species. Treatment with antibiotics (**Table 3**) after culture and sensitivity testing is advised. Antibiotics, especially in small rodents,

Table 3
Antibiotics in small rodent patients (be advised that culture and sensitivity testing is recommended)[42,48]

	Dose	Contraindication
Enrofloxacin	5–10 mg/kg PO or IM q 12 h or 5–20 mg/kg PO or SC q 24 h In drinking water: 50–200 mg/L	Do not use in juvenile patients, or patients with impaired renal function
Ciprofloxacin	7–20 mg/kg PO q 12 h	Do not use in juvenile patients, or patients with impaired renal function
Sulfadiazine/ Trimethoprim	15–30 mg/kg PO q 12 h; or 30 mg/kg IM q 12 h	Use with caution in patients with diminished renal or hepatic function, or urinary obstruction and urolithiasis
Chloramphenicol	30–50 mg/kg PO q 12 h	Avoid using it in patients with hematologic disorders, pregnancy, neonates, hepatic failure, renal failure
Florfenicol	30–50 mg/kg PO q 12 h	

Data from Hawkins MG, Graham JE. Emergency and critical care of rodents. Vet Clin North Am Exot Anim Pract 2007;10:501–31; and Jakab C, Rusvai M, Biró N, et al. Claudin-5-positive angioleiomyoma in the uterus of a degu (*Octodon degus*). Acta Vet Hung 2010;58:331–40.

require adequate spectrum and dosing to prevent unwanted side effects. Formulations therefore should be ordered from a special compounding pharmacy, or, if not available, require dilution.[4]

VAGINAL AND UTERINE TUMORS

Neoplastic changes of the genital tract in degus are rare. At presentation, hemorrhagic vaginal discharge or a soft tissue swelling can be found in the urogenital area. Neoplastic changes are described to be in the uterus or vagina. The described tumors are leiomyomas, leiomyosarcomas, and angioleiomyomas.[9,65,66] Surgical intervention should be planned carefully based on age and the general health status of the patient. Bloodwork and whole-body radiographs should be performed, along with fine-needle aspiration of

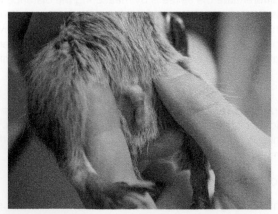

Fig. 16. A fur ring around the penis of a degu. Early recognition is the key to a positive outcome.

the tumor for in-house analysis, if accessible. If the patient is healthy enough to undergo surgery, premedicate with buprenorphine (0.01–0.05 mg/kg subcutaneously, intramuscularly, or intravenously) and meloxicam (0.2–1 mg/kg by mouth or subcutaneously). Induction and maintenance can be performed with sevoflurane or isoflurane. Body temperature control and support with electrolytes are crucial in small rodents. Postoperative pain medications should be used and can prevent self-mutilation when used at adequate doses. Prognosis is generally good for vaginal/uterine tumors in degus.

PENILE PROLAPSE

Similar to chinchillas, fur rings can occur in degus and cause a penile prolapse or preputial inflammation.[9] Males should be examined for fur rings regularly. In severe cases, this condition can lead to penile or preputial ulceration (**Fig. 16**).

REFERENCES

1. Weir BJ. The management and breeding of some more histricomorph rodents. Lab Anim 1970;4(83):83–97.
2. Donnelly T, Brown C. Guinea pig and chinchilla care and husbandry. Vet Clin Exot Anim 2004;7:351–73.
3. Hong C, Armstrong M. Ectopic pregnancy in 2 guinea-pigs. Lab Anim 1978;12: 243–4.
4. Donnelly TM. Ferrets, rabbits, and rodents: clinical medicine and surgery. In: Quesenberry KE CJ, editor. Disease problems of small rodents. St Louis (MO): WB Saunders; 2004.
5. Nuget-Deal J. Performing quality anesthesia on ferrets, rabbits and rodents. Proceedings of the North American Veterinary Conference 2010;75–8.
6. Donnelly TM. Introduction to small mammal anaesthesia. Proceedings of the BSAVA Congress 2015;148–9.
7. Broadbelt D, Blissitt K, Hammond R. The risk of death: the confidential enquiry into perioperative small animal fatalities. Vet Anaesth Anal 2008;35:365–73.
8. Minarikova A, Hauptman K, Jeklova E. Diseases in pet guinea pigs: a retrospective study in 1000 animals. Vet Rec 2015;22:177–200.
9. Jekl V, Hauptman K, Knotek Z. Diseases in pet degus: a retrospective study in 300 animals. J Small Anim Pract 2011;52:107–12.
10. O'Malley B. Clinical anatomy and physiology of exotic species. In: O'Malley B, editor. Guinea pigs. Germany: Elesevier Limited; 2005.
11. Quesenberry K, Donnelly T, Hillyer E. Ferrets, rabbits, and rodents. In: Quesenberry K, Carpenter J, editors. Biology, husbandry, and clinical techniques of guinea pigs and chinchillas. 2nd edition. St Louis (MO): WB Saunders; 2004.
12. Hsu CC, Chan MM, Wheler CL. Laboratory Animal Medicine. In: Fox JG, Anderson LC, Otto G, editors. Biology and diseases of chinchillas. Elsevier; 2015.
13. Brown SA. Ferrets, rabbits, and rodents: clinical medicine and surergy. In: Quesenberry K, Carpenter J, editors. Basic anatomy, physiology and husbandry. 2nd edition. St Louis (MO): WB Saunders; 2004.
14. Funk RS. Ferrets, rabbits and rodents: clinical medicine and surgery. In: Quesenberry K, J. Carpenter, editors. Medical management of prairie dogs. 2nd edition. St Louis (MO): WB Saunders; 2004.
15. Ness RS. Ferrets, rabbits, and rodents: clinical medicine and surgery. In: Quesenberry K, Carpenter J, editors. Sugar Gliders. 2nd edition. St Louis (MO): WE Saunders; 2004.

16. Bihun C. Ferrets, rabbits, and rodents: clinical medicine and surgery. In: Quesenberry K, Carpenter J, editors. Basic anatomy, physiology, husbandry, and clinical techniques. 2nd edition. St Louis (MO): WB Saunders; 2004.
17. Quesenberry, K.E. and K.R. Boschert. Guinea pigs Breeding and Reproduction of Guinea Pigs [cited 2016 October 6].
18. Shomer NH, Holcombe H, Harkness JE. Laboratory Animal Medicine. In: Fox JG, Anderson LC, Otto G, editors. Biology and diseases of guinea pigs. 3rd edition. Elsevier; 2015.
19. Gao CQ, Kaufman JM, Eertmans F. Difference 495 in receptor-binding contributes to difference in biological activity between the unique guinea pig GnRH and mammalian GnRH. Neurosci Lett 2012;507:124–6.
20. Girling S. Basic small mammal anatomy and physiology. In: Girling S, editor. Veterinary nursing of exotic pets. Oxford (United Kingdom): Blackwell Publishing; 2003. p. 195–223.
21. Guilmette J, Langlois I, Helie P. Comparative study of 2 surgical techniques for castration of guinea pigs (Cavia porcellus). Can J Vet Res 2015;79:323–8.
22. Pliny A. Ovarian cystic disease in guinea pigs. Vet Clin Exot Anim 2014;17:69–75.
23. Burns RP, Paul-Murphy J, Sicard GK. Granulosa cell tumor in a guinea pig. JAVMA 2001;218:726–8.
24. Bean AD. Ovarian Cysts in the Guinea Pig (Cavia porcellus). Vet Clin Exot Anim 2013;16:757–76.
25. Beregi A, Zorn S, Felkai F. Ultrasonic Diagnosis of Ovarian Cysts in Ten Guinea Pigs. Vet Radiol Ultrasou 1999;40:74–6.
26. Erwingmann A, Gloeckner B. Leitsymptome bei Meerschweinchen. Chinchilla und Degu. Tierarztl Prax K H 2006;34:274.
27. Kohutova S. Diagnostics and therapy of endocrine active reproductive tract diseases in a pet guinea pig (Cavia aperea f. porcellus), in University of Veterinary and Pharmaceutical Sciences Brno. Brno (Czech Republic): University of Veterinary and Pharmaceutical Sciences Brno; 2016.
28. Schuetzenhofer G, Goericke-Pesch S, Wehrend A. Effects of deslorelin implants on ovarian cysts in guinea pigs. Schweiz Arch Tierheilkd 2011;153(9):416–7.
29. Riggs SM. Guinea pigs. In: Tully T, Mitchell M, editors. Manual of exotic pet practice. St Louis (MO): WB Saunders; 2009. p. 456–73.
30. Rogers JB, Blumenthal HT. Studies of guinea pig tumors i. report of fourteen spontaneous guinea pig tumors, with a review of the literature. Cancer Res 1960;20:191–7.
31. Field J, Griffith JW, Lang CM. Sponaneous reproductive tract leiomyoas in aged guinea-pigs. J Gtimp Path 1989;101:287–94.
32. Andrews EJ. Mammary neoplasia in the guinea pig (Cavia porcellus). Cornell Vet 1976;66:82–96.
33. O'Rourke D. Disease problems of guinea pigs. In: Quesenberry K, Carpenter J, editors. Ferrets, rabbits, and rodents: clinical medicine and surgery. St Louis (MO): WB Saunders; 2004. p. 245–54.
34. Bishop CR. Reproductive medicine of rabbits and rodents. Vet Clin Exot Anim 2002;5:507–35.
35. Suarey-Bonnet A, Martín de Las Mulas J, Millan MY. Morphological and Immunohistochemical Characterization of Spontaneous Mammary Gland Tumors in the Guinea Pig (Cavia porcellus). Vet Pathol 2010;47:298–305.
36. Donnelly, T.M. Guinea Pigs. [cited 2016 August 3]; Available at: http://www.merckvetmanual.com/mvm/exotic_and_laboratory_animals/rodents/guinea_pigs.html?qt=Guinea%20pig&alt=sh.

37. Mayer J. Rodents. In: Carpenter JW, editor. Exotic animal formulary. St Louis (MO): WB Saunders; 2013. p. 477–513.
38. Golden JG, Hughes HC, Lang CM. Experimental toxemia in a pregnant guinea pig (*Cavia porcellus*). Lab Anim Sci 1980;30:174–83.
39. Martinho F. Dystocia Caused by Ectopic Pregnancy 544 in a Guinea Pig (*Cavia porcellus*). Vet Clin Exot Anim 2006;9:713–6.
40. Hawkins MG, Graham JE. Emergency and Critical Care of Rodents. Vet Clin Exot Anim 2007;10:501–31.
41. Richardson VCG. The reproductive system. In: Rabbits health, husbandry and diseases. Oxford (UK): Blackwell Science Ltd; 2000. p. 44–58.
42. Plumb DC. Plumb's veterinary drug handbook. Ames (IA): Blackwell Publishing Professional; 2008.
43. Fossum TW. Surgery of the reproductive and genital systems. 3rd ed. Small animal surgery. St Louis (MO): WB Saunders; 2007.
44. Clercq ED, Kalmar I, Vanrompay D. Animal Models for Studying Female Genital Tract Infection with Chlamydia trachomatis. Infect Immun 2013;81:3060–7.
45. Schmidt S, Schrag D, Giese B. Ultrasonic diagnosis in gynecology in small animals. Tierarztl Prax 1986;14:123–64.
46. Engelhardt ABv. Behandlung des Endometritis/Pyometrakomplexes eines Meerschweinchens - ein Fallbericht. Prakt Tierarzt 2006;87:14–7.
47. Pisu MC, Andolffato A, Veronesi MC. Pyometra in a six-month-old nulliparous golden hamster (*Mesocricetus auratus*) treated with aglepristone. Vet Q 2012; 32:179–81.
48. Adamcak A, Otten B. Rodent therapeutics. Vet Clin North Am Exot Anim Pract 2000;3:221–37.
49. Plummer P, Sahin O, Burrough E. Critical Role of LuxS in the Virulence of *Campylobacter jejuni* in a Guinea Pig Model of Abortion. Infect Immun 2012; 80:585–93.
50. Abramowitch S, Feola A, Zegbeh J. Tissue mechanics, animal models, and pelvic organ prolapse: a review. Eur J Obstet Gynecol Reprod Biol 2009;144:S146–58.
51. V, J. 2016.
52. Buzo JM, Ponzio MF, F.d. Cuneo M. Reproduction in chinchilla (*Chinchilla lanigera*): Current status of environmental control of gonadal activity and advances in reproductive techniques. Theriogenology 2012;78:1–11.
53. Jarrett CL, Jarrett RT, Harvey SB. The uterus duplex bicollis, vagina simplex of female chinchillas. J Am Assoc Lab Anim Sci 2016;55:155–60.
54. Mans C, Donnelly TM. Update on diseases of chinchillas. Vet Clin Exot Anim 2013;16:383–406.
55. Celiberti S, Gloria A, Contri A. Sexual hormone fluctuation in chinchillas. Vet Clin Exot Anim 2013;16:197–209.
56. Klaphake E. Common rodent procedures. Vet Clin Exot Anim 2006;9:389–413.
57. Becker, A. 2010.
58. Donnelly TM. Disease problems of chinchillas. In: Quesenberry K, Carpenter J, editors. Ferrets, rabbits, and rodents: clinical medicine and surgery. St Louis (MO): WB Saunders; 2004. p. 255–65.
59. Brower M. Practitioner's guide to pocket pet and rabbit theriogenology. Theriogenology 2006;66:618–23.
60. Granson HJ, Carr AP, Parker D. Cystic endometrial hyperplasia and chronic endometritis in a chinchilla. JAVMA 2011;239:233–6.
61. Jenkins JR. Diseases of geriatric guinea pigs and chinchillas. Vet Clin Exot Anim 2010;13:85–93.

62. Lee TM. *Octogon degus*: a diurnal, social and long-lived Rodent. ILAR Journal 2004;45:14–24.
63. Palacios AG. Husbandry and Breeding in the *Octodon degus* 594 (Molina 1782). Cold Spring Harb Protoc 2013;350–4.
64. Contreras L, Bustos-Obregón E. Anatomy of reproductive tract in *Octodon degus* Molina: a nonscrotal rodent. Arch Androl 1980;4:115–24.
65. Skoric M, Fictum P, Jekl V. Vaginal leiomyosarcoma in a degu (*Octodon degus*): a case report. Veterinarni Medicina 2010;55:409–12.
66. Jakab C, Rusvai M, Biró N. Claudin-5-positive angioleiomyoma in the uterus of a degu (*Octodon degus*). Acta Vet Hung 2010;58:331–40.

Reproductive Medicine in Ferrets

Vladimir Jekl, DVM, PhD, DECZM (Small Mammal)*, Karel Hauptman, DVM, PhD

KEYWORDS

- Ferret • Reproduction • Estrus • Hyperestrogenism • Neoplasia • Contraception
- Sterilization • Deslorelin

KEY POINTS

- Similarly to tomcats, ferrets' testicles are located beneath the anus, and the prostate gland is the only accessory sexual gland in male ferrets.
- The ferret uterus is bicornuate, and the ovaries are embedded in the ovarian bursa.
- Ferrets are seasonally polyestrous animals; initiation and the end of the gonadal activity depend on the light-dark cycle.
- Ovulation is induced by pressure on the cervix by mating with male ferrets.
- In vaginal lavages of intact female ferrets, the presence of neutrophils is common during all stages of the estrous cycle. Presence of erythrocytes and bacteria is uncommon except during estrus, when they are associated only with superficial cells.

REPRODUCTIVE ANATOMY AND PHYSIOLOGY OF FERRETS

The body of male ferrets is generally larger than that of female ferrets. Males tend to have more body muscle and much larger, wider, rounder heads. Females tend to have narrower, daintier heads, with thinner, pointier noses. Both female and male ferrets have 8 nipples.

Selected biological and reproductive data are summarized in **Table 1**.

Male Anatomy

Testicles are located beneath the anus, similarly to tomcats (**Fig. 1**). The epididymis is composed of a convoluted spermatic duct, which is divided into head, body, and tail and is located on the dorsal aspect of the testis as it lies in the scrotal sac. The ductus deferens is accompanied by the deferent artery and vein and the main testicular artery and vein, which, with the nerve and lymphatic system vessels, form the

---

Disclosure: The authors have nothing to disclose.
Avian and Exotic Animal Clinic, Faculty of Veterinary Medicine, University of Veterinary and Pharmaceutical Sciences Brno, Palackeho tr. 1946/1, 61242 Brno, Czech Republic
* Corresponding author.
E-mail address: jeklv@vfu.cz

Table 1
Selected biological and reproductive data in ferrets

Parameter		Range
Lifespan (y)		5–9
Weight (kg)	Female	0.5–1.0
	Male	1.0–2.3
Rectal temperature	°C	37.8–40.0
	°F	100–104
Heart rate (Beats/min)		180–250
Respiration (Breaths/min)		30–35
Puberty (mo)		4–9
Gestation (d)		39–42
Newborn weight (g)		8–12
Litter size		4–14
Eye opening (d)		28–37
Weaning (wk)		39–42

Data from Refs.[1–3]

spermatic cord. The testis, epididymis, and spermatic cord are covered by the vaginal tunic, the visceral part of which is a continuation of the abdominal peritoneal membrane. Deep to the vaginal tunic is the tunica albuginea, a dense, white, fibrous capsule. The testis and epididymis are connected to the parietal vaginal tunic with the caudal ligament of the epididymis. The spermatic cord passes cranially through the inguinal canal into the abdomen and then opens into the urethra at the level of the prostate.[1]

Testicles descend into the scrotum at the age of 10 weeks. However, they can be located within the scrotum during the breeding season and then can be located more in the inguinal canal.

The os penis (**Fig. 2**) can be palpated easily caudal to the preputial opening, which is located midline on the caudoventral abdomen. The base of the os penis

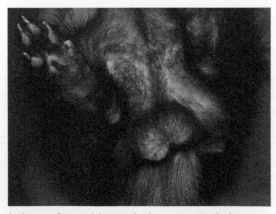

Fig. 1. Testicles in hobs are located beneath the anus, similarly to tomcats. (*Courtesy of* Vladimir Jekl, DVM, PhD, DECZM and Karel Hauptman DVM, PhD, Brno, Czech Republic; with permission.)

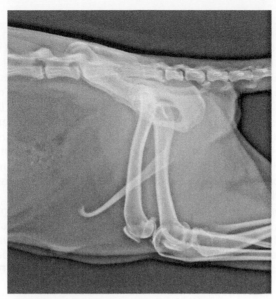

Fig. 2. Radiograph of the ferret caudal abdominal and pelvic area. The typically J-shaped os penis is easily seen. (*Courtesy of* Vladimir Jekl, DVM, PhD, DECZM and Karel Hauptman DVM, PhD, Brno, Czech Republic; with permission.)

is embedded in a tendon that passes under the pelvis and is attached to the caudal edge of the 2 pubic bones. The groove on the bone supports the urethra, maintaining patency during coitus. The distal aspect of the penile bone is J shaped, curves dorsally, and supports the glans penis. The urethral orifice is a slit-like opening on the ventral surface of the glans (**Fig. 3**) approximately 2 to 4 mm proximal to its tip.[2]

The prostate gland is the only accessory sexual gland in ferrets and surrounds the urethra at the base of the urinary bladder.

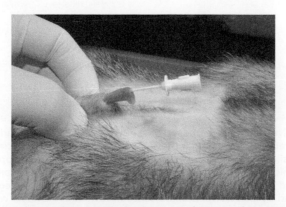

Fig. 3. Ferret in dorsal recumbency with the tomcat catheter in place. Note the small glans penis with typical J-shaped appearance. (*Courtesy of* Vladimir Jekl, DVM, PhD, DECZM and Karel Hauptman DVM, PhD, Brno, Czech Republic; with permission.)

Female Anatomy

Ovaries are located in the dorsal aspect of the abdomen caudal to both kidneys. The left ovary is attached by the ligamentum suspensorium to the abdominal wall close to the middle of the 13th rib (**Fig. 4**A). The right ovary is attached by the ligamentum suspensorium to the abdominal wall near the middle of the last rib (14th). Ferret ovaries are almost completely enveloped within the ovarian bursa, a pouch formed by the mesosalpinx and the mesovarium that encloses the infundibulum of the uterine tube and the ovary (**Fig. 5**).

The ferret uterus is bicornuate.[1] The uterus has short body and 2 long uterine horns (see **Fig. 4**A and B). Blood supply is provided by ovarian and uterine arteries and veins. The vagina lies in the pelvic canal and is split to 2 parts: a cranial part with the uterine neck and a caudal part, the vestibulum. The urethral orificium lies on the ventral floor of the vaginal vestibule. The vulva consists of the vestibule, clitoris, and labia, and is located in the perineum ventral to the anus.[3]

The genital opening (vulva) of the female ferret is located in the region just beneath the animal's anus. The vulva of the female ferret appears as a vertical slitlike opening. If the ferret is not in heat, the skin of the vulval opening is flat and flush with the surrounding skin. When the ferret is in estrus, the skin of the vulval opening becomes swollen and edematous, rising well above the level of the surrounding skin (**Fig. 6**).

REPRODUCTION AND HORMONAL CONTROL

Initiation of the gonadal activity depends on the light-dark cycle, which stimulates or inhibits reproduction through transmission of information about the day length to the brain.[4] Ferrets need alternating periods of increasing duration of daylight (long days), and days of decreasing duration of daylight (short days).

Under natural conditions, if the length of light per day is sufficient (12–14 h/d), males become sexually mature at 6 to 8 months and females at 4 months. Ferrets born the previous summer reach puberty by the following spring at the age of 8 to 12 months.[66]

During the breeding season, both males and females have greasier skin and stronger body odor.

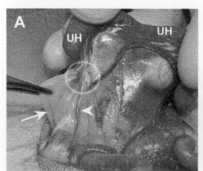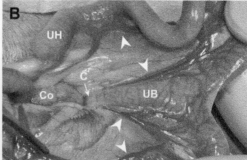

Fig. 4. Perioperative photographs of a ferret reproductive organs. (*A*) Ovaries are located in a dorsal aspect of abdomen caudally to the both kidneys. The ovary (*encircled*) is attached to the abdominal wall by ligamentum suspensorium ovarii (*arrow*). Blood supply is provided by ovarian artery, which, together with ovarian vein, is embedded by fat (*arrowhead*). (*B*) Uterine horns (UH) and uterine body (UB) are thickened because of pseudopregnancy. Vascularization is provided by uterine veins and arteries (*arrowheads*). Uterine cervix (C) is more whitish than surrounding tissue. In close vicinity of the uterine body is the colon (Co). (*Courtesy of* Vladimir Jekl, DVM, PhD, DECZM and Karel Hauptman DVM, PhD, Brno, Czech Republic; with permission.)

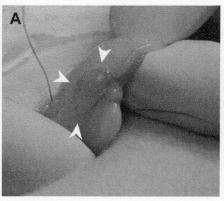
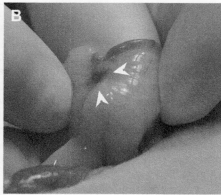

Fig. 5. Perioperative views of a ferret left ovary, which is almost completely enveloped within the ovarian bursa (*arrowheads*). (*A*) Parietal, and (*B*) visceral views. (*Courtesy of* Vladimir Jekl, DVM, PhD, DECZM and Karel Hauptman DVM, PhD, Brno, Czech Republic; with permission.)

Male Ferrets (Hobs)

Males come into breeding condition a little earlier in the spring than jills. The testosterone negative feedback inhibition of the hypothalamic secretion of gonadotropin-releasing hormone (GnRH) controls puberty and seasonality of reproduction in the male.[5]

Jallageas and colleagues[6] described a stimulation of the pulsatile liberation of luteinizing hormone (LH) reflecting the pulsatile activity of the GnRH system when daylight was equal to or in excess of light hours/dark hours 8:16.

Moreover, a high correlation was found to exist between testis size and plasma testosterone concentrations during the annual reproductive cycle of the male ferret. From August to December (out of season) testicles are smaller (mean length, 12 ± 1 mm) and the plasma testosterone concentration is low (mean, 33 ± 0.6 ng/dL; 1.2 ± 0.21 nmol/L). Peak values of testis size (mean length, 20 ± 0.2 mm) and plasma testosterone concentrations (mean, 475 ± 20 ng/dL; 16.5 ± 0.69 nmol/L) are reached in April to June.[7]

During the breeding season, the length of spermatogenesis in the ferret was estimated to be 52 to 58.5 days. Spermatogenesis is classified into 8 stages and the duration of 1 cycle is 13 days in ferrets in breeding condition.[8]

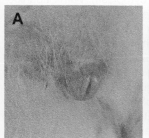
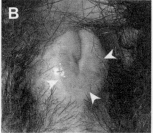
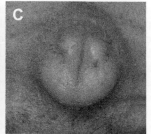

Fig. 6. (*A–C*) If the ferret is in estrus, the skin of the vulval opening is swollen and edematous, rising well above the level of the surrounding skin. Perivulvar skin urine staining (*A*) and superficial erosions (*B*, *arrowheads*) associated with vulvar licking can be also seen. (*Courtesy of* Vladimir Jekl, DVM, PhD, DECZM and Karel Hauptman DVM, PhD, Brno, Czech Republic; with permission.)

Female Ferrets (Jills)

Ferrets are seasonally polyestrous animals, but jills show a constant estrus between March and August if they are not bred. If they ovulate, they have multiple estrous cycles. The estradiol concentrations are responsible for controlling the female reproductive tract and the development of secondary sexual characteristics. Estradiol creates the tonic inhibition of LH secretion by the anterior pituitary during both prepubertal life and anestrus. Estradiol secreted by the follicles controls vulval swelling, uterine development, changes in vaginal cells, and sexual receptivity.[9] Estrus onset is not associated with increased serum follicle-stimulating hormone (FSH) levels.

Estrus is easily detectable. The vulva becomes enlarged, swollen, and congested, sometimes with clear or thick white vaginal discharge (see **Fig. 6**). Jills eat less and are more sensitive.

The vulva is smaller during anestrus (5–16 mm). During proestrus its size and turgidity increase (11–18 mm), with its maximum in estrus (17–33 mm). The vulva usually remains enlarged, swollen, and congested to its maximal state (see **Fig. 6**) until mating or ovulation. During the time of maximal swelling, a variable amount of clear serous or yellowish mucous discharge, which can wet the hair of the perineal area, is usually present. In conjunction with the vulval swelling, there is a thickening of the uterine endometrium, and follicles develop in the ovaries.[9]

VAGINAL CYTOLOGY
Vaginal Cytology During Estrous Cycle

Vaginal lavages are obtained using sterile plastic l-mL insulin syringes and plastic 100-μL pipette tips that have the tip edges slightly rounded by heat and the hub cut to fit on the syringe,[10] or using laboratory pipets. The tip is gently inserted approximately 1.0 to 1.5 cm into the vagina until it meets slight resistance, and 0.05 to 0.1 mL of sterile physiologic saline is flushed and aspirated several times. Contents of the syringe are expelled onto a clean glass slide, sprayed with cytologic fixative, or/and allowed to air dry. Papanicolaou-stained[10] or May-Grunwald-Giemsa Romanovsky vaginal lavages are viewed by light microscopy at 100 and 200 times magnification. Vaginal epithelial cells are categorized as parabasal, intermediate, superficial intermediate, or superficial cells. Subjective assessments of numbers of neutrophils, erythrocytes, and bacteria are made for each lavage.

Vaginal epithelial cells in ferrets are morphologically similar to those described in dogs.[10] Parabasal cells are rarely observed. Occasionally, parabasal and intermediate cells are vacuolated and/or contain neutrophils within the cytoplasm. With Papanicolaou stain, superficial intermediate cells are basophilic (blue-green) or acidophilic (pale pink to red). The superficial cells are large with angular cytoplasmic margins and degenerative nuclear changes consisting of pyknosis or rhexis, or absence of nuclei. During anestrus and proestrus, superficial cells are either basophilic or acidophilic and are rarely orangeophilic (indicating keratinization). Staining of superficial cells changes as estrus progresses. For the first 3 to 5 days of estrus, superficial cells show mixed staining properties (basophilic, acidophilic, and orangeophilic) and contain degenerated nuclei. After 4 to 6 days, lavages contain highly keratinized, generally anucleate cells. Papanicolaou stain shows these changes more clearly than Wright stain.

Most vaginal epithelial cells from pet ferrets in anestrus are intermediate and superficial intermediate (up to 30% of cells; range, 1%–36%) cells. In proestrus, the number of superficial cells increases up to 87% (range, 15%–87%), and the number of neutrophils and bacteria (large bacilli) increase slightly as well. In estrus, the superficial cells are highly keratinized in more than 90% (range, 71%–100%).[10]

Vaginal Cytology During Pregnancy and Pseudopregnancy

During pregnancy, a little yellowish mucus containing a few leukocytes is frequently observed within the vulva.

Numerous bacteria, neutrophils, cellular debris, and some erythrocytes were observed in a few females that experienced prolonged estrus.[10]

The large epithelial cells, present in vaginal lavages several days after mating or in cases of pseudopregnancy, can be confused with neoplastic cells. These cells are probably derived from the uterine symplasma formed during pregnancy or pseudopregnancy in ferrets.[11]

MATING, OVULATION, IMPLANTATION, AND GESTATION PERIOD

Jills are reflex ovulators, and a coital stimulus is required to trigger the ovulation. In ferrets, preintromission events do not lead to any increase in ovulatory hormones and do not induce ovulation.[12]

The best time for breeding is during 2 consecutive days of the second week of the jill's heat. Females and males copulate many times and for prolonged periods of time (may last from 15 minutes to 3 hours), therefore male and female are left together for 2 consecutive days.[13] The hook at the distal part of the os penis provides a hard substrate that is used to stimulate the nerve-rich portion of the female ferret's vagina and cervix, which helps induce ovulation (odor and neck biting also help). Copulation is accompanied in female mustelids by an increase in the level of LH, which causes ovulation.

After mating, the swelling and turgidity of the vagina gradually decrease after 3 to 4 days and it regains its normal size in 2 to 3 weeks after ovulation, and for the remainder of pregnancy or pseudopregnancy it as small as during anestrus. If the vulva does not recede, ovulation has probably not taken place.

If not mated with a male, about one-half of unmated females remain in heat, and blood estrogen concentration remains high for the remainder of the breeding season. Jills can die from anemia associated with hyperestrogenism (discussed later).

An average of 12 oocytes (5–13) per female are ovulated into the ovarian bursa 30 to 40 hours after copulation. Between days 12 and 13 after mating, the embryos have become implanted in the endometrium.

The total gestation period lasts 39 to 42 days, and in multiparas it is usually 42 days. Pregnancy consist of a long preimplantation period of 10 to 12 days and an active gestation period of 30 days.[11,14] Ferret preimplantation embryos experience a prolonged period of oviductal residence; from day 10 onward, embryos can be recovered only from uteri. Implantation in the ferret is central, with rapid invasion of the uterine epithelium by the trophoblast over a broad area that eventually becomes a zonary band of endotheliochorial placenta.[14]

Corpus luteum starts to secrete progesterone immediately after ovulation, with the progesterone peak in days 12 to 14 during the period of implantation. Progesterone concentrations decline continuously between day 24 and parturition at day 42. Jills display a protracted decline in circulating progesterone level, and progesterone levels reach basal concentrations around 7 days after parturition.[9] The conceptuses have no effect on the duration of the luteal phase, because pregnancy and pseudopregnancy are indistinguishable.[13]

The pregnant uterus can be confirmed from day 12 of pregnancy and from 14 to 16 days by palpation. Skeletons can be visible on radiographs from day 30 of pregnancy.[5] Kitten birth weight is 10 g (range, 8–12 g; **Fig. 7**) with a litter size of 4 to 14, reducing with the age of the jill. Kits can hear from 32 days and the eyes open at 4 to 5 weeks. They can be weaned at 6 to 8 weeks.[1] During pregnancy and lactation,

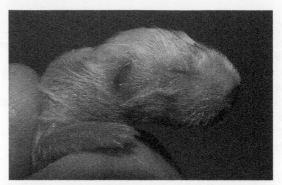

Fig. 7. Ferret kits are born completely dependent on the mother (nidicolous animals). They are born toothless and with sealed ears and eyelids. (*Courtesy of* Vladimir Jekl, DVM, PhD, DECZM and Karel Hauptman DVM, PhD, Brno, Czech Republic; with permission.)

mother ferrets are susceptible to stress and can have problems with parturition or can present cannibalism.

The recurrence of estrus after pregnancy has been found to vary according to whether or not the young were suckling. Jills return to heat 2 weeks after weaning a litter if the photoperiod is right. Some jills with small litters come into heat while still nursing the kits. If kittens are born dead, the estrus can recur within 9 to 17 days.[13] Under natural light conditions, jills can have 2 litters a year.

MANAGEMENT OF REPRODUCTION
Estrus Induction

Light cycle–induced estrus
A change in light conditions every 2 months causes 3 periods of gonadal activity a year.[15] A nonstimulatory photoperiod should be used 6 wk/y to rest the ferret and preserve maximum fertility; a maintenance diet can be given at this time. Jills return to estrus approximately 3 weeks after reinstitution of the longer photoperiod.[15,16]

Drug-induced estrus
Follicle-stimulating hormone Administration of 0.25 mg of FSH twice per day until the signs of estrus appeared, with the injection of 5 IU of human chorionic gonadotropin (hCG) once each day when vaginal cornification exceeded 75% and continued until estrus, was the best hormone regimen tested. This treatment was highly successful (86%) for inducing estrus and supporting pregnancy as far as blastocyst implantation.[17] However, only 23% of the ferrets so treated gave birth to kits, none of which survived for more than 3 days, which may have been caused by insufficient prolactin secretion and thus inadequate luteal maintenance and milk production, because these females were maintained on a short-day photoperiod.[17]

Gonadotropin-releasing hormone, gonadotropin-releasing hormone agonists
The deslorelin implant first stimulates FSH and LH release, and it induces estrus within 3 to 4 days after treatment.[18,19] Estrus lasts for approximately 10 days[19] and then is terminated. So far, there are no references describing deslorelin implant removal and further ferret breeding.

ARTIFICIAL INSEMINATION IN FERRETS

Kidder and colleagues[20] described transcervical artificial insemination using a fiber optic endoscope in conjunction with a specially designed speculum and catheter that permitted cervical catheterization and intrauterine insemination. Sperm were collected from the epididymides of 10 discarded breeder males; the number of sperm in diluted samples used for insemination ranged from $4.4 \times 10^6/100$ μL to $13.6 \times 10^6/100$ μL with progressive motility of sperm ranging from 40% to 60%. Sperm collected from each male were diluted with an egg-yolk extender and used to inseminate 8 to 12 females, with deposition of sperm transcervically into the uterine body. Insemination 24 hours after hCG administration resulted in pregnancy in 79% of jills. The vaginal inseminations were unsuccessful in all cases.

EMBRYO TRANSFER IN FERRETS

Embryo transfer to recipient females is a foundational strategy for several assisted reproductive technologies. Ferrets are used as an experimental animal for embryo transfer, which is then applied to human medicine and for conservation of the endangered species of the family Mustelidae.[21–23] Surgical and nonsurgical methods of embryo transfer in ferrets were developed. In the nonsurgical method, specially designed transcervical catheters were used together with a fiber optic endoscope to visualize and then catheterize the ferret cervices.[23] Ten consecutive transcervical uterine flushes in each of 37 female ferrets 145 to 178 hours after an ovulatory injection of hCG resulted in the retrieval of 324 embryos, an average of 8.76 embryos per ferret. A total of 251 embryos from 27 donors were nonsurgically transferred to the uteri of 31 recipients, and resulted in 65 young (26%). Twenty-eight of the recipients (90%) were initially pregnant, as indicated by postpartum necropsies, and 22 ferrets (71%) produced young. The average litter size was 2.95 (range, 1–7). Transfer of blastocysts had a higher degree of success than transfer of zygotes (90% vs 71%).[24] Transuterine migration of embryos following unilateral or bilateral transfer is common.

CONTRACEPTION
Contraception in Male Ferrets

Surgical sterilization
Orchidectomy Hobs can be positioned in a sternal or dorsal recumbency and the scrotal area aseptically prepared for sterile surgery. The testicle is immobilized with fingers and a cranial to caudal skin incision, which is parallel to the scrotal septum, is made over each testicle (**Fig. 8**). The testicle is pushed out of the scrotum; the parietal tunica is incised; and testicle, epididymis, ductus deferens, and spermatic cord vessels are exteriorized outside of the tunica. Spermatic cord and testicular vein and arteries are ligated with suture; however, other techniques used for feline orchiectomy (use of hemoclips, an overhand hemostat technique, figure-of-eight hemostat technique[25]) can be also used. The cord is transected 2 to 4 mm distal to the ligation and checked for possible bleeding. The distal part of the parietal tunica can be prepared, ligated, and excised. The technique is repeated for the remaining testicle. Skin wounds are left to heal by second intention. Analgesia (meloxicam 0.2 mg/kg orally every 12 hours) is continued for 3 to 5 days after surgery.

Cryptorchid testicles are approached via an inguinal or abdominal approach based on the particular testicle location. Cryptorchid testicles can be found at the area between the inguinal canal and the caudal pole of the kidney or by following the ductus deferens (**Figs. 9** and **10**). Spermatic cord and testicular artery and vein are ligated separately and the testicle is excised. Abdominal wall is closed routinely in 2 layers.

Deferentectomy/vasectomy Hobs are positioned in a sternal or dorsal recumbency and the prescrotal area is aseptically prepared for sterile surgery. A vaginal tunica

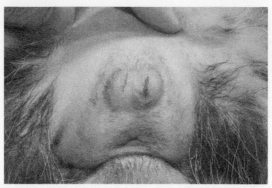

Fig. 8. Orchidectomy in a hob. Two parallel skin incisions are made, 1 over each testicle. (*Courtesy of* Vladimir Jekl, DVM, PhD, DECZM and Karel Hauptman DVM, PhD, Brno, Czech Republic; with permission.)

is approached via skin inguinal incision. The spermatic cord is palpated and a 5-mm incision is made in the vaginal tunica. The vas deferens is separated from veins and arteries with care to avoid damaging the vascular supply, which can lead to ischemic testicle/epididymal necrosis. The vas deferens typically appears to have cross-striations as it zigzags tightly.[26] After distal and proximal deference duct ligation, a segment of approximately 0.5 to 1 cm is excised using 5-0 (1.5 M) monofilament or polyfilament absorbable suture material (the authors prefer polyglactin 910). The tissue that has been excised can be submitted to a pathology laboratory for examination to confirm that the right tissue was removed. The proximal part of the vas deference can be sutured to the vaginal tunica from the outside to prevent possible deference duct reunion, but this seems to be very rare. Then, vaginal tunica and skin are closed using single interrupted sutures.

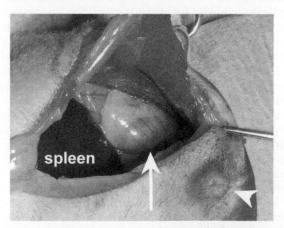

Fig. 9. Orchidectomy in a 2-year-old cryptorchid ferret at the breeding season. Cryptorchid testicles (*arrow*) were localized on the midway between the caudal part of the kidney and inguinal canal. The intra-abdominal approach was preferred, with skin incision made parallel to the prepuce (*arrowhead*). (*Courtesy of* Vladimir Jekl, DVM, PhD, DECZM and Karel Hauptman DVM, PhD, Brno, Czech Republic; with permission.)

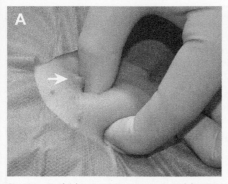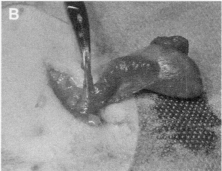

Fig. 10. Orchidectomy in a 1-year-old cryptorchid ferret in the breeding season. (*A*) The cryptorchid testicle was palpated caudosagittally to the preputial opening (*arrow*). Prescrotal approach was used (*B*) because the cryptorchid testicle was located close to the inguinal canal. (*Courtesy of* Vladimir Jekl, DVM, PhD, DECZM and Karel Hauptman DVM, PhD, Brno, Czech Republic; with permission.)

The vasectomized male (hoblet) becomes sterile approximately 6 to 7 weeks after bilateral vasectomy.

HORMONAL CONTRACEPTION IN MALE FERRETS
Deslorelin Acetate Implant

A slow-release depot GnRH-agonist implant containing 9.4 mg of deslorelin suppresses plasma FSH and testosterone concentrations, testis volume, and spermatogenesis. Moreover, the musky odor in the ferrets that had received a deslorelin implant was less than that in the ferrets that were either surgically castrated or had received a placebo implant.[27] Neal and colleagues[7] and Schoemaker and colleagues[27] also found a positive correlation between testis volume and testosterone concentrations, which is of practical use in the clinical setting when owners can see once the testes size starts to increase, which is the indication for another implant placement. The contraception lasted for at least 173 days, but the experiment was ended at that time.

Vinke and colleagues[28] also showed that chemical castration with the 9.4-mg deslorelin implant results in a decrease in the occurrence of aggressive behavior between male ferrets both in the presence and absence of a receptive female. In addition, it reduced aggression more than surgical castration, and reduced sexually motivated behavioral patterns in male-female confrontations. In deslorelin-treated ferrets there was also an increase in play behavior, which might indicate improved welfare of the ferrets.

Deslorelin in the form of 4.7-mg implant was effective in hobs for 969 ± 53 days (range, 865–1072 days for 95% confidence interval [CI]).[19] In a similar study, the mean time to return to fertility in hobs was 937 ± 41 days (range, 489–1080 days).[29] The results were based partly on a telephone survey and client questionnaire. To guarantee continuous gonadal suppression, van Zeeland and colleagues[19] recommended replacing the implant annually, although biannual replacement may be sufficient in most ferrets. At the authors' clinic the adrenal gland panel is measured and the volume of the testis evaluated 1 year after implant administration and then at intervals of 3 to 6 months to allow the implant to be as efficient as possible and to establish which animals need to be reimplanted. The results indicate that the deslorelin implant effectively prevents reproduction and the musky odor of intact male ferrets and it is therefore considered a suitable alternative for surgical castration in these animals (**Box 1**).

Box 1
Desexing vs adrenal gland disease

- Orchidectomy and ovariectomy/ovariohysterectomy at any age, combined with the artificially prolonged photoperiod experienced by indoor pet ferrets, and a possible genetic component, lead to the adrenal gland disease

- Desexing-related increased LH concentrations caused by loss of negative feedback in the hypothalamopituitary-gonadal axis is the underlying reason for adrenocortical hyperplasia and tumor formation

- Adrenal gland disease is more common in ferrets treated by gonadectomy at an early age (5–6 weeks).

Data from Refs.[30–32]

CONTRACEPTION IN FEMALE FERRETS
Surgical Sterilization

The indications for ovariohysterectomy in ferrets are similar to those for other companion animals. In addition, to prevent estrogen toxicity hyperestrogenism, nonbreeding female ferrets should be spayed at 4 to 8 months of age. The midline approach is preferred by the authors. The skin and also the abdominal wall is incised midway between the umbilicus and cranial part of the pubis. The ovarian ligaments are very loose, which makes exteriorization of the ovaries and ovarian pedicle ligation easy (**Fig. 11**A and B). Ovarian ligament and ovarian vessels can be ligated separately or as 1 unit, depending on the amount of fat (see **Figs. 4** and **11**B). Ovarian bursa (see **Fig. 5**) should not be penetrated to prevent ovarian remnant tissue. he uterus is ligated in its cervix (or distal part of the uterine body) with transfixing ligations together with uterine vessels (**Fig. 11**C and D).

Ovariectomy is not recommended because of adrenal gland disease and sexual hormonal dysbalance, which can negatively affect the uterus.

Hormonal Contraception in Female Ferrets (Anestrous Ferrets/Estrus Prevention)

Regarding hormonal treatment, the use of progestins for reproduction control in ferrets has been described in the literature for long-term hormonal contraception.[18,33,34]

Gonadotropin-releasing hormone agonists
GnRH agonists inhibit the synthesis of LH and FSH via negative feedback. Continued exposure to a GnRH agonist abolishes the pulsatile secretion of LH as a result of downregulation of GnRH receptors in gonadotrophic cells. This process results in an impaired pituitary response to endogenous GnRH and in decreased synthesis and release of LH and FSH, thereby effectively reducing estrogen and androgen production, and in the case of entire females preventing follicular development. Because of the LH and FSH release inhibition, the depot GnRH agonists (leuprolide acetate, deslorelin) are widely used in the prevention and treatment of adrenocortical diseases (ACDs) in ferrets.

Because leuprolide is used mostly in cases of ACD prevention/treatment, for contraceptive purposes, an intramuscular (IM) dose of 100 μg at monthly intervals, with ferrets heavier than 1 kg receiving 200 μg per month (depot leuprolide acetate 3.75 mg), was suggested by Schoemacher.[35]

Depot deslorelin acetate in the form of a subcutaneous implant currently seems to be the best option for nonsurgical sterilization. In female ferrets, the effects of 4.7-mg implant last for 1034 ± 44 days (range, 949–1121 days for 95% CI).[19] In addition, about one-third of treated jills become calmer, suggesting behavior changes. In a study by Prohaczik and colleagues,[18] the duration of the ovarian quiescence was 698 ± 122 days.

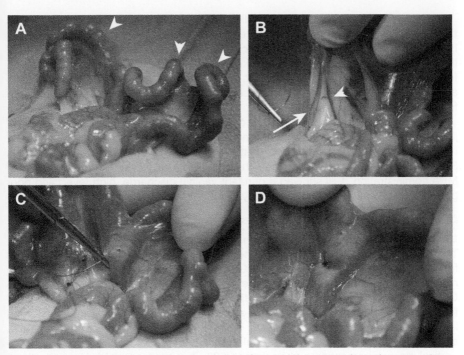

Fig. 11. Ovariohysterectomy in a 1.5-year-old ferret. (*A*) Note enlarged uterine horns (*arrowheads*) associated with pseudopregnancy. (*B*) Ovarian ligament (*arrow*) and ovarian vessels (*arrowhead*) can be ligated separately or as 1 unit, depending on the amount of fat. (*C* and *D*) Uterine cervix or the distal part of the uterine body is ligated using transfixing ligations. (*D*) Uterine vessels are included in the ligation. Two overlapping ligations of the uterus or 1 transfixing and then encircling ligation can be used based on the amount of tissue that needs to be ligated. (*Courtesy of* Vladimir Jekl, DVM, PhD, DECZM and Karel Hauptman DVM, PhD, Brno, Czech Republic; with permission.)

Because the deslorelin implant first stimulates FSH and LH release, it induced estrus within 3 to 4 days after treatment.[18,19] Estrus lasted for approximately 10 days, and pseudopregnancy was seen in 16% of jills.[19]

Side effects include minor local adverse reactions (redness, alopecia) in the site of deslorelin placement. If the treated jills were mated at the first posttreatment estrus, none of them became pregnant. However, mating in cases of second estrus was successful.[18] To guarantee continuous gonadal suppression, yearly replacement is advised, although biannual replacement may be sufficient in most ferrets.

Progestogens

To prevent estrus, long-acting forms of synthetic gestagens, medroxyprogesterone acetate (MPA) and proligestone, were used in ferrets. MPA (15 mg) and proligestone (40 mg) subcutaneously administered in February suppress the ovarian activity for 94 ± 18 days and for 99 ± 40 days, respectively.[18] The fertility at the first estrus after treatment, expressed as the proportion of ferrets mated in each group at the first estrus that subsequently produced a litter, was 75% in the MPA group and 60% in the proligestone group.[18]

In a report by Oxenham,[33] to suppress the estrus for whole breeding season, the proligestone (50 mg subcutaneously pro toto) in some jills needs to be administered twice. The fertility in the year following the injection seemed to be unaffected.

It seems that if the treatment with proligestone is started in late March, it increases the probability that jills will not show estrus in the subsequent breeding season, because the end of the period of efficacy of the gestagen coincides with the end of the breeding season. However, ferrets kept in an artificial environment and exposed to a stimulating photoperiod throughout the year may return to estrus 3 to 5 months after the treatment, implying that a second treatment would be needed each year for long-term breeding control.[18]

A small area of alopecia occurred at the injection site in 5.3% (7 out of 131 animal) of jills, which remained for a variable length of time.[33] Prohaczik and colleagues[18] recorded in 2 ferrets (MPA and proligestone) progressive alopecia around the vulva 33 and 45 days after treatment, and this resolved in 5 weeks. As a side effect of MPA administration, 1 jill showed a purulent vaginal discharge, high fever, and poor general condition when it aborted at day 37 of pregnancy.

Other Possible Contraceptive Techniques

Gonadotropin-releasing hormone vaccination

The immunocontraceptive GnRH vaccine was developed as a reproductive inhibitor for wildlife and consists of numerous GnRH peptides conjugated in a systematic manner to a mollusk hemocyanin protein.[36] Because of the reduction in available GnRH, in many mammalian species,[37] the secretion of LH and FSH is reduced and follicular development, ovulation, and estrus are inhibited; in males, testosterone levels are reduced, testicular size and aggressive behavior decrease significantly, and no interest is shown in estrous females. In ferrets, the vaccine is used for adreno-cortical disease prevention and treatment (500 µg subcutaneously). However, there are only a few reports about its use in intact female or male ferrets. Schoemaker[35] recorded severe adverse effects, so its possible use as a contraceptive in ferrets needs further studies.

- A limited light regimen and administration of melatonin are not effective in inhibiting the hypothalamus-pituitary-gonadal axis in ferrets.[37]
- Use of GnRH receptor antagonists, immunization with LH, and LH receptors were not studied in ferrets.[35]

REPRODUCTIVE TRACT DISEASES IN FERRETS

In the United States, desexing is performed routinely in ferrets at the age of 6 weeks.[30] However, in Europe, most ferrets are desexed when they are several months old or they are kept as intact animals. For this reason, diseases of the reproductive organs and a prolonged estrus are far more frequent in Europe.[38] A review of reproductive diseases/anomalies is given later for both sexes, and reproductive tract disorders related to partial sex are described.

Hermaphroditism

There is only 1 report of true hermaphroditism, in a 9-month-old male ferret that was presented with bilateral nonpruritic alopetia.[39] A bilateral cryptorchidism with fully developed uterus and ovaries was seen by laparoscopy and confirmed by histopathologic examination of all the tissues. Complete desexing was curative.

Urogenital Abnormalities

Urinary and genital systems both derive from intermediate mesoderm in early fetal life and are closely associated embryologically and anatomically. The paramesonephric (müllerian) duct in males and the mesonephric (wolffian) duct in females regress and only certain portions may be salvaged by a new organ. During the conversion of the primordial urogenital system into a postnatally functional system, the ducts are resorbed completely before or shortly after birth or may persist in vestigial forms into adulthood. Incomplete resorption of these ducts and/or postnatal regrowth of the vestigial remnants results in a heterogeneous group of urogenital anomalies. Frequently, the vestigial remnants become fluid-filled cystic structures of variable size and shape along the urogenital tracts or in the retroperitoneal and/or pelvic cavities.[40] A congenital müllerian duct abnormality (vestibulovaginal constriction) was reported by Jekl and colleagues.[41] The anomaly was defined as the failure of caudal paramesonephric ducts to fuse with the urogenital sinus with consequent absence of anatomic continuity between the cranial vagina and the vestibule (**Fig. 12**). Mucometra and cystic endometrial hyperplasia were confirmed by histopathologic examination.

Cysts on the dorsal bladder neck or trigone can also be urinary bladder diverticula, which are lined with the same epithelium as the urinary bladder.

Bladder duplication may result from doubling of the endodermal allantoic analogue with the development of the midsagittal wall (1 bladder for each ureter).

Cystic urachal remnants are localized at the urinary bladder apex.

Diagnosis is based on abdominal palpation, where the fluid-filled masses can be palpated caudally to kidneys, mostly in the area of the urinary bladder. Ultrasonography reveals cystic structures that can communicate with the urinary outflow tract or with the prostate gland. Intravenous pyelography can reveal the presence of the contrast medium in these structures, and can confirm possible communication with the urinary system. Final diagnosis is based on histopathologic examination of the cystic structure. Diagnostics are also directed at hormone active diseases, such as adrenal gland disease, ovarian tumors, ovarian remnant tissue, or Sertoli cell testicular tumors.

Because many of the structures are diagnosed parallel to adrenal gland disease, treatment with synthetic GnRH analogues (eg, deslorelin) is advocated by the authors. Clinical impact of the cystic mass needs to be assessed for every case and changes in the size are monitored by ultrasonography. In indicated cases, therapy includes total mass excision.

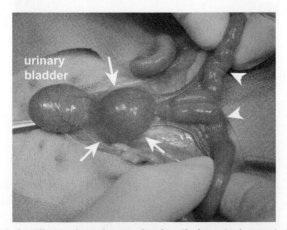

Fig. 12. A congenital müllerian duct abnormality (vestibulovaginal constriction) in a 1.5-year-old ferret. Because of the absence of anatomic continuity between the cranial vagina and the vestibule, the mucus and fluid had accumulated in the cranial vagina (*arrows*). Uterine changes (uterine wall thickening [*arrowheads*]) were associated with cystic endometrial hyperplasia. (*Courtesy of* Vladimir Jekl, DVM, PhD, DECZM and Karel Hauptman DVM, PhD, Brno, Czech Republic; with permission.)

REPRODUCTIVE DISORDERS IN MALE FERRETS
Congenital Disorders

Cryptorchidism

Cryptorchidism is a condition characterized by incomplete or nonexistent descent of 1 or both testicles (retained testicles), which can be located in the inguinal canal or in the abdominal cavity (**Fig. 13**). Bodri[42] reported a 0.75% (12 individuals from 1597 males) incidence of cryptorchidism in ferrets. There are no reports describing a hereditary cause in ferrets, but all breeding animals from the same family should be monitored. The affected testicle is usually smaller than the healthy one, but in older ferrets it commonly becomes neoplastic and more distinct on palpation.

Diagnostics are based on palpation and ultrasonography, which determine the location, size, and possible neoplastic disease.

The affected ferret should not be bred and it is recommended to perform orchidectomy via caudal midline laparotomy or via skin and vaginal tunic incision over the inguinal canal of the retained testicle.

Congenital penile deviation

Congenital penile deviations are very rare, and are associated with penile bone deformations (**Fig. 14**). Clinical symptoms are associated with urine staining. Treatment consists, if clinical signs are present, of penile amputation and perineal ureterostomy.

Orchitis

Orchitis in ferrets is a very rare condition even in intact males. A ferret diagnosed with orchitis and epididymitis/scrotal abscess was presented to the authors' clinic because of scrotal swelling associated with scrotal bite trauma. Orchidectomy, antibiotic

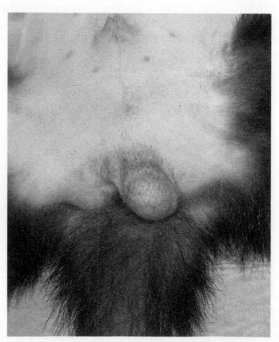

Fig. 13. Unilateral cryptorchidism in a 1-year-old ferret. (*Courtesy of* Vladimir Jekl, DVM, PhD, DECZM and Karel Hauptman DVM, PhD, Brno, Czech Republic; with permission.)

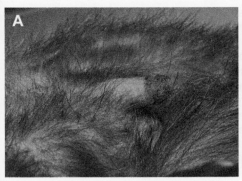
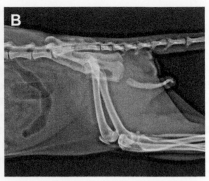

Fig. 14. (A and B) Congenital penile deviation in a 4-month-old ferret. (A) Paraphimosis and penile self-mutilation were also present. (B) Lateral radiograph showing penile bone deformation and opposite penile bone direction. (Courtesy of Vladimir Jekl, DVM, PhD, DECZM and Karel Hauptman DVM, PhD, Brno, Czech Republic; with permission.)

therapy (amoxicillin-clavulanate 15–25 mg/kg by mouth every 12 hours for 7 days), and analgesia (meloxicam 0.1 mg/kg by mouth every 12 hours) were curative.

Testicular neoplasia

Considering that neutering of male ferrets is a common practice to prevent reproduction and to reduce interspecies aggression, the prevalence of reproductive tumors may be difficult to define. In one study,[43] the incidence of testicular tumors in all submitted neoplasms was 1.1% (17 testicular tumors out of a total of 1525 submitted neoplastic tissues).

There are only few reports of unilateral testicular tumors in intact male ferrets, including interstitial cell tumors (Leydig cell tumors), Sertoli cell tumors, a mixed Sertoli cell tumor with an interstitial cell tumor (Fig. 15), seminoma, benign peripheral nerve sheath tumor, and carcinoma of the rete testis.[44–48] In addition, a testicular fibrosarcoma was diagnosed at the authors' clinic.

In cryptorchid ferrets, apart from interstitial cell tumors, seminomas, and Sertoli cell tumors, a testicular leiomyosarcoma and a mixed germ cell–sex cord–stromal tumor with a concurrent interstitial cell tumor were reported.[43,49,50]

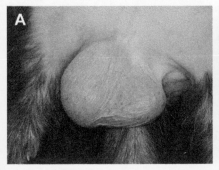
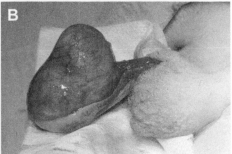

Fig. 15. (A and B) A mixed Sertoli cell tumor with an interstitial cell tumor in a 5-year-old male ferret. (A) Right testicular enlargement. (B) Orchidectomy was curative. (Courtesy of Vladimir Jekl, DVM, PhD, DECZM and Karel Hauptman DVM, PhD, Brno, Czech Republic; with permission.)

Testicular tumors have been reported in middle-aged to older ferrets and are commonly incidental findings or the ferret is presented with an enlarged scrotum. Macroscopically, the affected testicle is larger, firm, and irregularly shaped. In contrast, the contralateral testicle is commonly smaller and hypofunctional/atrophic. Alopecia and pruritus may be seen in cases of interstitial cell hyperplasia/tumor or Sertoli cell tumors.[49,51] Gonadal hormone levels are rarely increased even in tumors with potential hormonal production (testosterone in cases of interstitial tumors, estradiol in cases of Sertoli cell tumors[52]). Male feminization, as was described in dogs,[52] is not seen in ferrets. Ultrasonography examination can reveal different hyperechoic masses within the parenchyma, sometimes with intratesticular cystic cavities. Changes in color, hemorrhages, necrosis, and adhesions within the testicular tunics can also be present.

Batista and colleagues[47] concluded that the testicular neoplasms developed without the existence of any other concomitant pathologic process. Because of the small number of reported cases, the biological behavior of these tumors is difficult to predict. Visceral metastasis to the liver was reported only in 1 ferret with a Sertoli cell tumor.[43]

Orchidectomy, sometimes complemented with scrotal ablation, is curative.

Prostatic hyperplasia and prostatitis

Prostatic disease in ferrets is commonly associated with adrenal gland disease. Because of estrogen and androgen stimulation, the prostate becomes markedly enlarged, hyperplastic, and may contain multiple cysts. Squamous metaplasia can lead to accumulation of keratin, squamous epithelial cells, and cellular debris within the acini, causing prostatic inflammation.[53] Ductal obstruction then occurs, leading to the development of single or multilobulated retention cysts filled with keratin debris and inflammatory cells.[51,54] Prostatomegaly can lead to partial or complete, life-threating urethral obstruction (**Fig. 16**).

The disease is clinically manifested by dysuria, stranguria, oliguria, pollakiuria, urine dibbling, preputial dermatitis, and/or preputial trauma. Owners commonly report the presence of tenesmus during defecation. Problems with defecation can be associated with compression of the rectum with a large prostate, or this symptom can be misinterpreted in ferrets presenting with stranguria. Concurrent symptoms may be

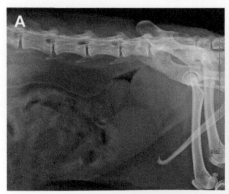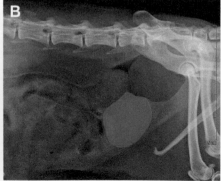

Fig. 16. (*A* and *B*) Lateral abdominal radiograph of a neutered male ferret with adrenal gland disease. Ferret was presented with urine straining associated with prostatomegaly (*B, blue*). Urinary bladder (*B, green*) and colon were distended. (*Courtesy of* Vladimir Jekl, DVM, PhD, DECZM and Karel Hauptman DVM, PhD, Brno, Czech Republic; with permission.)

associated with adrenal gland disease or kidney failure (anorexia, apathy, lethargy, posterior weakness, alopecia, and/or pruritus).

Other differential diagnoses for ferrets presenting with dysuria or anuria include urolithiasis, urinary tract infection, kidney failure, extensive penile/urethral trauma, and bladder neoplasm. Dysuria in male ferrets can also be present congenital urogenital disorders; for example, mesonephric or paramesonephric duct cysts, urinary bladder diverticula, bladder duplication, or urachal cysts.[40]

On clinical examination, discharge from the urethra can be present and prostatic masses can be palpated dorsally or dorsocaudally to the urinary bladder. Large prostatic cysts may be palpated cranially to the bladder. Large prostatic masses may be present and the distended bladder can be painful on palpation. If adrenal gland disease is present, alopecia is present (**Fig. 17**) and adrenal glands may be palpated.

Diagnosis is based on abdominal radiographic (see **Fig. 16**) and ultrasonographic examination. Ultrasonography is of particular use, because it can also reveal adrenal gland disorder.[55] The prostatic capsule is a hyperechoic structure that can be identified all around the prostate gland. Several hypoechoic or anechoic rounded or ovoid structures can be identified in the prostate or around the prostate gland. The walls of abscesses commonly have irregular margins. Contents of the hypoechoic structures can be aspirated with ultrasonography guidance and then cytologically examined to differentiate cysts from abscesses.

Hematology and plasma chemistry can determine overall health status and evaluate kidney function, because azotemia is very common. Levels of estradiol, androstenedione, and 17a-hydroxyprogesterone can be measured by a validated sex steroid serum panel. These androgens are normally found in minute quantities in neutered ferrets, but levels may be pathologically increased in ferrets with adrenocortical disease.[56]

Urinalysis should be one of the standard diagnostic methods used in cases of stranguria. It may reveal increased numbers of erythrocytes and leukocytes, and also bacteria. The presence of bacteria, especially in leukocytes (phagocytosis), indicates primary or secondary bacterial prostatic or urinary infections; therefore, bacterial culture and antibiotic susceptibility testing should be performed.

Therapeutic choices for the urethral obstruction include urethral catheterization, cystocentesis, and/or tube cystostomy.[54] Urethral catheterization can be difficult in ferrets and has a high complication rate of blockage and self-induced removal.[54] The urethral orifice is a very small slit in the ventral penis and is difficult to visualize.

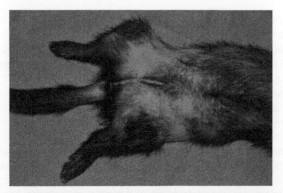

Fig. 17. Alopecia in a ferret with adrenal gland disease and associated prostatomegaly. (*Courtesy of* Vladimir Jekl, DVM, PhD, DECZM and Karel Hauptman DVM, PhD, Brno, Czech Republic; with permission.)

However, based on the authors' experience, after a little training the orifice can be found within a minute. Cystocentesis can be used during surgery or when catheterization is unsuccessful until more appropriate drainage by spontaneous urination, urinary catheterization, or tube cystostomy is established. Urethral catheterization requires anesthesia. The authors use tomcat catheters with 1-mm to 1.3-mm lumens. The stylet is removed when the catheter reaches the caudal part of the pubis.

Surgical techniques for managing large prostatic cysts and abscesses in ferrets include surgical excision, marsupialization, and prostatic abscess omentalization. Complete resection of prostatic cysts and abscesses is difficult because of adhesions to the urinary tract and prostate. During exploratory surgery, prostatic abscess or cyst is isolated from surrounding tissues, the contents are aspirated, and part of the capsule is excised. Any communications to the bladder or urethra should be identified and closed to prevent urine leakage and peritonitis. Samples of the abscess or cyst wall should be submitted for cytology, bacterial culture, and histopathology for further screening and optimal antibiotic treatment. After thorough debridement and isotonic fluid flushing, the abscess is omentalized or marsupialized to the lateral or ventral part of the body wall. Omentalization is preferred to marsupialization because more complications can occur with marsupialization (continual infection, continued secretion, septic peritonitis, urine leakage, peritonitis, additional surgery).[51]

Adrenal gland disease should be addressed simultaneously with the prostatic disease treatment. Adrenocortical disease can be addressed surgically (adrenalectomy) and/or using hormonal treatment. The depot formulation of the synthetic GnRH agonist, leuprolide acetate, is most commonly used (100–250 μg/kg/mo IM).[57] In many individuals, high-dose leuprolide acetate administration causes prostatic tissue to shrink within 12 to 48 hours so that the ferret may even begin to urinate around the urethral catheter.[58] Deslorelin acetate implant (4.5 mg) was shown to be an effective and safe treatment of adrenocortical disease and should be considered when surgical intervention carries significant risk.[59] However, because of the flare-up effect (up to 2 to 3 weeks) and also based on author (VJ) experience, the effect on prostate size is much slower. In cases of high estrogen levels, anastrozole (0.1 mg/kg by mouth every 24 hours) is recommend as an adjunct therapeutic drug to the leuprolide.[60] Other hormonal treatments include the use of antiandrogens (flutamide 10 mg/kg by mouth every 12–24 hours, bicalutamide 5 mg/kg every 24 hours, or finasteride 5 mg/kg by mouth every 24 hours),[58] which are used to decrease prostatic size.

Paraphimosis

Os penis is a slender, grooved bone with a hook at the proximal end and an inflated base at the other, which gives it typical J-shaped appearance. The hook can be caught on wire cages or the lips of hard, sharp surfaces, or some parts of the substrate or other material can be introduced into the prepuce, which prevents the penis from retracting into the prepuce.

Diagnosis is based on clinical examination and evaluation of the penis and prepuce under general anesthesia. The entire penis should be pulled out of the prepuce and examined for any superficial or deep injuries, foreign bodies, and inflammatory changes. Radiography can reveal penile bone fractures.

Therapy includes debridement of the entire penis and prepuce and flushing with sterile Ringer or saline. Any foreign material should be gently removed and the penis retracted into the prepuce. Local anesthetics, eye drops, or lidocaine spray can be used to alleviate pain. Use of meloxicam (0.1 mg/kg orally/subcutaneously every 12 hours) is recommend for at least 2 to 3 days. Use of antibiotics is mostly not necessary. In cases of inflammation, amoxicillin-clavulanate or sulfonamides can be used.

Fractures of os penis

Completely healed penile bone fractures are common incidental findings on survey abdominal radiographs (**Fig. 18**). If severe penile trauma is present, blood and nerve supply distally to trauma and damage of the urethra must be evaluated by adspection, palpation, and radiography. If urethral obstruction is present, contrast cystography or intravenous pyelography is indicated. In cases of severe urethral trauma, temporary urethral catheterization or perineal urethrostomy is performed.

Penile bone tumors

There are no published reports of penile bone tumors in ferrets. However, the authors have diagnosed an osteosarcoma of the os penis in a hob.

TUMORS OF THE APOCRINE GLANDS OF THE PREPUCE

Tumors of the apocrine glands of the prepuce (also referred to as preputial glands) have a profoundly increased incidence of malignancy; approximately 75% of preputial neoplasms are malignant, showing aggressive infiltration of local tissues (**Fig. 19**), metastasis to local lymph nodes, and occasionally pulmonary metastasis.[19,61,62] Moreover, these tumors tend to recur at excision sites and readily and quickly metastasize.

Ferrets are usually presented with acute onset of preputial swelling or mass. Apathy, anorexia, and posterior limb weakness can also be present. Dyspnea can be associated with lung metastases. Preputial tumors are firm on palpation and can reach more than 4 cm in diameter. Final diagnosis is based on histopathologic examination of the mass. Apart from the overall health screening, the focus should be on detection of possible metastases (thoracic radiographs, abdominal ultrasonography) and adrenal gland evaluation; Bulliot and colleagues[63] mentioned a potential role of hyperadrenocorticism in the cause and reappearance of ferret preputial tumors.

Complete surgical excision of preputial tumors is difficult because of their rapid and aggressive growth as well as the possibility of presurgical metastasis, so any masses in the preputial region should be submitted to histopathologic examination as soon as possible. Surgical excision with wide surgical margins (at least 5 mm, but >1 cm is better) is recommend with partial[64] (the authors' –preference is complete) penile amputation and perineal urethrostomy. Use of advanced skin flaps for wound closure is often necessary. Radiation therapy and chemotherapy may aid in the elimination of any local

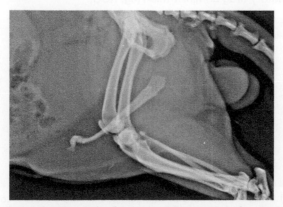

Fig. 18. Lateral abdominal radiograph of a 5-year-old intact male ferret with deformation of the distal part of the os penis. No urinary problems were noted. (*Courtesy of* Vladimir Jekl, DVM, PhD, DECZM and Karel Hauptman DVM, PhD, Brno, Czech Republic; with permission.)

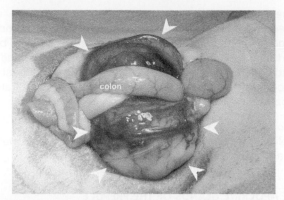

Fig. 19. A 5-year-old male ferret with metastases of the preputial gland adenocarcinoma into the lumbar lymph nodes (*arrowheads*). Because of the disease severity, the ferret was euthanized. (*Courtesy of* Vladimir Jekl, DVM, PhD, DECZM and Karel Hauptman DVM, PhD, Brno, Czech Republic; with permission.)

residual tumorous cells and in decreasing the risk of metastases, but the risk of remission still seems to be high.[65]

REPRODUCTIVE TRACT DISEASES IN FEMALE FERRETS
Congenital Diseases/Anomalies

Congenital diseases associated with the mesonephric (wolffian) duct is discussed earlier.

Different location or number of mammary teats is commonly seen in female ferrets (**Fig. 20**). This anomaly has no clinical impact on the female ferret or kittens; however, in cases of higher numbers of kittens, a small number of teats/mammary glands can potentially affect the milk feeding by neonates.

Pseudopregnancy

Pseudopregnancy in ferrets can develop following a sterile mating, as a result of hormonal imbalance caused by reduced light intensity 1 month before breeding, or as a result of pro-ovulatory drug administration (eg, hCG).

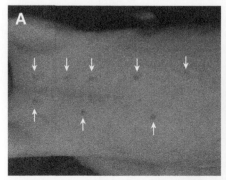
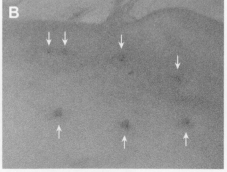

Fig. 20. (*A* and *B*) Different locations or numbers of mammary teats is common in female ferrets (*arrows*). The normal number of teats and mammary glands is 8. (*Courtesy of* Vladimir Jekl, DVM, PhD, DECZM and Karel Hauptman DVM, PhD, Brno, Czech Republic; with permission.)

The duration of the luteal phase in cases of pseudopregnancy is identical to that of pregnancy (40–42 days). Progesterone concentrations decline continuously between day 24 and day 42.[9]

The endometrium breaks down between day 35 and day 40, and resembles the anestrous state by day 45. Histologic changes in the endometrium are the same in the pregnant and pseudopregnant uterus. Features of the endometrium in these cases include dilated glands containing large amounts of secretory material, marked enlargement of luminal and glandular epithelial cells with extreme karyomegaly, symplasma formation, and sloughing of symplasmic masses into the uterine lumen. There are also small accumulations of neutrophils within some dilated glands. Symplasma formation occurs as the most superficial hypertrophied epithelial cells lose their integrity and form masses of protoplasm containing whole or fragmented nuclei.[66] These features are similar to the appearance of the endometrium 20 to 25 days following breeding and may resemble neoplastic proliferation (see **Figs. 4** and **11**).

Hyperestrogenism

Hyperestrogenism, also known as estrogen toxicosis or prolonged estrus, in jills is associated with prolonged estrus. Ferrets are induced ovulators and when they are not bred, especially when kept alone or together with other females or neutered males, can remain in estrus for extended periods. An incidence of 50% of jills showing hyperestrogenism and a mortality of 40% was reported by Sherrill and Gorham.[67] The high levels of estrogen can cause various degrees of bone marrow hypoplasia and decreased splenic extramedullary hematopoiesis. Hematological findings include initial thrombocytosis and leukocytosis followed by thrombocytopenia, leukopenia, and anemia. If not treated, ferrets die from exhaustion or cell asphyxia, or they can bleed to death. In the study by Sherrill and Gorham,[67] hemorrhagic anemia caused by thrombocytopenia was the most common cause of death and the mortality was 40%.

Nonspecific clinical symptoms include apathy, general weakness, dehydration, anorexia, and progressive weight loss. Clinical signs are associated with enlarged vulva, behavior signs of estrus, symmetric hypotrichosis/alopecia around the perianal area, anemic mucosal membranes (**Fig. 21**), and petechial mucosal bleeding. In severe cases, general alopecia and/or melena can be present.

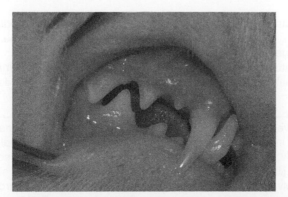

Fig. 21. Anemic mucosal membranes of the oral cavity associated with hyperestrogenism (prolonged estrus) in an intact 2-year-old female ferret. (*Courtesy of* Vladimir Jekl, DVM, PhD, DECZM and Karel Hauptman DVM, PhD, Brno, Czech Republic; with permission.)

Diagnosis is based on history of prolonged estrus and vulvar enlargement. Hematology shows different stages of nonregenerative anemia, thrombocytopenia, and/or leukopenia.

Blood transfusion is recommended when the hematocrit value decreases to less than 0.2 L/L. However, dehydration status should be also evaluated and each case assessed individually. Ferrets do not have blood groups, so a good donor is commonly a large male. The amount of blood that can be obtained from healthy ferret is about 0.8% of body weight. At the authors' clinic, the blood is obtained from the cranial vena cava and immediately mixed with sodium citrate in a ratio of 6:1 and then slowly administered to the recipient. Sometimes more than 1 donor is needed to reestablish normal hematocrit.

In addition, the estrus is terminated and ovulation is induced, with the administration of hCG at the dose of 100 IU/kg intramuscularly pro toto.[17] Two injections in an interval of 7 days may be needed to induce ovulation. The preovulatory LH surge can also be indirectly mimicked by the stimulating endogenous LH release by the administration of GnRH (20 IU) given intramuscularly 10 days after the onset of estrus.[35] hCG and GnRH should stimulate ovulation and induce pseudopregnancy in 95% of jills 35 hours after treatment.[35]

Alternatively, to suppress estrus, a deslorelin acetate implant (4.7 mg) can be administered subcutaneously. This method was successfully used in 7 ferrets, which displayed typical estrous signs for 4 to 6 weeks. After 4 weeks of the deslorelin treatment, the vulva was obviously less swollen and the owners reported an obvious decrease in the intensity of odor from week 1 after treatment.[68] Food intake was increased from 5 to 7 weeks after treatment in all animals. In those cases, suppression of estrus remained for 22 to 35 months after treatment.[68] Based on the author's experience (VJ), it is recommended to use deslorelin implants in jills that are in estrus just for 1 to 2 weeks, because panmyeloid suppression can be noted if deslorelin is administered after 4 to 6 weeks of estrus. If the estrus is terminated using hCG, the ferret will start to gain weight within 4 to 7 days after hCG administration (authors' personal experience in more than 200 ferrets).

For estrus suppression, the use of proligestone (50 mg subcutaneously pro toto) is also reported.[33] When a jill in estrus was injected with proligestone, the signs subsided over 3 to 4 days. No ill effects were reported.

Tamoxifen has estrogenic effect in ferrets, so it is contraindicated.

A limited photoperiod and administration of melatonin is not effective in suppressing estrus in jills.[33]

Definitive treatment is ovariohysterectomy. However, ferret sterilization can be associated with the development of adrenocortical hyperplasia and possible neoplastic changes.

A so-called natural technique used to suppress estrus in jills is to mate them with a vasectomized male, which induces ovulation with subsequent pseudopregnancy.

Vaginitis

Vaginitis can develop in pregnant jills; after mating as a result of vaginal trauma; in jills after delivery; or in cases of prolonged estrus, ovarian tumors, adrenal gland disease, and pyometra.[69,70] Poor husbandry and inadequate sanitation may also promote vaginitis in breeding jills kept on particulate bedding when hay, straw, or shavings adhere to the swollen vulva during estrus.[58] Vaginitis is associated with overgrowth of bacteria such as Escherichia coli, Staphylococcus, Streptococcus, Proteus, or Klebsiella.[69] Vaginitis should be differentiated from the swelling associated with estrus by history, vaginal cytology, and the presence of mucopurulent vaginal discharge. Concurrent pyometra/metritis can be present. Ascending vaginitis can also lead to a secondary cystitis and rapid formation of cystoliths.[69]

Mucoid, mucopurulent, or purulent vaginal discharge and associated perineal staining/superficial dermatitis, and vulvar licking can be the only clinical signs. In cases of metritis/pyometra, anorexia, apathy, fewer, abdominal pain, and abdominal distension can be present. Diagnosis is based on vaginal cytology and vaginoscopy, if necessary. Diagnosis of ascendant urinary tract infection requires urine collection by cystocentesis, because free-catch samples are contaminated with vaginal contents. Abdominal ultrasonography can reveal urogenital as well as adrenal gland disorder. Hematology and blood chemistry are unremarkable in cases of vaginitis alone.

Treatment of vaginitis consists of removal of the foreign material from the vagina and resolving the underlying hormonal dysbalance (hCG administration, ovariohysterectomy, ovarian tumor/remnant removal, adrenal gland treatment [adrenalectomy, deslorelin implant]). Gentle local washing with dilute chlorhexidine (0.2% at maximum) and/or saline helps to dilute bacterial overload and remove inflammatory detritus. Some cases of vaginitis can resolve spontaneously with time, and conservative therapy is recommended. If the only clinical signs are those that are found incidentally, treatment is commonly not necessary. Systemic antibiotics are recommended in cases of metritis/pyometra or in cases of immunosuppression (leukocytopenia associated with bone medulla suppression).

Pyometra

Pyometra is uncommon in clinical practice in the United States, where the ferrets are spayed at the age of 6 weeks. It is reported that pyometra can be a major disease in intact pseudopregnant jills, stemming from a possible prolonged estrus. At the authors' clinic, pyometra is diagnosed more commonly in ferrets after parturition or in referral ferrets with inadequate ovarian excision during spay (**Figs. 22** and **23**); in intact ferrets, even with prolonged estrus, pyometra is seen only on rare occasions. Stump pyometra was also reported in spayed ferrets with adrenal gland disease.[71] Bacterial culture of the uterine contents can reveal infection with *E coli*, staphylococci, streptococci, or with *Corynebacterium* sp. Final diagnosis of pyometra/metritis should be

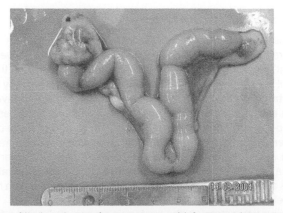

Fig. 22. The uterus filled with pus from a 4-year-old ferret with pyometra. (*Courtesy of* Vladimir Jekl, DVM, PhD, DECZM and Karel Hauptman DVM, PhD, Brno, Czech Republic; with permission.)

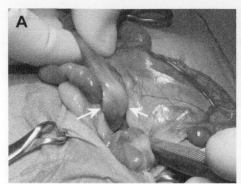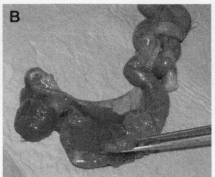

Fig. 23. A ferret with vaginal abscess and pyometra (*A*) associated with suspected vaginal damage during coitus. (*B*) Postoperative view of the uterus. *E coli* was cultivated from both vaginal abscess and uterine content. Recovery was uneventful. (*Courtesy of* Vladimir Jekl, DVM, PhD, DECZM and Karel Hauptman DVM, PhD, Brno, Czech Republic; with permission.)

based on histopathologic examination, because the presence of brownish fluid in the uteri is commonly a consequence of cystic endometrial hyperplasia and/or hydrometra.[72]

The clinical presentation is similar to that in dogs and ferrets may show an open pyometra with purulent vaginal discharge or closed pyometra. Ferrets are apathetic, anorectic, dehydrated, and may be febrile, anemic, and alopetic. On abdominal palpation, distended uterus can be palpated in the midabdomen and caudal abdomen. Abdominal ultrasonography reveals hypoechoic tubular structures dorsal and cranial to the bladder. Hematology and plasma chemistry can detect anemia, leukocytopenia/leukocytosis, and other organ involvement.

Medical management includes rehydration, antibiotics, and prostaglandin F2-alpha administration (Lutalyse, Pharmacia and Upjohn, MI; 0.1–0.5 mg IM), followed in 1 hour by oxytocin (5–10 IU IM) to stimulate myometrial contraction and expulsion of pus.[69] Definitive treatment involves ovariohysterectomy or surgical removal of infected stump. In cases of the simultaneous presence of adrenal gland disease, adrenalectomy and/or deslorelin implant administration is recommended. In cases of aplastic anemia, blood transfusion is indicated.

Cystic Endometrial Hyperplasia, Hydrometra

Hydrometra is the accumulation of aseptic fluid within the uterus in the presence of persistent corpora lutea. Hydrometra associated with hormonal active ovarian tumors is one of the most frequently diagnosed uterine diseases of ferrets in the authors clinic (>20 cases) and it is especially common after incomplete ovariectomy (**Figs. 24–26**).[73] High levels of estrogen in the blood serum probably influence the development of the hydrometra. The endometrium may, in such cases, respond to the estradiol stimulation by increasing the number of endometrial glands. At a later stage of development, the originally sterile uterus may become infected, and a pyometra may develop. Hydrometra and cystic endometrial hyperplasia were also described in ferrets with segmental atresia of the uterus, adrenal gland disease, and congenital defects.[47,73,74] Uterine torsion is also seen by the authors and it was associated with hydrometra and ovarian tumor (see **Fig. 26**).

Hence an ovariohysterectomy is the preferred means of desexing female ferrets. If estrus signs appear in a ferret following desexing, it is imperative that the clinician thoroughly investigates possible causes and institutes appropriate therapy.

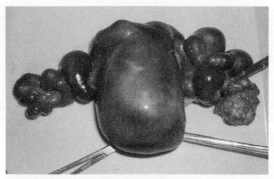

Fig. 24. Hydrometra associated with hormonal active ovarian leiomyoma in a 6-year-old ferret. The ferret was incompletely spayed by another practitioner 5 years before the surgery. Ovariohysterectomy was curative. (*Courtesy of* Vladimir Jekl, DVM, PhD, DECZM and Karel Hauptman DVM, PhD, Brno, Czech Republic; with permission.)

Reproductive Tract Tumors in Intact Females

In a retrospective study of 4774 ferrets (1968–1997) only 2.3% of the 639 tumors recorded involved the reproductive system.[75] Within the reproductive system, the ovary is the organ most frequently affected by neoplastic proliferation. Ovarian leiomyoma Is the most common tumor reported, although granulosa cell tumors, thecomas, fibromyomas, arrhenoblastoma, luteoma, undifferentiated carcinomas, and ovarian teratoma have also been described.[46,72,73,75–79] Ovarian leiomyomas are well-defined unilateral or bilateral tumors and may reach 1 to 8 cm in diameter, but they are generally much smaller. High number of ovarian tumors were seen by the authors in referral ferrets after incomplete ovariectomies, in which the remaining ovarian tissue became neoplastic (see **Figs. 24–26**; **Fig. 27**).

Ovarian tumors can be found incidentally during clinical examination or the ferrets can be presented with hormonal alopecia, chronic weight loss, and signs of estrus (changes in behavior, edematous vulva, mucous vaginal discharge) caused by increased levels of sexual hormones.

Increased estradiol and/or progesterone levels may also be associated with hydrometra, cystic endometrial hyperplasia, or other uterine disorders.

Abdominal palpation and ultrasonography seem to give better information than radiography (see **Fig. 27**). Hormonal analysis can show increased levels of sexual

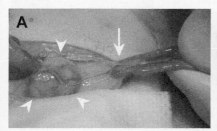
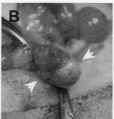
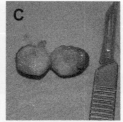

Fig. 25. Ovarian granulosa cell tumor (*arrowheads*) and uterine tube cystic changes (*arrow*) in a 4-year-old ferret associated with incomplete spay, referral case (*A–C*). Detailed perioperative (*B*) and postoperative (*C*) views of the ovarian tumor. Ferret was presented with alopecia. Ovariohysterectomy was curative. (*Courtesy of* Vladimir Jekl, DVM, PhD, DECZM and Karel Hauptman DVM, PhD, Brno, Czech Republic; with permission.)

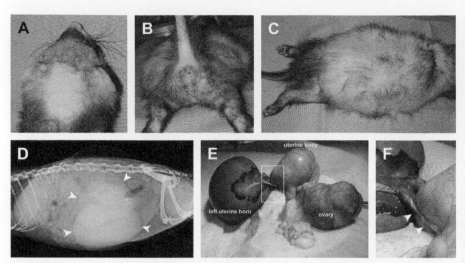

Fig. 26. Ovarian granulosa cell tumor in a ferret after incomplete spay, referral case. Ferret was presented with alopecia (*A–C*) and distended abdomen (*C*). Abdominal radiography revealed large abdominal masses of soft tissue radio-opacity (*D, arrowheads*). (*E*) Perioperative view of the granulosa cell tumor of the right ovary, uterine mucometra, and uterine torsion. (*F*) Detailed view of the uterine torsion (*arrowheads*). Ovariohysterectomy was curative. (*Courtesy of* Vladimir Jekl, DVM, PhD, DECZM and Karel Hauptman DVM, PhD, Brno, Czech Republic; with permission.)

hormones. The anticipated inhibition of bone marrow activity is not a common finding in ovarian tumors, despite the increased level of estradiol.[38,73] Adrenal gland disease, a common cause of alopetic changes in ferrets, can be rule out by adrenal gland ultrasonography and decreased postoperative levels of sexual hormones.

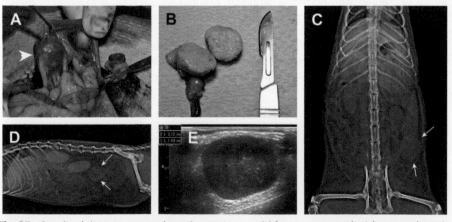

Fig. 27. Ovarian leiomyosarcoma in an intact 4-year-old ferret presented with general weakness. Perioperative (*A, arrowhead*) and postoperative (*B*) view of the ovarian tumor. (*C* and *D*) Abdominal radiographs of the ferret. Ovarian tumor was soft tissue opacity (*arrows*) and was localized caudally to the left kidney and spleen. Kidneys are marked green (*D*). (*E*) Ultrasonography revealed soft tissue hypoechoic mass of 2.2 × 1.6 cm. Ovariohysterectomy was curative. (*Courtesy of* Vladimir Jekl, DVM, PhD, DECZM and Karel Hauptman DVM, PhD, Brno, Czech Republic; with permission.)

Therapy includes fluid support, easily digestible diet, and ovariohysterectomy.

Uterine Neoplasia

Uterine tumors in ferrets are extremely rare. Uterine leiomyoma, uterine leiomyosarcoma, and malignant mixed müllerian tumor in the uterus were reported.[46,75,78,80]

Implantation sites in the ferret uterus are unique findings that may be seen during gestation or even during pseudopregnancy. Microscopically the marked pleomorphism of the decidual epithelium (presymplasma) strongly resembles a malignant neoplasm to pathologists unfamiliar with this normal finding.[78]

Pregnancy Toxemia

Pregnancy toxemia (also called gestational ketosis) in ferrets is a clinically relevant metabolic disease that is caused by negative energy balance in the late period of gestation and is potentially fatal for the jill and kits. In rare cases, pregnancy toxemia can develop even in ferrets after parturition, when part of the placenta remains in the uterine lumen and becomes necrotic (**Figs. 28** and **29**).

Fetal nutritional demand (fat, carbohydrates) exceeds maternal supply during the last trimester of pregnancy, leading to excess fatty acid mobilization, which leads to variable degrees of hyperlipidemia, hypoglycemia, ketosis, and hepatic lipidosis.

In the ferret, pregnancy toxemia usually occurs between days 32 and 42 of gestation, especially just before the whelping date. It is more common in primiparous female ferrets or females carrying average litters and fed adequate diets, but when an accidental fast occurs during this period.[81] Even 1 overnight fast can induce toxemia in females with a large litter. Batchelder and colleagues[82] reported that pregnancy toxemia is seen in at least 75% of jills carrying 8 or more kits that are deprived of food for 24 hours during the last week of gestation. More than 50% of jills carrying more than 15 kits develop toxemia even if not deprived of food, but these may respond to supplemental feeding alone. Most jills carrying 18 to 20 kits develop toxemia even when consuming an excellent diet. This finding may be caused in part by limitations of the abdominal capacity, which on gross inspection appear insufficient for the kits and the volume of food necessary to meet energy demands.

Pregnancy toxemia can also develop in older ferrets under conditions that initiate an imbalance in energy metabolism, such as a change to a lower-energy diet late in pregnancy, temporary lack of access to water, or the stress of illness or shipping.

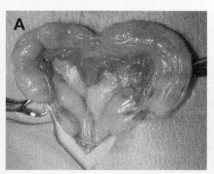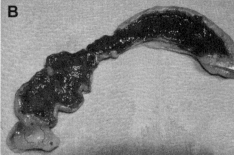

Fig. 28. Two-year-old ferret was presented with general weakness 2 days after the parturition of 4 dead fetuses. Perioperative (A) and postoperative (B) views of distended uterus. Pregnancy toxemia associated with placental necrosis and intrauterine hemorrhages was the final diagnosis. Ovariohysterectomy was curative. (Courtesy of Vladimir Jekl, DVM, PhD, DECZM and Karel Hauptman DVM, PhD, Brno, Czech Republic; with permission.)

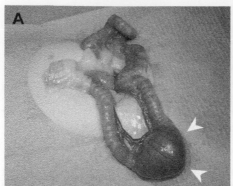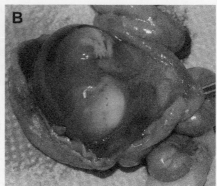

Fig. 29. Dystocia in a ferret that was presented with vaginal bleeding. The exact day of mating was not known. (*A*) Perioperative view of a ferret gravid uterus with 1 fetus (*arrowheads*). (*B*) Detailed view of a normally developing fetus. The reason for the dystocia remained unknown. Ovariohysterectomy was curative. (*Courtesy of* Vladimir Jekl, DVM, PhD, DECZM and Karel Hauptman DVM, PhD, Brno, Czech Republic; with permission.)

Clinical symptoms and signs include a sudden onset of lethargy, dehydration, hypothermia, hair loss, distended abdomen, and diarrhea. Melena may be also present. Abdominal palpation reveals gravid uterus. Dyspnea, sternal recumbency, and icterus may also be present and sudden death may occur. Abdominal radiography and ultrasonography can confirm the high number of fetuses and their viability. Abdominal free fluid is also a common finding at the authors' clinic. Hematological and plasma/serum chemistry can reveal different stages of anemia, leukocytosis or leukopenia, hypoproteinemia, hypoalbuminemia, azotemia, high activity of liver enzymes, and hyperbilirubinemia. Hyponatremia, hypochloremia, and hyperkalemia can be also detected. Blood glucose concentration tends to be low early in the disease (usually <50 g/dL, <2.8 mmol/L), but when the disease progresses may increase to more than 144 mg/dL (8 mmol/L).[82,83]

Metabolic acidosis with the presence of ketones can be proved using acid-base balance evaluation. Also, high levels of beta-hydroxybutyrate (normal values 2.6 ± 0.21 mg/dL, 0.25 ± 0.02 mmol/L), hypoinsulinemia, and decreases in the T4 and T3 concentrations can be detected.[83] Urinalysis shows proteinuria, aciduria, and ketonuria.

At necropsy, multiple well-developed fetuses are found within the gravid uterus. Petechial bleeding is commonly present at the serosal surface of the abdominal organs, especially the uterus. The liver is enlarged, brownish to yellowish color, and it is fragile, suggesting liver lipidosis. Stomach ulcers are also common.

The disease must be treated as soon as the clinical signs develop because pregnancy toxemia is progressive and can be fatal in 24 to 48 hours. The therapy is intended to increase energy intake and metabolic acidosis/ketoacidosis with subsequent dehydration, circulatory changes (eg, hypovolemia), and gastric ulcerations. This treatment includes intravenous fluid therapy with electrolytes and glucose, frequent feeding with a high-energy and high-protein diet (eg, Emeraid Carnivore, Emeraid, Cornell, IL; Royal Canin Convalescence Support Clinical Canine/Feline Instant, Royal Canin, France), despite liver dysfunction and stomach mucosa protectants (ranitidine 24 mg/kg IM every 12 hours; famotidine 0.5 mg/kg by mouth or subcutaneously every 24 hours; or omeprazole 4 mg/kg by mouth every 24 hours). Cesarean section should be considered as soon as the ferret is stabilized.

Ferrets that recover are not predisposed for recurrence. Kittens need to be force fed or preferably introduced to another nursing jill, because agalactia is common. Gravid ferrets should be fed a high-quality diet (at least 35% of crude protein, 20% fat) and closely monitored while gravid.

OTHER DISEASES

In periparturient jills, the reproductive disorders, apart from pregnancy toxemia, include dystocia (**Fig. 29**), agalactia, and mastitis.

In large groups of breeding jills, dystocia was described in 1% of the jills.[58] In pet ferrets, dystocia seems to be very rare.[84]

Mastitis in ferrets should be treated aggressively because peracute disease and septicemia can be present.[85] Acute infection often becomes gangrenous within a few hours. Chronic infection commonly develops insidiously 2 to 3 weeks after parturition. Potential causal agents include *Staphylococcus* sp and hemolytic *E coli*.[58,85] Clinical signs include firm swelling of 1 or more mammary glands and discoloration of the overlying skin. Mucopurulent or bloody discharge with milk discoloration can also be present.

Treatment consists of fluid therapy, antibiotics (amoxicillin-clavulanate, marbofloxacin, and metronidazole), analgesia, and nutritional support combined with wide surgical excision of the affected mammary gland. Administration of antibiotics should be based on the results of bacteriology and antibiotic testing of the samples from the affected mammary gland. The kits could transmit mastitis to another ferret if they nurse, so they should be hand raised (in the case of older kits) or provided with additional nutritional support.[58] Affected jills should be isolated from other animals.

Agalactia can be associated with various reproductive or systemic/environmental conditions,[70] so the aim of the diagnostics is to find and treat underlying disorder.

SUMMARY

To understand disorders of the reproductive tract and associated organs a thorough knowledge of the anatomy and physiology of reproduction is necessary. Many reproductive tract diseases, estrogen toxicosis included, are life-threatening conditions in intact females; therefore, surgical or hormonal contraception is recommended in all nonbreeding jills. In hobs, the most severe disease is associated with prostatic enlargement (caused by adrenal gland disease) and preputial gland adenocarcinoma.

REFERENCES

1. Lewington J. Ferrets. In: O'Malley, editor. Clinical anatomy and physiology of exotic species: structure and function of mammals, birds, reptiles and amphibians. St Louis (MO): Elsevier; 2005. p. 237–61.
2. Orcutt CJ. Ferret urogenital diseases. Vet Clin North Am Exot Anim Pract 2003;6: 113–38.
3. Powers LV. Basic anatomy, physiology, and husbandry. In: Quesenberry KE, Carpenter JV, editors. Ferrets, rabbits, and rodents: clinical medicine and surgery. 3rd edition. St Louis (MO): Elsevier; 2012. p. 1–12.
4. Turek FW, Van Cauter E. Rhythms in reproduction. In: Knobil E, Neill JD, editors. The physiology of reproduction. New York: Raven Press; 1998. p. 1789–830.
5. Marini RP, Otto G, Erdman S, et al. Biology and diseases of ferrets. In: Fox JG, Andreson LC, Loew FM, et al, editors. Laboratory animal medicine. 2nd edition. San Diego (CA): Elsevier; 2002. p. 483–517.

6. Jallageas M, Boissin J, Mas N. Differential photoperiodic control of seasonal variations in pulsatile luteinizing hormone release in long-day (ferret) and short-day (mink) mammals. J Biol Rhythms 1994;9(3–4):217–31.

7. Neal J, Murphy BD, Moger WH, et al. Reproduction in the male ferret: Gonadal activity during the annual cycle; recrudescence and maturation. Biol Reprod 1977;17(3):380–5.

8. Nakai M, Van Cleeff JK, Bahr JM. Stages and duration of spermatogenesis in the domestic ferret (Mustela putorius furo). Tissue and Cell 2004;36:439–46.

9. Lindeberg H. Reproduction of the female ferret (Mustela putorius furo). Reprod Dom Anim 2008;43(Suppl 2):150–6.

10. Williams ES, Thorne ET, Kwiatkowski DR, et al. Comparative vaginal cytology of the estrous cycle of black-footed ferrets (Mustela nigripes), Siberian polecats (M. eversmanni), and domestic ferrets (M. putorius furo). J Vet Diagn Invest 1992;4(1):38–44.

11. Buchanan GD. Reproduction in the ferret (Mustela furo). I. Uterine histology and histochemistry during pregnancy and pseudopregnancy. Am J Anat 1966;118(1): 195–216.

12. Amstislavsky S, Ternovskaya Y. Reproduction in mustelids. Anim Reprod Sci 2000;60–61:571–81.

13. Hammond J, Marshall FHA. Reproductive biology and management of captive black-footed in the ferret. Proc R Soc Lond B Biol Sci 1930;105:607–30.

14. Enders AC, Schlafke S. Implantation in the ferret: epithelial penetration. Am J Anat 1972;133:291–316.

15. Herbert J. Light as a multiple control system on reproduction in mustelids. In: Seal US, Thorne ET, Bogan MA, et al, editors. Conservation biology and the black-footed ferret. London: Yale Univ. Press; 1989. p. 38–159.

16. Mayer J, Marini RP, Fox JG. Biology and diseases of ferret. In: Fox JG, Anderson LC, Otto G, et al, editors. Laboratory animal medicine. 3rd edition. San Diego (CA): Elsevier; 2015. p. 577–622.

17. Mead RA, Neirinckx S. Hormonal induction of oestrus and pregnancy in anoestrous ferrets (Mustela putorius furo). J Reprod Fertil 1989;86:309–14.

18. Prohaczik A, Kulcsar M, Trigg T, et al. Comparison of four treatments to suppress ovarian activity in ferrets (Mustela putorius furo). Vet Rec 2010;166:74–8.

19. van Zeeland YR, Pabon M, Roest J, et al. Use of a GnRH agonist implant as alternative for surgical neutering in pet ferrets. Vet Rec 2014;175(3):66.

20. Kidder JD, Foote RH, Richmond ME. Transcervical artificial insemination in the domestic ferret (Mustela putorius furo). Zoo Biol 1998;17:393–404.

21. Mead RA, McRae M. Is estrogen required for implantation in the ferret? Biol Reprod 1982;27(3):540–7.

22. Mead RA, Joseph MM, Neirinckx S, et al. Partial characterization of a luteal factor that induces implantation in the ferret. Biol Reprod 1988;38(4):798–803.

23. Kidder JD, Roberts PJ, Simkin ME, et al. Nonsurgical collection and nonsurgical transfer of preimplantation embryos in the domestic rabbit (Oryctolagus cuniculus) and domestic ferret (Mustela putorius furo). J Reprod Fertil 1999;116(2): 235–42.

24. Li Z, Sun X, Chen J, et al. Factors affecting the efficiency of embryo transfer in the domestic ferret (Mustela putorius furo). Therineology 2006;66(2):183–90.

25. Towle HA. Testes and scrotum. In: Tobias KM, Johnston SA, editors. Veterinary surgery: small animal. St Louis (MO): Elsevier Saunders; 2012. p. 1903–16.

26. Lewington JH. Ferret vasectomy, orthopaedics and cryosurgery. In: Lewington JH, editor. Ferret husbandry, medicine and surgery. 2nd edition. Philadelphia: Elsevier Saunders; 2007. p. 440–7.
27. Schoemaker NJ, van Deijk R, Muijlaert B, et al. Use of a gonadotropin releasing hormone agonist implant as an alternative for surgical castration in male ferrets (*Mustela putorius furo*). Theriogenology 2008;70(2):161–7.
28. Vinke AM, Van Deijk R, Houx BB, et al. The effects of surgical and chemical castration on intermale aggression, sexual behaviour and play behaviour in the male ferret (*Mustela putorius furo*). Appl Anim Behav Sci 2008;115:104–21.
29. Bulliot C, Mentré V, Berthelet A, et al. Intern use of a gonadotropin releasing hormone agonist implant containing 4.7 mg deslorelin for medical castration in male ferrets (*Mustela putorius furo*). J Appl Res Vet Med 2014;12(1):67–75.
30. Schoemaker NJ, Schuurmans M, Moorman H, et al. Correlation between age at neutering and age at onset of hyperadrenocorticism in ferrets. J Am Vet Med Assoc 2000;216:195–7.
31. de Jong MK, ten Asbroek EE, Sleiderink AJ, et al. Gonadectomy-related adrenocortical tumors in ferrets demonstrate increased expression of androgen and estrogen synthesizing enzymes together with high inhibin expression. Domest Anim Endocrinol 2014;48:42–7.
32. Goericke-Pesch S. An alternative to surgical desexing in ferrets. Vet Rec 2014; 175(3):64–5.
33. Oxenham M. Oestrus control in the ferret. Vet Rec 1990;126(6):148.
34. Risi E. Control of reproduction in ferrets, rabbits and rodents. Reprod Dom Anim 2014;49(Suppl 2):81–6.
35. Schoemaker NJ. Hyperadrenocorticism in ferrets. Thesis Universiteit Utrecht. Universiteit Utrecht: Faculteit Diergeneeskunde; 2003. p. 1–176.
36. Miller LA, Fagerstone KA, Wagner RA, et al. Use of a GnRH vaccine, GonaCon, for prevention and treatment of adrenocortical disease (ACD) in domestic ferrets. Vaccine 2013;31(41):4619–23.
37. Fagerstone KA, Miller LA, Killian G, et al. Review of issues concerning the use of reproductive inhibitors, with particular emphasis on resolving human-wildlife conflicts in North America. Integr Zool 2010;5:15–30.
38. Hauptman K. Clinical diagnostics in small mammals [PhD Thesis]. Brno (Czech Republic): University of Veterinary and Pharmaceutical Sciences Brno; 2005 [in Czech].
39. Bertheled A. A case of true hermaphroditism in a ferret. Proceedings of the International Conference on Avian and Herpetological and Exotic Mammal Medicine, ICARE 2015. Paris, April 18–23, 2015. p. 447.
40. Li X, Fox G, Erdman SE, et al. Cystic urogenital anomalies in ferrets (*Mustela putorius furo*). Vet Pathol 1996;33:150–8.
41. Jekl V., Skoric M., Hauptman K. First case of a vaginal split in a ferret. Proceedings of the 1st International Conference on Avian, Herpetological and Exotic Mammal Medicine. Wiesbaden, Germany, April 20–26, 2013. p. 276.
42. Bodri MS. Theriogenology question of the month. J Am Vet Med Assoc 2000; 217(10):1465–6.
43. Williams BH, Weiss CA. Ferrets: neoplasia. In: Quesenberry KE, Carpenter JW, editors. Ferrets, rabbits, and rodents: clinical medicine and surgery. 2nd edition. Philadelphia: WB Saunders; 2003. p. 91–106.
44. Dillberger JE, Altman NH. Neoplasia in ferrets: eleven cases with a review. J Comp Pathol 1989;100:161–76.
45. Meschter CL. Interstitial cell adenoma in a ferret. Lab Anim Sci 1989;39(4):353–4.

46. Beach JE, Greenwood B. Spontaneous neoplasia in the ferret (*Mustela putorius furo*). J Comp Pathol 1993;108:133–47.
47. Batista-Arteaga M, Suárez-Bonnet A, Santana M, et al. Testicular neoplasms (interstitial and Sertoli cell tumours) in a domestic ferret (*Mustela putorius furo*). Reprod Domest Anim 2011;46(1):177–80.
48. Hohšteter M, Smolec O, Gudan Kurilj A, et al. Intratesticular benign peripheral nerve sheath tumor in a ferret (*Mustela putorius furo*). J Small Anim Pract 2012; 53:63–6.
49. Kammeyer P, Ziege S, Wellhöner S, et al. Testicular leiomyosarcoma and marked alopecia in a cryptorchid ferret (*Mustela putorius furo*). Tierarztl Prax Ausg K Kleintiere Heimtiere 2014;42(6):406–10.
50. Inoue S, Yonemaru K, Yanai T, et al. Mixed germ cell-sex cord-stromal tumor with a concurrent interstitial cell tumor in a ferret. J Vet Med Sci 2015;77(2):225–8.
51. Powers LV, Winkler K, Garner MM, et al. Omentalization of prostatic abscesses and large cysts in ferrets (*Mustela putorius furo*). J Exot Pet Med 2007;16:186–94.
52. Peters MA, Rooij DG, Teerds KJ, et al. Spermatogenesis and testicular tumours in ageing dogs. J Reprod Fertil 2000;120:443–52.
53. Coleman GD, Chavez MA, Williams BH. Cystic prostatic disease associated with adrenocortical lesions in the ferret (*Mustela putorius furo*). Vet Pathal 1998;35(6): 547–9.
54. Nolte DM, Carberry CA, Gannon KM, et al. Temporary tube cystostomy as a treatment for urinary obstruction secondary to adrenal disease in four ferrets. J Am Anim Hosp Assoc 2002;38(6):527–32.
55. Neuwirth L, Collins B, Calderwood-Mays M, et al. Adrenal ultrasonography correlated with histopathology in ferrets. Vet Radiol Ultrasound 1997;38:69–74.
56. Chen S. Advanced diagnostic approaches and current medical management of insulinomas and adrenocortical disease in ferrets (*Mustela putorius furo*). Vet Clin North Am Exot Anim Pract 2010;13(3):439–52.
57. Wagner RA, Bailey EM, Schneider JF, et al. Leuprolide acetate treatment of adrenocortical disease in ferrets. J Am Vet Med Assoc 2001;218:1272–4.
58. Pollock CG. Disorders of the urinary and reproductive systems. In: Quesenberry KE, Carpenter JW, editors. Ferrets, rabbits, rodents clinical medicine and surgery. 3rd edition. Philadelphia: WB Saunders; 2012. p. 46–61.
59. Lennox AM, Wagner R. Comparison of 4.7 mg deslorelin implants and surgery for the treatment of adrenocortical disease in ferrets. J Exot Pet Med 2012;21:332–5.
60. Johnson-Delaney CA. Medical therapies for ferret adrenal disease. Semin Avian Exot Pet Med 2004;13:3–7.
61. Pinches MDG, Liebenber G, Stidworthy MF. What is your diagnosis? Preputial mass in a ferret. Vet Clin Path 2008;37:443–6.
62. Antinoff N, Williams BH. Neoplasia. In: Quesenberry KE, Carpenter JW, editors. Ferrets, rabbits, and rodents: clinical medicine and surgery. 3rd edition. St Louis (MO): WB Saunders; 2012. p. 103–21.
63. Bulliot C, Mentré V, Bonnefont C. Trois cas de tumeurs des glandes préputiales chez des furets associées à une maladie surrénalienne. Point Vet 2012;43: 48–52 [in French].
64. van Zeeland YR, Lennox A, Quinton JF, et al. Prepuce and partial penile amputation for treatment of preputial gland neoplasia in two ferrets. J Small Anim Pract 2014;55(11):593–6.
65. Miller TA, Denman DL, Lewis GC Jr. Recurrent adenocarcinoma in a ferret. J Am Vet Med Assoc 1985;187(8):839–41.

66. Fox JG, Bell JA. Growth, reproduction and breeding. In: Fox JG, editor. Biology and diseases of the ferret. 2nd edition. Baltimore (MD): Williams and Wilkins; 1998. p. 211–27.
67. Sherrill A, Gorham J. Bone marrow hypoplasia associated with estrus in ferrets. Lab Anim Sci 1985;35(3):280–6.
68. Goericke-Pesch S, Wehrend A. The use of a slow release GnRH-agonist implant in female ferrets in season for oestrus suppression. Schweiz Arch Tierheilkd 2012;154(11):487–91.
69. Lewington JH. Reproduction and genetics. In: Lewington JH, editor. Ferret husbandry, medicine and surgery. 2nd edition. Philadelphia: Elsevier Saunders; 2007. p. 86–121.
70. Fisher PG. Ferrets: urogenital and reproductive system disorders. In: Keeble E, Meredith A, editors. BSAVA manual of rodents and ferrets. Quedgeley (United Kingdom): BSAVA; 2009. p. 1–12.
71. Martinez-Jimenez D, Chary P, Barron HW, et al. Cystic endometrial hyperplasia-pyometra complex in two female ferrets (*Mustela putorius furo*). J Exot Pet Med 2009;18(1):62–70.
72. Cotchin E. Smooth-muscle hyperplasia and neoplasia in the ovaries of domestic ferrets (*Mustela putorius furo*). J Pathol 1980;130(3):169–71.
73. Jekl V, Hauptman K, Jeklova E, et al. Hydrometra in a ferret – case report. Vet Clin North Am Exot Anim Pract 2006;9(3):695–700.
74. Baumgärtner W, Juchem R. Aplastic anemia in ferrets. Tierarztl Prax 1987;15(3): 333–5 [in German].
75. Li X, Fox JG, Padrid PA. Neoplastic diseases in ferrets: 574 cases (1968-1997). J Am Vet Med Assoc 1998;212(9):1402–6.
76. Rodríguez JL, de las Mulas JM, de los Monteros JL, et al. Ovarian teratoma in a ferret (*Mustela putorius furo*): a morphological and immunohistochemical study. J Zoo Wildl Med 1994;25(2):294–9.
77. Hauptman K, Jekl V, Dorrestein GM, et al. Comparison of estradiol and progesteron serum levels in ferrets suffering from hyperoestrogenism and ovarian neoplasia. Vet Med (Czech) 2009;11:532–6.
78. Fox JG, Muthupalami S, Kiupel M, et al. Neoplastic diseases. In: Fox JG, Marini RP, editors. Biology and diseases of the ferret. 3rd edition. Hoboken (NJ): Wiley Blackwell; 2014. p. 587–626.
79. Patterson MM, Rogers AB, Schrenzel MD, et al. Alopecia attributed to neoplastic ovarian tissue in two ferrets. Comp Med 2003;53:213–7.
80. Schaeffner J, Virnich A, Laik C, et al. Malignant mixed Muellerian tumour in the uterus of an ovariectomised ferret. Kleintierpraxis 2012;57(2):63–6.
81. Bell JA. Periparturient and neonatal diseases. In: Hillyer EV, Quesenberry KE, editors. Ferrets, rabbits and rodents: clinical medicine and surgery. Philadelphia: WB Saunders; 1997. p. 53–62.
82. Batchelder MA, Bell JA, Erdman SE, et al. Pregnancy toxemia in the European ferret (*Mustela putorius furo*). Lab Anim Sci 1999;49:372–9.
83. Prohaczik A, Kulcsar M, Huszenicza GY. Metabolic and endocrine characteristics of pregnancy toxemia in the ferret. Vet Med (Czech) 2009;54(2):75–80.
84. Garrigoua A, Huynh M, Pignon C. Dystocia in a young ferret (*Mustela putorius furo*) with a possible "single kitten syndrome". Revue Vétérinaire Clinique 2014; 49:63–6.
85. Liberson AJ, Newcomer CE, Ackerman JI, et al. Mastitis caused by hemolytic *Escherichia coli* in the ferret. J Am Vet Med Assoc 1983;183(11):1179–81.

Reproduction of Rescued Vespertilionid Bats (*Nyctalus noctula*) in Captivity

Veterinary and Physiologic Aspects

Jiri Pikula, MVDr, PhD, DECZM (Wildlife Population Health)[a],*,
Hana Bandouchova, MVDr, PhD, DECZM (Wildlife Population Health)[a],
Veronika Kovacova, MSc[a], Petr Linhart, MSc[a],
Vladimir Piacek, MVDr[a], Jan Zukal, PhD[b]

KEYWORDS

- Bat • Fertilization • Captive birth • Euthanasia • Ethics • Blood profile
- Thermoregulation • Torpor

KEY POINTS

- Wildlife veterinarians make responsible decisions on animal euthanasia based on chances of survival in the wild and quality of life in captivity.
- Consideration of adult female reproductive status is an important ethical aspect when considering euthanasia of wildlife casualties.
- Although vespertilionid bats of temperate regions mate before the winter, ovulation and fertilization are stimulated by homeothermy after emergence from hibernacula in the spring.
- Due to delayed fertilization, the authors argue that handicapped mated insectivorous female bats should be allowed to give birth in captivity.
- High standards of veterinary care are only possible for insectivorous bats when their annual life cycle and costs of reproduction are taken into consideration.

CHALLENGES IN WILDLIFE MEDICINE

Wildlife clinicians practicing zoologic medicine face a wide range of challenges related not only to species diversity but also to differences in the medical issues associated with captive and free-ranging wild animals. Veterinary practitioners must have

Disclosure Statement: The authors have nothing to disclose.
This study was supported by the Internal Grant Agency of the University of Veterinary and Pharmaceutical Sciences Brno (239/2015/FVHE).
[a] Department of Ecology and Diseases of Game, Fish and Bees, University of Veterinary and Pharmaceutical Sciences Brno, Palackeho tr. 1946/1, 612 42 Brno, Czech Republic; [b] Institute of Vertebrate Biology, Academy of Sciences of the Czech Republic, Kvetna 8, 603 65 Brno, Czech Republic
* Corresponding author.
E-mail address: pikulaj@vfu.cz

extensive knowledge and wide experience in many specialties to offer a high standard of care in a medical field where most patients are nontraditional species that are treated only infrequently. Although the best available medical care can be provided to wildlife species on an individual basis, much research is still needed regarding conservation, ecosystem, and population health in many declining and extinction-threatened species.[1]

It is imperative that veterinary practitioners minimize distress and pain in wild animals. When addressing medical, welfare, and ethical issues related to wildlife casualties, practitioners tend to follow a decision tree with 3 main outcomes: release of successfully treated specimens, permanent captivity of nonreleasable animals, or euthanasia.[2] Euthanasia is considered an appropriate decision when animals have no chance of survival in the wild and/or a poor disposition for life in captivity. The most stressful ethical dilemma, however, concerns adult female bats due to their gravidity or possibility of giving birth to healthy offspring.

ANNUAL CYCLE OF INSECTIVOROUS NOCTULE BATS, INCLUDING REPRODUCTIVE PATTERN

In the Holarctic temperate zone, the annual cycle of insectivorous bats is influenced by seasonal climatic changes and invertebrate food availability. During their active period, female vespertilionid bats gather at summer maternity roosts where they give birth to and raise their young. Male bats remain solitary during this period. After the young are weaned and become independent, both male and female bats migrate to swarming sites, where mating takes place in the autumn.[3] Mating tends to be polygynous and promiscuous. Although copulation takes place before the winter hibernation, female bats store sperm in their uteri throughout the hibernation period, which usually lasts from December to April. On emergence from the hibernacula in the early posthibernation period, ovulation and fertilization are stimulated by homeothermy (ie, thermoregulation to maintain stable body temperature higher than the environmental temperature). This reproduction strategy is known as delayed fertilization and is of immense importance for veterinary management of bats. Female bats injured in the autumn are usually kept in homeothermic conditions, which may result in the onset of gravidity and subsequent birth of bat pups in midwinter, 2 months later.[2] To avoid such out-of-season births, wildlife rehabilitators need to simulate the natural annual cycle of insectivorous bats using artificial hibernacula.

AN ETHICAL ISSUE RELATED TO REPRODUCTION IN HANDICAPPED VESPERTILIONID BATS

The authors report a case of female noctule bats (Nyctalus noctula; family Vespertilionidae) that were nonreleasable due to traumatic injury but nevertheless kept in captivity rather than being euthanized because they were still capable of giving birth to healthy offspring. Although the species is classified as of least concern in the International Union for Conservation of Nature Red List of Threatened Species,[4] it is protected under international law by the Bonn (Agreement on the Conservation of Populations of European Bats [EUROBATS]) and Bern conventions.

Noctule bats, common in Europe, are a synanthropic species using human-modified habitats. They form dense hibernation clusters in hollow thick-walled city park trees and in crevices of buildings and bridges. Noctule bats are among the most common bat species brought for veterinary treatment due to injuries sustained during tree felling or reconstruction of buildings.[2]

In November 2015, a group of 68 female noctule bats was sent to the rescue center at the University of Veterinary and Pharmaceutical Sciences in Brno, Czech Republic, for examination and treatment because their hibernaculum inside a fallen park tree had been destroyed. All animals were in need of urgent care and rehydration therapy on presentation and some suffered from open contaminated limb fractures (**Fig. 1**). Disruption of blood supply to the distal extremities made limb amputation the treatment of choice. The decision to keep nonreleasable handicapped species is mainly based on the possibility of using the specimen for educational purposes. In this case, the decision was ruled by the mated state of female bats at this time of the year. The authors argue that, due to the peculiar reproduction pattern of hibernating bats, being mated is the same as being pregnant. Hence, bats were provided with therapy, and veterinary diagnostic and physiologic techniques were used to monitor state of health of the female bats and to evaluate their likelihood of successfully producing offspring for subsequent release.

HOUSING AND DIET OF NOCTULE BATS IN CAPTIVITY

During the period of treatment, the bats were housed either individually or as a group in plastic boxes equipped with soft netting to enable roosting, a piece of cloth to hide in, and dishes to supply drinking water and food. The plastic boxes (500 mm × 400 mm × 400 mm) allowed easy cleaning and replacement of paper bedding. Noctule bats were kept euthermic under room conditions (21°C [69.8°F]) and supplied with nutrition on a daily basis during the period of therapy. The bats soon learned to feed themselves[5,6] on mealworms (*Tenebrio molitor* larvae) and crickets (*Acheta domestica*). They were also trained for hand-feeding with a complete commercial recovery instant diet (Convalescence Support, Royal Canin, Aimargues, France) administered as a gruel from a syringe. After successful treatment, the bats were fattened up until they had sufficient fat stores for hibernation, after which they were fasted for a day or 2 to empty their gastrointestinal tract. The bats were then transferred to a chamber with temperature regulated at 7°C (44.6°F). Here they stayed from early December to late March. During the hibernation period, the boxes were regularly checked to make sure they had enough drinking water and a high humidity level (greater than 80%). The bats were also inspected for signs of torpor (without arousing them) on a weekly basis

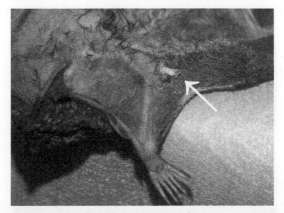

Fig. 1. Femoral fracture in a noctule female bat. Most fractures in specimens as small as vespertilionid bats, such as this one close to the knee joint (*arrow*), are open and contaminated by the time they are presented for treatment.

because nontorpid bats quickly burn off their fat stores at low temperatures and may die. After hibernation, noctule bats fit to be released were let free. Any permanently handicapped bats were kept under the same conditions as in the autumn. Although no adaptation of the diet was necessary prior to delivery, lactating female bats were fed only with the commercial diet (discussed previously) fortified with calcium gluconicum 10% (B. Braun, Melsungen, Germany), 5 mg/kg of body weight, and given plain water and/or Rehydration Support (Royal Canin), as desired.

GESTATION PERIOD, DELIVERY, AND BIRTHWEIGHT OF THE YOUNG

Under natural conditions, hundreds of pregnant female noctule bats gather at nursery roosts, where pups are delivered synchronously from approximately mid-June. Vespertilionid bat gestation lasts approximately 2 months. With the 8 captive female bats, the period from termination of hibernation in the artificial hibernacula to birth ranged from 64 days to 71 days. Because ovulation was not determined in the early posthibernation period by measuring progesterone, the exact duration of the gestation period is not known.[5]

Exposure of pregnant female bats to torpor-inducing cold temperatures and food scarcity may extend the length of the gestation period.[7] Lowered body temperature in torpid female bats induces a profound reduction in metabolism, heart rate, and oxygen and nutrient supply to tissues,[8] which may jeopardize prenatal development. As in other vertebrates, decreased embryonic heart rate at lower intrauterine temperatures is likely to increase the time necessary to reach the total number of heartbeats necessary for embryogenesis and embryonic growth.[9]

Pregnancy diagnosis in mammalian species as small as noctule bats is difficult. In the authors' opinion, use of radiography is obsolete in gravid female bats. As an alternative, ultrasound effectively distinguished developing twins of 18 mm and 19 mm in a noctule female bat 14 days prior to delivery (**Fig. 2**). Aside from a reduction in feed consumption, no other signs of preparation for parturition were noticed.

Natural pup-bearing postures described for noctule bats[7] include (1) a vertical head-up position with pelvic limbs spread apart, with the uropatagium forming a pouch to catch the young; (2) a horizontal sloth-like position characterized by the female bat holding the ceiling of the roost with both pelvic limb feet and both thumb claws of thoracic limbs, the young being born onto the abdomen and uropatagium; and (3) a dog-sitting position on the floor of the roost with pelvic limbs spread apart with the

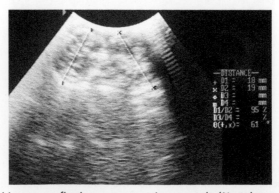

Fig. 2. Ultrasound image confirming pregnancy in a noctule (*Nyctalus noctula*) female bat. Two fetuses of equal size are discernable 14-days prior to delivery.

uropatagium forming a pouch to catch the young. Although handicapped noctule bats without amputated limbs had problems taking these natural birth postures, they were capable of giving birth, mostly using the dog-sitting position. Four captive female noctule bats were video-recorded while giving birth. All births occurred during the day. The first stage of labor could not be recognized externally. The second stage, that is, expulsion of the fetus in breech presentation, took approximately 2 to 3 minutes. It seems that the neonate bat actively helps itself to get out of the birth canal by using its large pelvic limb feet, whereas the female bat licks and cleans the fluids from the pup during the expulsion process. Although still attached to the placenta by the umbilical cord, the neonate climbs up its mother's body until it gets hold of the thoracic nipple, whereupon it seats itself under the respective flight membrane. The pup's birth is finished within minutes after expulsion of the fetal membranes, which are disconnected and eaten by the mother. The birth of twin pups largely takes the same course. Audible vocalization and social cross-talk between the mother and its young starts immediately after birth.

The noctule bat gives birth to 1 litter annually, with 1 or 2 pups per litter. The authors' group of 8 captive noctule female bats produced 14 pups born as twins and 1 single birth. The birthweight of bat pups surviving to weaning and release (mean ±SD, 4.24 ± 0.42 g; n = 11) was higher than that of stillborn pups or pups that died within 2 days (3.09 ± 0.72 g; n = 4). In a previous study by Kleiman,[7] the mean noctule birthweight was 5.7 g, although Kleiman mostly observed single-born pups rather than the twins observed in the study. Newborn noctule pups averaged 14.98 ± 2.08% (range 10.76%–17.15%) of maternal body weight. Vespertilionid bats that produce twins are known to invest more in terms of litter mass.[10]

LACTATION, POSTNATAL GROWTH, FOOD CONSUMPTION, AND WEANING

Noctule bats are a typical altricial species. They are born naked and without hair and have closed eyelids and external ears (cf. **Fig. 3**). Bat pups have to be cared for by their mother until they grow to at least 90% of adult wing size and 70% of adult postpartum body weight[11] (adult postpartum body weight in the captive noctule female bats was 28.9 g ± 3.89 g; n = 8). Separation of eyelids occurred on average at 7.50 days ± 0.77 days. Eruption of hair was first noticed on day 13.4 ± 1.52. Deciduous teeth replacement by permanent teeth started at 21.8 days ± 0.26 days postpartum.

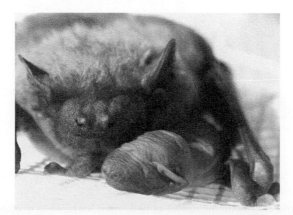

Fig. 3. Noctule female with a pup. The nakedness and closed eyelids of this 3-day-old pup are clearly visible.

Bat pups remain attached to their mother throughout the first 2 weeks and suckle without restriction. Newborn bats have a set of deciduous teeth, which are used to grip the mother's nipple. Later, the mothers remove the pups and deposit them in the roost. Each bat pup has its own nipple. Although lactation occurs within both the right and left mammary glands in female bats that give birth to twins, only 1 side is turned on at a time and continues to produce milk for a single pup. Lactation was not initiated in one of noctule female bats. Both her pups starved to death because the other female bats repulsed the young and could not be forced to take over nutrition of pups from another female bat. These starving neonates had no interest in suckling from a female bat other than their mother.

The growth rate of the young bats was high, with birthweight doubling in 10 days (**Fig. 4**). The daily body weight increase per pup ranged from 0.26 g to 0.62 g over 4 weeks. Healthy growth of captive-born noctule bats was documented by smoothly increasing growth curves (see **Fig. 4**). Checking early postnatal growth twice daily proved life-saving for 1 pup from a female bat suffering from mastitis, the problem first recognized through the pup's weight loss. The female in question only allowed its pup to suckle when tightly held. The disorder resolved itself, however, within a day and the pup survived to weaning.

The rapid growth of young noctule bats was supported by the high food consumption of the mothers (**Fig. 5**). Up to day 16 of lactation, twice-daily body weight measurements of breast-feeding noctule female bats showed high fluctuations in the food load that female bats took for physiologic maintenance and milk production (see **Fig. 5**), with the daily consumption of instant diet per female ranging from 8 mL to 15.91 mL during the 4 weeks of lactation. After weaning, 5 mL to 6 mL of the diet was sufficient for each female bat to maintain its body weight (see **Fig. 5**). Female bats during peak lactation required enormous quantities of drinking water (ie, up to 2.5 mL per female prior to the feeding event). Reduced milk production from approximately day 28 of lactation resulted in a considerable drop in drinking water

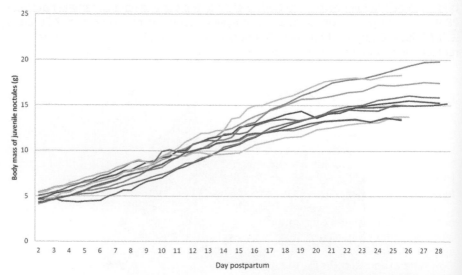

Fig. 4. Early postnatal growth, measured as body mass, in juvenile noctule bats (*Nyctalus noctula*) during the first 4 weeks of life. The figure is based on twice-daily measurements of 11 bat pups.

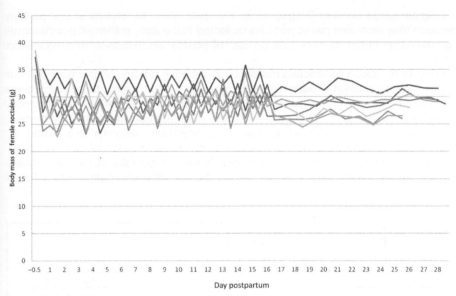

Fig. 5. Body mass changes in breast-feeding female noctule bats (*Nyctalus noctula*). The figure is based on twice-daily measurements of 7 bats until day 16 of lactation. The female bats were weighed once a day from day 17 postpartum, thus disguising any fluctuations of body weight associated with food consumption.

consumption (ie, down to 0.5 mL per female bat per day). Like their pups, peak-lactating female noctule bats were not observed in torpor.

Additional food had to be supplied to the pups from day 28 after a drop in their body weight. Where pups also displayed lowered body temperature, feeding was delayed until they warmed up using shivering thermogenesis. Although weaning using insects, such as mealworms, was difficult, pups readily changed to the instant liquid diet, consuming up to 3 mL at a time. Because the digestive tract had to adapt to the different diet, the amount given over several days was gradually increased. Food consumption by both female bats and their young seemed to reflect outside ambient conditions, with cold and rainy weather inducing a reduction in food consumption.

BLOOD PROFILES OF NOCTULE FEMALE BATS

Although some studies have described the blood physiology and hematology of bats,[12–18] reference ranges in the strict sense of the meaning have only been published for a few megachiropteran species.[19] Blood profile studies for insectivorous bats have increased in number recently due to the need to understand their physiologic adaptations to extreme hibernation conditions and response to pathogenic infections, such as white-nose syndrome.[20,21]

To determine the physiologic and biochemical state of health of captive handicapped noctule female bats, a microchiropteran species, blood was sampled after skin disinfection with alcohol from the uropatagial vessel using a 30-G ½-in Omnican syringe (B. Baun) to perform tests with 2 diagnostic analyzers, that is, VetScan VS2 Complete Diagnostic Profile (Abaxis, Union City, California) and VetScan i-STAT 1 EC8+ cartridge (Abaxis). These state-of-the-art hematology, chemistry, electrolyte, and blood gas analyzers deliver data from just 90 μL to 100 μL of whole blood, thus overcoming limitations of small body size.

Despite based on only 7 specimens, the data allow for statistical comparison because they represent paired samples collected in the early euthermic posthibernation period and from lactating bats on day 16 postpartum (Mann-Whitney-Wilcoxon test).

Many of the blood parameters measured in lactating noctule female bats differed significantly from those in early euthermic posthibernation female bats, which were considered a control group (**Table 1**). Although blood pH did not alter significantly, decreased partial pressure carbon dioxide, total carbon dioxide, bicarbonate, and base excess demonstrate compensated metabolic acidosis (see **Table 1**). There was a significant increase in blood plasma potassium in lactating female bats, probably also associated with acidosis as redistribution hyperkalemia. Increased levels of sodium and chlorides indicate dehydration. Euthermic bats demonstrated

Table 1
Venous blood profiles of healthy noctule bats at different life stages

Parameters	Units	Euthermic (n = 7)	Lactating (n = 7)
Na	(mmol/L)	155.28 ± 5.02	166.60 ± 8.29[a]
K	(mmol/L)	6.57 ± 1.13	7.94 ± 0.94[a]
Cl	(mmol/L)	119.00 ± 2.44	124.00 ± 6.19[a]
Ca	(mmol/L)	2.46 ± 0.13	2.15 ± 0.09[b]
P	(mmol/L)	2.25 ± 0.72	1.86 ± 0.78
pH		7.24 ± 0.05	7.23 ± 0.05
pCO$_2$	(kPa)	6.23 ± 1.04	4.86 ± 1.44[a]
tCO$_2$	(mmol/L)	21.73 ± 2.14	16.14 ± 3.38[b]
HCO$_3$	(mmol/L)	20.27 ± 2.00	15.05 ± 3.01[b]
BE	(mmol/L)	−7.00 ± 2.28	−12.57 ± 2.29[b]
AnGap	(mmol/L)	19.30 ± 2.11	17.20 ± 4.54
Hct	(L/L)	58.33 ± 2.87	60.28 ± 7.13
Hb	(g/L)	198.33 ± 9.74	205.00 ± 24.17
GLU	(mmol/L)	4.95 ± 1.37	4.77 ± 1.99
BUN	(mmol/L)	11.10 ± 2.35	17.65 ± 6.33[b]
CRE	(μmol/L)	49.85 ± 8.49	35.00 ± 16.46
TP	(g/L)	61.28 ± 5.08	58.40 ± 2.40
ALB	(g/L)	28.71 ± 4.92	8.25 ± 4.64[b]
AMY	(μkat/L)	8.32 ± 2.38	26.64 ± 4.42[b]
TBIL	(μmol/L)	6.28 ± 1.38	3.60 ± 0.54[b]
ALT	(μkat/L)	3.62 ± 0.89	2.28 ± 0.48[a]
ALP	(μkat/L)	0.74 ± 0.53	0.38 ± 0.16

Values represent mean ±SD.

Abbreviations: ALB, albumin; ALP, alkaline phosphatase; ALT, alanine aminotransferase; AMY, amylase; AnGap, anion gap; BE, base excess; Ca, calcium; Cl, chloride; CRE, creatine; Euthermic, healthy euthermic noctule female bats; GLU, glucose; Hb, hemoglobin; HCO$_3$, bicarbonate; Hct, hematocrit; K, potassium; Lactating, lactating noctule female bats on day 16 postpartum; Na, sodium; P, phosphorus; pCO$_2$, partial pressure carbon dioxide; pH, pH value; BUN, blood urea nitrogen; TBIL, total bilirubin; tCO$_2$, total carbon dioxide; TP, total protein.

[a] $P<.05$.
[b] $P<.01$ when comparing lactating female bats against the nonlactating group.

hyperphosphatemia. Lactating female bats generally had lower levels of calcium. These changes in phosphorus and calcium level may be due to excessive dietary supply of phosphorus or inadequate supply or intake of calcium, the latter in association with an increased need for calcium due to milk production. Milk production and breastfeeding also resulted in hypoproteinemia and significant hypoalbuminemia. Serum urea nitrogen, which, as in other insectivorous bats, is normally relatively high in noctule bats, increased in lactating female bats (see **Table 1**). Elevated levels of hematocrit and hemoglobin were associated with dehydration. Elevation of amylase, which catalyzes hydrolysis of polysaccharides, was probably due to mobilization of energy to maintain normoglycemia. Blood profile responses similar to those described previously were also observed in free-ranging greater mouse-eared bat (*Myotis myotis*) female bats in a summer breeding colony (authors' own unpublished data, 2016).

To conclude, blood profile changes in lactating noctule female bats document physiologic costs of reproduction that may represent fitness trade-offs.[22] By checking the blood profiles of lactating female bats, the authors were able to make dietary adjustments to improve quality of nutrition during the high-performance period of lactation.

BODY TEMPERATURE OF LACTATING NOCTULE FEMALE BATS AND EARLY POSTNATAL THERMOREGULATION

Regulation of body temperature is an important aspect of vertebrate evolution that allows an animal to maintain homeostasis in its physiologic functions. Temperate vespertilionid bats have adapted to seasonal changes in climate food availability by becoming heterothermic, that is, their body temperature varies with that of the environment.[23] While active, their body temperature is kept at levels similar to that of homeothermic mammals; when their body temperature drops close to the ambient temperature of the hibernaculum, however, bats enter seasonal hibernation. Homeothermy is energetically costly and bats use torpor to save energy. Repeated cycles of torpor and arousal during hibernation can result in profound alterations to a bat's metabolic rate and oxygen consumption, along with other physiologic changes at the organism, organ, cellular, and molecular levels.[8,24,25] Bats are also known to use daily torpor to save energy and water in cold ambient temperatures or to cope with food scarcity during the active and/or reproductive season.[26–28]

Daily thermal profiles were undertaken to evaluate the physiologic condition of the captive female noctule bats during lactation and the pups during early postnatal growth (**Figs. 6–8**). Because torpid bats are incapable of digesting food (the gut contents ferment, resulting in bloating and eventual mortality), the thermal profiles allowed selecting the appropriate food supply strategy for each bat's physiologic condition.[2] Fur surface body temperature, which is correlated with core body temperature, was measured using a Guide M8 thermocamera (Wuhan Guide Infrared, Wuhan, China). Thermal imaging during the 4 weeks postpartum revealed a mean temperature for lactating noctule female bats of 34°C (see **Fig. 6**), with some variation in the thermal profiles of individual female bats. Female noctule bats were observed lowering their body temperature and using daily torpor when weaning the young. This finding is in line with previously observed daily torpor patterns of free-ranging female Daubenton's bats that adopted this thermoregulatory behavior to optimize juvenile development.[26]

Neonatal thermoregulation development depends on interaction between the mother and its young. Isolation of the pups from their mother for 10 minutes enabled measurement and analysis of thermal development without disruption of the social bond. Comparison of lactating female thermal profiles with those of young attached to or isolated from their mothers allowed determining when neonates achieve adult

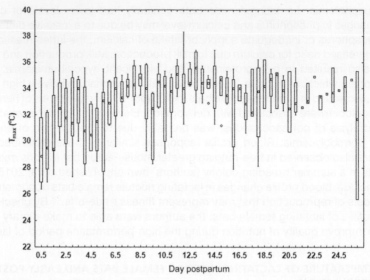

Fig. 6. Temperature of lactating female noctule bats (*Nyctalus noctula*). The mean temperature of lactating female noctule bats during the 4-week monitoring period was 34°C (93.2°F). T_{max}, maximum temperature.

thermal competence. Young bats were incapable of thermoregulation for at least 6 days postpartum (note the drop in body temperature of young isolated from their mothers at up to 6 days of age [see **Fig. 8**; **Fig. 9**]); after 6 days, however, high body temperature and competent homeothermic thermoregulation resulted in rapid growth in the young (see **Fig. 4**). Juvenile noctule bats seem capable of torpor, that

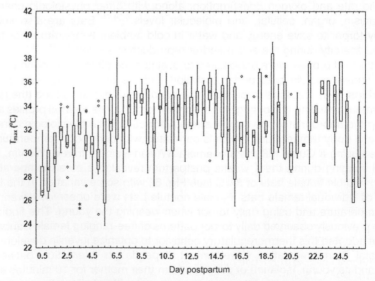

Fig. 7. Temperature of juvenile noctule bats (*Nyctalus noctula*) attached to their mothers. The temperature of the young bat follows the thermal profile of the female bat. T_{max}, maximum temperature.

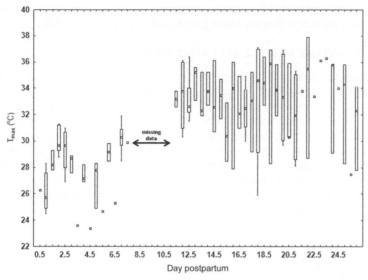

Fig. 8. Temperature of growing juvenile noctule bats (*Nyctalus noctula*) 10 minutes after removal from the mother. As shown by the drop in body temperature, young bats are incapable of thermoregulation for at least 6 days postpartum. T_{max}, maximum temperature.

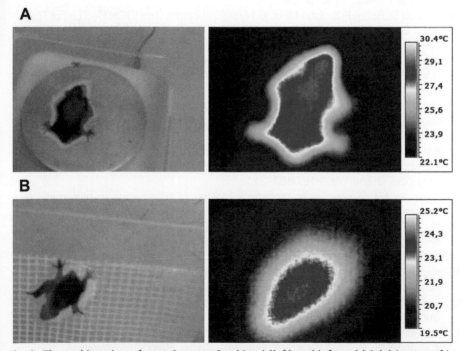

Fig. 9. Thermal imaging of noctule pups. Combined (*left*) and infrared (*right*) images of juvenile bats. (*A*) A 1.5-day-old female bat, shortly after separation from its mother (T_{max} 29.5°C [84.5°F]); (*B*) a 1-day-old bat, 10 minutes after separation from its mother for hand-feeding (T_{max} 24.5°C [75.2°F]). Longer separation from the mother bat quickly resulted in the pup's body temperature drop.

is, active lowering of body temperature, from approximately days 20 to 25, which coincides with a reduction in body mass growth rate (see **Figs. 7** and **8**).

RELEASE OF JUVENILE NOCTULE BATS AFTER WEANING

Because vespertilionid bats learn which summer, winter, and transitory roosts and foraging sites to use by social interaction, the question arises as to whether a successful release of captive-reared juveniles can be achieved. According to Dietz and colleagues,[29] young noctule bats practice foraging without the help of their mothers. The authors describe the case of a flightless captive female and a juvenile that became free-ranging in the autumn and returned to the artificial site where it had been reared the next year. Prior to release, the young bats had learnt self-feeding[6] on mealworms and crickets. Gebhard[30] noted that, if possible, placement of 2-compartment roost boxes close to an existing colony of wild bats yielded the best results for releasing vespertilionid juveniles without their mother.

REFERENCES

1. Sleeman JM. Has the time come for big science in wildlife health? Ecohealth 2013;10:335–8.
2. Hajkova P, Pikula J. Veterinary treatment of evening bats (Vespertilionidae) in the Czech Republic. Vet Rec 2007;161(4):139–40.
3. Altringham JD. Bats. Biology and behaviour. Oxford (United Kingdom): Oxford University Press; 1996. p. 262.
4. Csorba G, Bates P, Stubbe M, et al. Nyctalus noctula. The IUCN Red List of Threatened Species 2008: e.T14920A22015682. IUCN Global Species Programme Red List Unit, Cambridge, United Kingdom. Available at: http://dx.doi.org/10.2305/IUCN.UK.2016-2.RLTS.T14920A22015682.en. Accessed July 31, 2016.
5. Racey PA. The breeding, care and management of vespertilionid bats in the laboratory. Lab Anim 1970;4:171–83.
6. Racey PA, Kleiman DG. Maintenance and breeding in captivity of some vespertilionid bats, with special reference to the noctule. International Zoo Yearbook 1970;10:65–70.
7. Kleiman DG. Maternal care, growth rate, and development in the noctule (*Nyctalus noctula*), pipistrelle (*Pipistrellus pipistrellus*), and serotine (*Eptesicus serotinus*) bats. J Zool 1969;157:187–211.
8. Andrews MT. Advances in molecular biology of hibernation in mammals. Bioessays 2007;29:431–40.
9. Du WG, Radder RS, Sun B, et al. Determinants of incubation period: do reptilian embryos hatch after a fixed total number of heart beats? J Exp Biol 2009;212: 1302–6.
10. Kurta A, Kunz TH. Size of bats at birth and maternal investment during pregnancy. Sym Zool Soc Lond 1987;57:79–106.
11. Kunz TH, Stern AA. Maternal investment and post-natal growth in bats. Sym Zool Soc Lond 1995;67:123–38.
12. Arevalo F, Perez-Suarez G, Lopez-Luna P. Hematological data and hemoglobin components in bats (Vespertilionidae). Comp Biochem Physiol A 1987;88: 447–50.
13. Arevalo F, Perez-Suarez G, Lopez-Luna P. Seasonal changes in blood parameters in the bat species *Rhinolophus ferrumequinum* and *Miniopterus schreibersii*. Arch Int Physiol Biochim 1992;100:385–7.

14. Bassett JE, Wiederhielm CA. Postnatal changes in hematology of the bat *Antrozous pallidus*. Comp Biochem Physiol A 1984;78:737–42.
15. Jurgens KD, Bartels H, Bartels R. Blood oxygen transport and organ weights of small bats and small non-flying mammals. Respir Physiol 1981;45:243–60.
16. Krutzsch PH, Hughes AH. Hematological changes with torpor in the bat. J Mammal 1959;40:547–54.
17. Riedesel ML. Blood physiology. In: Wimsat WA, editor. Biology of bats, vol. 3. New York: Academic Press; 1977. p. 485–517.
18. Wolk E, Bogdanowicz W. Hematology of the hibernating bat: *Myotis daubentoni*. Comp Biochem Physiol A 1987;88:637–9.
19. Heard DJ, Whittier DA. Hematologic and plasma biochemical reference values for three flying fox species (*Pteropus* sp.). J Zoo Wildl Med 1997;28:464–70.
20. Hecht AM, Braun BC, Krause E, et al. Plasma proteomic analysis of active and torpid greater mouse-eared bats (*Myotis myotis*). Sci Rep 2015;5:16604.
21. Warnecke L, Turner JM, Bollinger TK, et al. Pathophysiology of white-nose syndrome in bats: a mechanistic model linking wing damage to mortality. Biol Lett 2013;9(4):20130177.
22. Speakman JR. The physiological costs of reproduction in small mammals. Philos Trans R Soc Lond B Biol Sci 2008;363:375–98.
23. Willis CKR. Daily heterothermy by temperate bats using natural roosts. In: Zubaid A, McCracken GF, Kunz TH, editors. Functional and evolutionary ecology of bats. New York: Oxford University Press Inc; 2006. p. 38–55.
24. Carey HV, Andrews MT, Martin SL. Mammalian hibernation: cellular and molecular responses to depressed metabolism and low temperature. Physiol Rev 2003;83: 1153–81.
25. Xu Y, Ch Shao, Fedorov VB, et al. Molecular signatures of mammalian hibernation: comparisons with alternative phenotypes. BMC Genomics 2013;14:567.
26. Dietz M, Kalko EK. Seasonal changes in daily torpor patterns of free-ranging female and male Daubenton's bats (*Myotis daubentonii*). J Comp Physiol B 2006; 176:223–31.
27. Lausen CL, Barclay RMR. Thermoregulation and roost selection by reproductive female big brown bats (*Eptesicus fuscus*) roosting in rock crevices. J Zool 2003; 260:235–44.
28. Wojciechowski MS, Jefimow M, Tegowska E. Environmental conditions, rather than season, determine torpor use and temperature selection in large mouse-eared bats (*Myotis myotis*). Comp Biochem Physiol A 2007;147:828–40.
29. Dietz C, Helversen O, Nill D. Bats of Britain, Europe & Northwest Africa. London: A&C Black; 2009. p. 400.
30. Gebhard J. Die Forschungsstation "Hofmatt" — Ein künstliches Fledermausquartier mit zahmen, in Gefangenschaft geborenen, freifliegenden und wilden, zugeflogenen Abendseglern (*Nyctalus noctula*). Myotis 1988;26:5–22.

Index

Note: Page numbers of article titles are in **boldface** type.

A

Vet Clin Exot Anim 20 (2017) 679–732
http://dx.doi.org/10.1016/S1094-9194(17)30008-7
1094-9194/17

vetexotic.theclinics.com

V

Printed and bound by CPI Group (UK) Ltd, Croydon, CR0 4YY

07/10/2024

01040506-0008